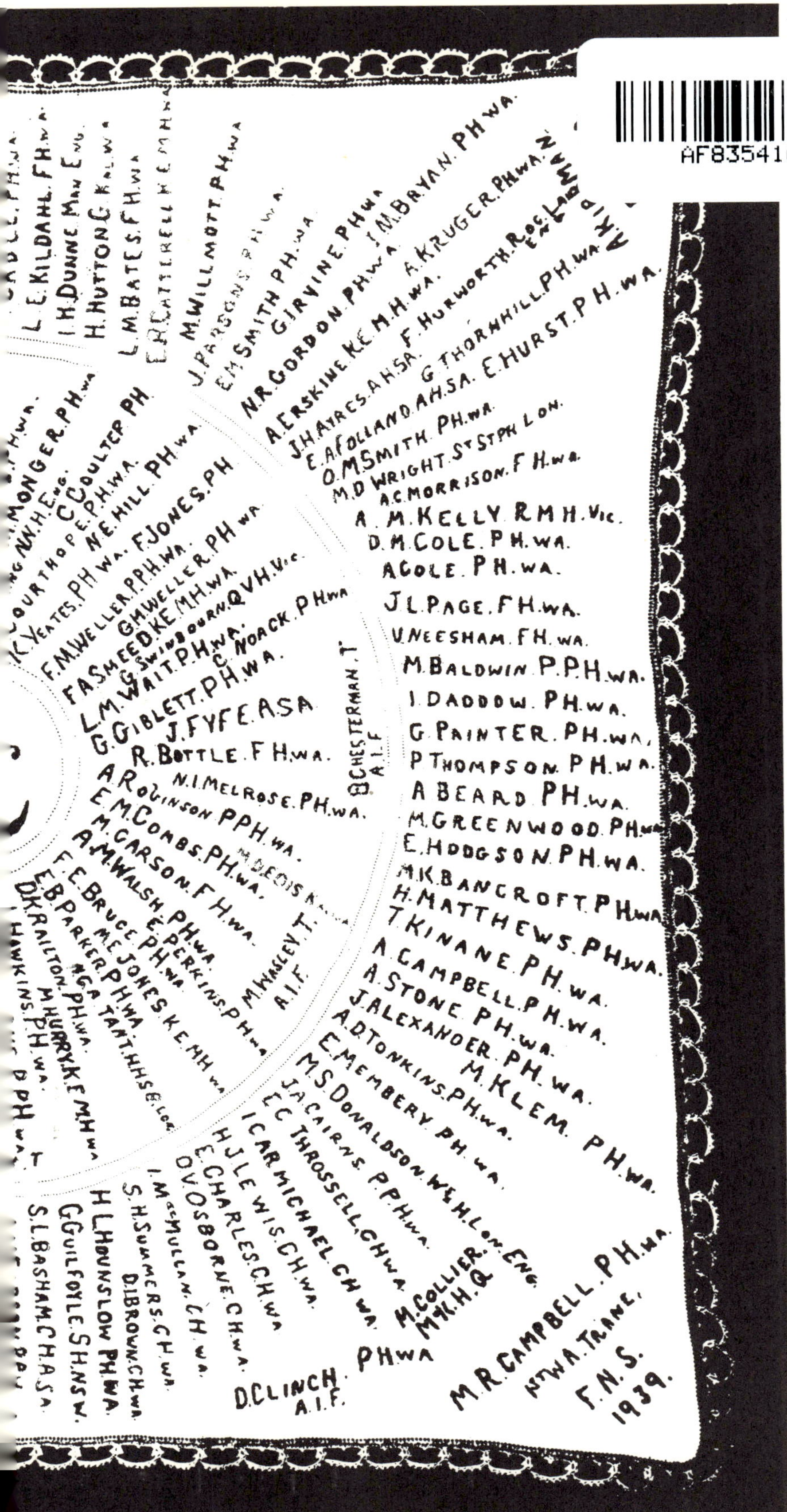
L. E. KILDAHL. F.H.wa.
I. H. DUNNE M.H. Eng.
H. HUTTON G. Kal. wa.
L. M. BATES. F.H. wa.
E. R. CATTERELL K.E.M.H. wa.
M. WILLMOTT. PH. wa.
J. PARSONS. P.H. wa.
E. M. SMITH. PH. wa.
G. IRVINE. PH. wa.
I. M. BRYAN. PH. wa.
N. R. GORDON. PH. wa.
A. KRUGER. PH. wa.
A. ERSKINE. K.E.M.H. wa.
F. HURWORTH. R.O.C. Eng.
J. H. AYRES. A.H.S.A.
G. THORNHILL. PH. wa.
E. A. FOLLAND. A.H.S.A.
E. HURST. P.H. wa.
O. M. SMITH. PH. wa.
M. D. WRIGHT. St Stph Lon.
A. C. MORRISON. F.H. wa.
A. M. KELLY. R.M.H. Vic.
D. M. COLE. P.H. wa.
A. COLE. PH. wa.
J. L. PAGE. F.H. wa.
V. NEESHAM. F.H. wa.
M. BALDWIN. P.P.H. wa.
I. DADDOW. PH. wa.
G. PAINTER. PH. wa.
P. THOMPSON. P.H. wa.
A. BEARD. PH. wa.
M. GREENWOOD. PH. wa.
E. HODGSON. PH. wa.
M. K. BANCROFT. P.H. wa.
H. MATTHEWS. PH. wa.
T. KINANE. PH. wa.
A. CAMPBELL. P.H. wa.
A. STONE. PH. wa.
J. ALEXANDER. PH. wa.
M. KLEM. PH. wa.
A. D. TONKINS. PH. wa.
E. MEMBERY. PH. wa.
M. S. DONALDSON. W.E.H. Lon. Eng.
J. A. CAIRNS. P.PH. wa.
E. C. THROSSELL. C.H. wa.
I. CARMICHAEL. C.H. wa.
H. J. LEWIS. C.H. wa.
E. CHARLES. C.H. wa.
O. V. OSBORNE. C.H. wa.
M. COLLIER. M.K.H.Q.
M. R. CAMPBELL. PH. wa.
N.T. W.A. Trane.
F.N.S. 1939.
D. CLINCH. A.I.F.
PH. wa.
I. McMULLAN. C.H. wa.
S. H. SUMMERS. C.H. wa.
D. BROWN. C.H. wa.
H. L. HOUNSLOW. PH. wa.
G. GUILFOYLE. S.H. N.S.W.
S. L. BASHAM. C.H. A.S.A.
MONGER. PH. wa.
C. COULTER. PH.
N. E. HILL. PH. wa.
F. JONES. PH.
K. YEATES. PH. wa.
F. M. WELLER. P.PH. wa.
G. M. WELLER. PH. wa.
F. A. SMEED. K.E.M.H. wa.
G. SWINBOURN. Q.V.H. Vic.
L. M. WAIT. PH. wa.
C. NOACK. PH. wa.
G. GIBLETT. PH. wa.
J. FYFE. A.S.A.
R. BOTTLE. F.H. wa.
B. CHESTERMAN. T. A.I.F.
N. I. MELROSE. PH. wa.
A. ROBINSON. P.PH. wa.
E. M. COMBS. PH. wa.
M. GARSON. F.H. wa.
A. M. WALSH. PH. wa.
E. PERKINS. P.H. wa.
M. WASLEY. T. A.I.F.
F. E. BRUCE. PH. wa.
M. E. JONES. K.E.M.H. wa.
E. B. PARKER. PH. wa.
N. G. A. TANT. H.H.S.B. Lon.
D. K. RAILTON. PH. wa.
M. HURRY. K.E.M.H. wa.
HAWKINS. PH. wa.

BUT WESTWARD LOOK

BUT WESTWARD LOOK

NURSING IN WESTERN AUSTRALIA
1829-1979

Victoria Hobbs

UNIVERSITY OF WESTERN AUSTRALIA PRESS
FOR THE ROYAL AUSTRALIAN NURSING FEDERATION
(W.A. BRANCH)

Hobbs, Victoria Alexandra May, 1907-
But westward look: nursing in Western Australia, 1829-1979.

Index
Bibliography
ISBN 0 85564 179 7

1. Nursing — Western Australia — History. I. Title.

610.73'09941

First published in 1980
by the University of Western Australia Press
for the Royal Australian Nursing Federation (W.A. Branch)

Agents: Eastern states of Australia and New Zealand: Melbourne University Press, Carlton South, Vic. 3053; U.S.A. and Canada: International Scholarly Book Services Inc., Box 555, Forest Grove, Oregon 97116.
Photoset by the University of Western Australia Press, printed by Frank Daniels Pty Ltd, Perth, and bound by Printers Trade Services, Belmont.

To Olive E. Anstey M.B.E.
President of the International Council of Nurses
1977-1981

FOREWORD

The nursing profession is indebted to the author for writing a book about the development of nursing in Western Australia. *But Westward Look* has been written as a chronological progression covering the first 150 years and places nursing in the context of the historical development of Western Australia.

The axiom that 'history repeats itself' is substantiated by the content of the book for it is a story of caring and struggle. It is about the people who cared for those who were unable, for whatever reason, to care for themselves and about the continuing struggle for improvement in the educational preparation and conditions of service for nurses in order to maintain and improve the quality of health care for the community. For example, the goal of tertiary level education for nurses was first mooted in Western Australia in 1935.

In 1980 nursing in Australia still does not have an undergraduate degree course for students entering nursing. The reasons for this anomaly in the educational preparation of health professionals have been related overtly by government to costs and funding. However, nursing must look to covert reasons and their influence on government decision-making, not least being concerns by individuals in some other health professions that their roles may be eroded rather than seeing a partnership arrangement developing, or, perhaps, to the traditional role placement of women in the workforce, for nursing is still a predominantly female vocation, and, not to be overlooked, are the traditional attitudes of many nurses about themselves and their own profession. That is not to suggest nurses and nursing should throw out all that is traditional as the struggle to improve nursing care standards through improved educational preparation continues.

In Western Australia nursing is indebted to its leaders past and present. Being a leader, such as those mentioned in this book, means a belief in nursing and self, being prepared to risk change, evaluating and accepting mistakes as well as achievements, modifying and moving forward again; in short, being committed and accountable. Nurses in general need to become more aware of their potential and power to influence decision-making at all levels of the health care system; an attribute of the late Florence Nightingale which has had insufficient emphasis and emulation! To use a system to effect change needs a knowledge and understanding of that system.

Nursing's future depends upon today's nurses. Let them learn from the foresight and tenacity of those who have preceded them and who have left a firm basis for the future development of nursing and nurses.

July 1980

WILMA GARDINER
SECRETARY/PRINCIPAL NURSING OFFICER,
R.A.N.F. (W. A. BRANCH)

CONTENTS

ILLUSTRATIONS

ACKNOWLEDGEMENTS

To thank individually all the people who have helped me in gathering the material for this book would require the writing of another volume. Their contributions have been vital and much appreciated.

I would, however, particularly like to thank the following: Alice Harris and Mollie Clarke for reading the A.T.N.A. and the W.A.N.A. minutes respectively; Hilda Jury, Jess Terry and Foreste Williams for the marathon indexing of the *Journals of the Western Australian Nurses*; Mollie Lukis, Margaret Medcalf, Robin South and the staff of the Battye Library; Vic Greaves and the staff of the University Press, and especially Naomi Zeffertt for her help and guidance.

I am also indebted to the following organizations which allowed me access to their archives: Royal Perth Hospital, Fremantle Hospital, Sir Charles Gairdner Hospital, King Edward Memorial Hospital, Western Australian School of Nursing, Medical Department, Nurses' Registration Board and the Royal Australian Nursing Federation.

V.H.

Say not the struggle naught availeth,
The labour and the wounds are vain,
The enemy faints not, nor faileth,
And as things have been they remain.

If hopes were dupes, fears may be liars;
It may be, in yon smoke concealed,
Your comrades chase e'en now the fliers,
And, but for you, possess the field.

For while the tired waves vainly breaking
Seem here no painfaul inch to gain,
Far back, through creeks and inlets making,
Comes silent, flooding in, the main.

And not by eastern windows only,
When daylight comes, comes in the light,
In front, the sun climbs slow, how slowly,
But westward, look, the land is bright!

Arthur Hugh Clough*

* Arthur Clough acted as secretary to the Nightingale Fund which was used to initiate the Nightingale School for Nurses at St Thomas's Hospital.

CHAPTER ONE

NINETEENTH CENTURY NURSING
1829-1899

It seems reasonable to assume that the earliest nursing in this country would have been by the indigenous people who for centuries had cared for their communities according to the dictates of tribal custom. Their story has yet to be written.

There are indications of skilled nursing aboard those ships which briefly brushed our shores, the French, Dutch, Portuguese and English. They came but did not linger, and departed, taking their stories with them, leaving behind only the ships whose wrecks are strewn along the coastline and their names commemorated in the islands, bays, headlands and wildflowers. However that there was skilled nursing can be surmised from the records of the survival rate of those on the long voyages, as well as the possible medical use of utensils found in these wrecks.

This history concerns the development of nursing in that part of the Australian continent now known as Western Australia, which had its beginnings as a permanent settlement at Albany, or Frederick Town as it was then called, when Major Edmund Lockyer of the brig *Amity* landed on Christmas Day 1826 to found the first British settlement on the western side of Australia. Later, in 1829, Captain Fremantle of H.M.S. *Challenger* took possession of the western part of the continent near the mouth of the Swan River and within a month was followed by Captain James Stirling, with his wife and family and an advance party of settlers for the new colony.

The Swan River Colony was a free settlement and the colonists were predominantly British. They brought with them their families, servants, possessions and the British way of life. The early musters list their names, trades and professions, which include surgeons and medical attendants, but no specific mention is made of nurses. The vastness of the area and sparseness of population made communication difficult, thus forcing people to use their initiative and previous experience when medical help was unavailable. This was an age when sickness, dangers of childbirth and infant mortality were accepted as part of everyday living. The task of caring for the sick was given to the womenfolk within the family unit and was consistent with the nursing pattern of their homeland.

In the first twenty years, hospitals were practically non-existent and limited to the military establishments. A few tents attached to the Perth Garrison in Barrack Street were designated as the Colonial Hospital, for the benefit of all civilian sick whatever their means.[1] This was the forerunner of the Perth Colonial Hospital, which later became today's Royal Perth Hospital.

The place for a sick person was in his own environment. Nursing was basic and aimed at the relief of symptoms; and diagnosis was made on the known course of a disease and changes observed, usually by the nurse, in the patient's physical appearance, his excretions and abnormal behaviour. Comparisons were made with familiar household commodities, such as 'pea soup', 'coffee grounds', 'red currant jelly' etc. The prognosis was mainly based on faith and folklore. Household products formed the basis of treatment, which was largely symptomatic, the only curative treatment being the somewhat crude surgery usually carried out on a patient in his bed or on the well-scrubbed kitchen table. Many of the household remedies persisted and were embodied in the nurses' training syllabus for the next hundred years, for example, starch poultice, mustard paste, soap and water enema etc. Medications were limited and dispensed by the doctor, the universal tranquillizer and analgesic being alcohol, brandy for the more affluent and gin for the poorer. In the latter part of the century the patent medicine widely advertised as a cure-all was firmly believed in. Patients whose physical appearance or behaviour made them unacceptable to the community were placed in custodial care, either privately or in an institution (until an asylum was built, the wrecked hulk of the *Marquis of Anglesea* was used for this purpose).[2]

Women who showed particular aptitude and willingness to undertake the nursing management of a very ill patient were invaluable to the medical practitioner, who would recommend them both verbally and in writing. Such a reference from a doctor would confer on its recipient the status and recognition of being an experienced nurse. This practice continued for a very long time, especially in the field of midwifery, and was one of the factors which retarded the formation of nursing associations and registration of nurses. Until a system of hospital instruction was introduced, one could say that all nurses practised midwifery in the course of their nursing duties and like Mrs Gamp went with equal zest to a lying in and a laying out.

Apart from the hospital, institutional nursing was practised in the infirmaries attached to the prisons and migrant holding centres, and as they arose, poorhouses, orphanages and lunatic asylums. Those in charge of these institutions were usually designated as master and matron, their duties being generally of a custodial nature, while the actual work was carried out by the inmates. The slow development of the colony was to some extent due to the absence of an adequate labour force, for as the assigned servants completed their terms of contract, they too took up holdings and became employers. An attempt to solve this problem was the introduction of juvenile migration under a scheme sponsored by welfare organizations in England. Under a special act of parliament, children, mostly boys from such institutions as Millbank and Parkhurst which were penetential reformatories, were brought out to be apprenticed to tradesmen or for domestic service.[3] The ages of these children ranged between nine and fifteen years and many suffered from malnutrition. It has been suggested that they might have been responsible for the introduction of some of the communicable diseases, e.g. chickenpox, and contributed to the high mortality rate among the juvenile population. However there appears to be no information as to where these children were accommodated or how they were nursed.

By the end of the 1840s the hard-pressed settlers had petitioned the imperial government for convicts to help buoy up the economy. There was some opposition to this as transportation to eastern Australia was being phased out and its introduction to Western Australia was considered a retrograde step. However it was stipulated that the convicts be male only and their crimes generally of a non-violent nature.

The first convicts for the colony arrived on 1 June 1850 on the *Scindian*; they were accompanied by pensioner guards and their families and some immigrants. On arrival they were assigned to farmers and tradesmen and employed on the construction of roads and much needed public buildings. As the imperial government accepted responsibility for housing the newcomers, the first buildings were convict depots, with attached infirmaries known as convict hospitals. In Fremantle a large gaol with a gaol hospital, a lunatic asylum and a pretentious house for the comptroller of convicts were built. This latter residence, 'The Knowle', eventually became the Fremantle Hospital and is still in use.[4] Patients and staff were transferred to the hospital from the pensioner establishment in Point Street in 1897.[5]

In Perth the Colonial Hospital, begun as a tent complex in 1830, was eventually relocated on a grant of land in Victoria Square and Murray Street (then part of Goderich Street). However, due to structural instability the hospital had to be rebuilt in 1855[6] and this building is in use today. The nearby poorhouse, which also functioned as a maternity home for the destitute and an orphanage, provided the hospital with domestic staff and laundry facilities. Its construction was of an earlier date and it no longer exists.

It is recorded that in 1853 a Miss or Mrs McLaughlin was appointed as nurse and cook to the Colonial Hospital,[7] and there are various references to the employment of matrons, nurses and medical attendants to the different institutions, but there is no indication that there was any attempt at organized nurse training. However the press of the 1880s carries numerous lengthy letters deploring the conditions under which the sick poor were being nursed and urging the introduction of lady probationers on a voluntary basis under a 'suitably qualified matron'. Pleas were also made for better hospital facilities in Fremantle and in the country areas where the convict hospitals provided the only care available to destitute patients, and then only if they were male.[8]

With the cessation of transportation in 1868 the imperial government handed over to the colonial government all buildings connected with the convict establishment, including depots, pensioner barracks etc. The Mount Eliza Depot, a former convict establishment situated in the vicinity of the Swan Brewery in Mounts Bay Road, had been converted into an old men's home. However its situation was considered undesirable by the nearby residents and the home was later moved to Dalkeith. It is now known as Sunset.[9]

In the country centres the infirmaries attached to the depots became known as colonial hospitals.[10] These were demolished as funds became available to build more substantial structures which became the government hospitals at Albany, Bunbury, Geraldton, Northam, Busselton and York. One of the earliest buildings was at Roebourne, but fears of cyclonic damage led to its replacement with one which has successfully withstood the cyclones over the years. Generally these early country hospitals reflect in their architecture the hospital care of the time, being two-storeyed structures of stone with long wards and no lifts, thereby creating problems for future nursing.

In 1886 a select committee was appointed to report on possible extensions to Perth Colonial Hospital.[11] The outcome of this was that it was decided that the hospital accommodation was adequate but could be improved by the addition of a six-bed operating ward. The field of surgery at this period was limited and operative procedures were carried out in the wards, often in full view of other patients. In the same report the suggestion of a maternity section for the hospital was not accepted on the grounds that the poorhouse adequately fulfilled this function.

Attitudes to the care of the chronically ill and disadvantaged are reflected in the medical reports of the colonial surgeon and the reports of government officers (1886-87).[12] Mrs Annear, matron of the poorhouse, Perth, stated that there had been an increase in the admissions of widows, deserted wives, and aged and infirm women. Josiah Dewers, master of the Mount Eliza Depot, reported that many of the inmates were unable to leave their beds and were unavailable for duties connected with the order and maintenance of the establishment. He was authorized to admit paupers chargeable to colonial funds. Margaret Walpole, whose husband, Dr Walpole, practised in Albany from 1883 to 1885, came to the colony fresh from her nursing experience at Barts and Great Ormond Street, London, and in her diary describes the plight of people in the district, especially the women in the outlying areas who could not get nursing care. She also describes the havoc caused by an epidemic of measles in the area.[13]

A major factor which contributed to the delay in commencing a hospital training system for nurses in Western Australia was the unique position of the colonial surgeon, who prior to the Hospitals' Act of 1894 had complete control of all government-supported hospitals and was answerable only to the colonial secretary. His autocratic attitude and refusal to allow certain private practitioners the use of the facilities of the hospitals or access to the patients or their records caused a great deal of dissatisfaction among medical men. (The last holder of the office, Dr Waylen, will go down in history for his refusal to sanction the connection of a telephone which in his opinion would serve no purpose as a messenger boy was employed.)

Although surgery was still carried out in the patient's home, advances in this field created a demand for hospital facilities and more experienced nurse assistants; it was realized that much of the preparation and aftercare of the patient could safely be left to the nurse who could be instructed in the use of equipment and the initiating of procedures which had previously been the responsibility of the surgeon. The result of this was the taking over of large houses as nursing homes, sponsored by doctors and managed by reliable women, the latter often chosen for their housekeeping ability rather than nursing experience. In some instances two or three members of a family would share the responsibility of running a hospital, assisted by so-called probationer nurses, and from this arose the practice of a nurse training in a private hospital under a qualified doctor.

The proclamation of responsible government in Western Australia in 1890, when parliament was formed in accordance with the Constitution Act of 1889, meant the phasing out of the previous system and the introduction of new titles and offices. In 1890, in anticipation of this, an attempt was made to change the accepted method of appointment of nursing staff to the Perth Colonial Hospital, and to introduce a type of nurse training. Previous to this the position of matron, which was an appointment approved by the governor, had been made on seniority and not specific qualifications, and carried privileges consistent with employment in the colonial service. In the absence of Dr Waylen, who was overseas on leave, the acting colonial surgeon, Dr Thomas Lovegrove, secured the appointment of Miss Mary Ann Nicolay to the position of matron in succession to Mrs Miles.[14] (Miss Nicolay's salary of £100 per annum was almost double that of her predecessor, which provoked criticism by the colonial surgeon on his return.)

In a letter to the nurses of the Children's Hospital, Miss Nicolay refers to the two female members of her staff as probationers, but they are not designated as such in the *Blue Books*, and although she gives some details of her own training, there is no indication of the type of instruction given in the hospital to these young women.[15] One of these, Miss Ada Rewell, had been at the hospital for about twelve months, and remained on the staff for about five years.[16] She was always spoken of very highly by her contemporaries. Miss Bates, the second nurse did not stay.

Miss Nicolay was not happy in her position and after six months tendered her resignation. On 1 July 1891 she wrote to Dr Waylen:

> I beg to place before you my resignation. I have tried to work this Hospital for six months and have utterly failed. Trusting you will be able to find another to fill my post in a month from this date, as I should prefer leaving at the expiration of my months notice, but I should not wish to put you to any inconvenience.

Dr Waylen wrote to the colonial secretary: 'Miss Nicolay has for some time past talked of finalizing and has now done so formally—with the present salary I dont think there will be any difficulty in filling her post', who replied: 'Miss Nicolays resignation will, I suppose have to be accepted. If possible a properly trained nurse should be appointed to her place.' These exchanges were also dated 1 July 1891.

On 13 July Dr Waylen wrote: 'Miss Nicolay—after due consideration now asks to be allowed to withdraw the letter tendering her resignation of the post of Matron of the Colonial Hospital—under all the circumstances I would ask that she be permitted to do so.'

There the matter rested till Miss Nicolay's letter to Dr Waylen on 22 September:

> I wish to tell you that when convenient to yourself I wish to leave this Hospital I do not date my resignation as I do not wish to put you to any inconvenience but if you will kindly tell me when you are suited with a Matron I shall be ready to leave.

Dr Waylen advised the colonial secretary: 'I think the accompanying letter of Miss Nicolay should be accepted as final', who replied, 23 September. 'Accept Miss Nicolay's resignation as soon as you can secure a suitable matron.'[17] So that contrary to general belief, Miss Nicolay's tenure as matron of the Colonial Hospital was brief, a matter of twelve months.

Mary Ann Nicolay is credited with having been at the Nightingale School in 1872 and with personally knowing Florence Nightingale and there is some evidence to suggest that there could have been family connections. The Nightingale School did not subscribe to the issuing of certificates to its graduates, which was a disadvantage as the onus of proof was on the individual.

Usually titled Sister Mary Ann Nicolay, this well-known figure in nursing circles for over fifty years has become almost legendary. After retirement she always wore the traditional outdoor nurses' uniform, navy-blue frock, bonnet with streamers and on occasions a long navy-blue cape. She was a dominant personality, fiercely pro-Nightingale and very vocal. Over the years she gave numerous accounts of her nursing experiences in interviews to the press,[18] but unfortunately there are contradictions in these which have led to much confusion in recounting nursing history. It is also unfortunate that historians have tended to confuse Mary Ann Nicolay with Mrs Mary Ann Nicholas,[19] who was the last matron of the Colonial Hospital during the transition period when it was becoming the Perth Public Hospital, with a three-year training school for nurses, in 1896.

Miss Nicolay's successor in 1891 was Miss E. M. Andrew and her appointment marked a return to the system of promotion according to seniority within the government service. Nurses were recruited mostly from the ranks of the young women who emigrated to Western Australia with government assistance and who were sponsored by the Girls' Friendly Society and other organizations in England. During the long voyage out, the matron in charge of the group assessed their capabilities and suitability for employment, and a few were recommended for employment as nurses at the Colonial Hospital.[20] There seems to have been no set term of service and they were required to do the domestic work as well as the nursing, Miss Andrew having dispensed with the services of the women from the poorhouse. These nurses referred to themselves as probationers and when they left the hospital they were given references stating that they had received experience in medical and surgical wards, but no hospital certificates were issued. Subsequently when employed in other areas they were recognized as being fully trained and given status and salary according to seniority.

It is difficult to know the extent of nursing care carried out by the male medical attendants and orderlies. The former are listed as being in charge of the medical posts which evolved from the convict hospitals, but the staff for the Colonial Hospital's male wards was in part obtained from the Mount Eliza Depot.

There is some evidence to support the fact that a two-year training for the General Nursing Certificate was introduced during the transition period of the administration of the Colonial Hospital from 1895 to 1897. This is referred to by Jessie Hurnall (Mrs Clifton) in an article in the *Perth Hospital Journal* in which she states that none of the nurses finished the course but had to leave because of 'alcohol and morphia habits'.[21] This is not strictly true, for at least one of those listed during that period finished the course and obtained a certificate. She was Margaret Coombe Birt,[22] who was decorated for her work as matron of the Red Cross Hospital at Huntington, England, during the First World War.[23] Efforts to find a certificate for the two year training period have so far proved unsuccessful.

Following the discovery of gold in the Kimberleys in 1885 Western Australia began to feel the effects of increased immigration, but it was the events of the 1890s which had an unprecedented effect on the nursing situation, for the state was ill prepared for the population explosion which followed further discoveries in the Eastern Goldfields. People came from far and wide, the eastern Australian states, the United Kingdom, Europe, Asia, the United States of America and South Africa. Ships, the only means of transport to Western Australia, were overcrowded and those passing through Asian ports brought contact with bubonic plague, smallpox and gastro-intestinal diseases. On arrival, unsatisfactory housing, poor sanitation and an inadequate water supply contributed to the spread of infection. The predominating disease was typhoid fever and in 1893 an outbreak of smallpox put the community into a state of panic.[24]

In her 'Reminiscences', Mrs Agnes Sadleir, who as Miss Seymour had joined the nursing staff of the Perth Colonial Hospital in 1892, describes the admission to the hospital of the first patient with smallpox and his subsequent removal with other patients and contacts to tents erected in a clearing in the bush about 1½ km from the Subiaco railway siding. Delegated to nurse the patient, Miss Seymour contracted the disease, but her vaccination seems to have stood her in good stead, for she was deemed well enough to care for some of the patients. Her reference to 'amateur nurses' seems to indicate that these were recruited from the ranks of anyone willing to nurse. She also speaks of the two priests, one Anglican and one Catholic, who voluntarily went into isolation with the patients, and their work in providing amenities for the convalescents and the large number of 'contacts'. Special mention is made of the day the first iron buildings were erected, the day that marks the beginning of the Victoria Hospital, West Subiaco, for many years known to the nurses of Perth Hospital as I.D.B. (Infectious Diseases Branch), and the forerunner of today's Royal Perth Rehabilitation Hospital, Shenton Park.

We are indebted to Miss Seymour for her description of the nursing care given to patients at the Colonial Hospital, of her experience as a community nurse in the Fremantle area as a member of the organization known as 'Sisters of the People' sponsored by the Methodist Church,[25] and of her further nursing experience when seconded to the staff of Coolgardie Hospital during the typhoid epidemic in the hectic years of the great discoveries of gold. Although she did not hold a hospital certificate, Miss Seymour was recognized as a professional nurse and appointed night superintendent of Coolgardie Hospital. Practical and quick thinking, she always showed initiative and, above all, concern for patients as people with recognition of their needs apart from physical care.

Not all the gold-seekers came through Perth. Many trekked overland from the ports of Albany and Esperance, but all converged on the rich, almost waterless empty country where everything had to be transported from the distant rail-head by coach or camel train. The erection of hotels and boarding-houses could not keep pace with the influx, and dwellings of hessian and cities of tents dominated, springing up in their hundreds at each new find. Inevitably there was disease. Typhoid fever swept through the community in epidemic proportions and the mortality was appalling.

At first the few women who had accompanied their husbands to the goldfields and those employed in hotels and boarding-houses endeavoured to care for the sick men. Some of these, like Mrs Penglase and Nurse Baseby,[26] had had previous nursing experience in hospitals and infirmaries, while the others carried on as best they knew how. The lack of facilities for skilled nursing care resulted in many deaths.

An appeal for nurses did not go unheeded especially in the eastern states, and many came to join their relatives or colleagues already in the west.[27] A large proportion were from Victoria and South Australia, but from Western Australia there were very few.

Their social and nursing backgrounds differed widely, but they worked side by side tirelessly, dedicated to the preservation of life; some succumbed to the fever which was rife and some died from other causes, including violence. Many married the young men they had nursed.

It is difficult to know just which was the first hospital on the goldfields as doctors and nurses had their own establishments, but Coolgardie had the first hospital of any size.[28] It began as a community hospital, administered by a committee which later became a board. The government did not accept responsibility for the venture until some time later, so the names of the early staff are not listed in the *Blue Books*. The hospital was of tent construction and it is recorded that in April 1894 Sister Margaret O'Brien and Nurse Leana Miller arrived by coach from Adelaide and Miss O'Brien was asked by Warden Finnerty to supervise the government patients for the time being.[29] They consented, not relinquishing their own idea of a private hospital.

In November 1894 both nurses resigned, seemingly because of criticism, and devoted their time to their own venture. The patients in the government hospital were left in the care of untrained nurses. Although the names of these have not been officially recorded it is known that at least one of them had had nursing experience at the Colonial Hospital in Perth.[30] This is the first indication that there was a difference in status between the certificated nurse and the nurse with a doctor's or hospital reference. Nevertheless, the efforts of those who carried on did not go unrewarded, and when Mercy Taylor, who became Mrs Gregory, met an untimely death some years later, a memorial fountain was erected to commemorate her work in the hospital.[31] This memorial is in the gardens at Coolgardie.

A description of Miss O'Brien's hospital is graphically given in a series of letters written by J. F. Marks to his wife, in June 1894:

> I had never been to see the place. It was rougher than I expected just tents and only blankets on the bunks no sheets. I had a stretcher given me, just a cornsack tacked to a frame, all the beds, such as they are, being occupied. Sleeplessness had set in by this time and I couldn't get a wink while my bones ached with lying cramped on the narrow bunk. I was feeling jolly bad and I got another blanket under me to soften the lying. The other beds were spring mattress stretchers but the mattresses to go over the wires hadn't arrived—like thousands of other things they were on the road somewhere. However they were very comfortable as I found when in three or four days a convalescent cleared out and I got his bunk. It was

> heaven after the cornsack. They dosed me with quinnine and I think arsnic at first.
>
> As I say, the hospital as a hospital is a pretty rough one. When the wind blows it comes through the flap door of the tent and the other available inlets and the nights were precious cold. The one redeeming feature, and I suppose that is really nearly everything, was the nursing. There are two of them, Sister O'Brien and Nurse Miller I was under the Sister's care and she certainly looked after me admirably. She appears to be a born nurse and is always cheerful and nice and ready to talk and have a laugh. . . . she evidently likes the work. She was in charge of the North Adelaide Hospital for a long time I believe.[32]

One of the earliest welfare organizations was the Salvation Army, which was well established in Coolgardie in 1893,[33] but additional help came, especially in the care of the sick, in 1897 from the Sisters of the People,[34] and Sisters of the Order of St John of God.[35] The former set up missions and worked as community nurses, and the latter established a hospital in Kalgoorlie, the forerunner of today's St John of God Hospitals which function in Perth, Kalgoorlie and other country centres. Members of the order also went farther north to Broome teaching and nursing, their outstanding service being in the care of patients with Hansen's disease, a work which they have continued until the present day.

The Sisters of St John of God did not have any formal training, although some of their number had been nursing for many years. Later, when they wanted to register their hospital as a training school for nurses within the order, they had to employ a secular matron.

The Sisters of the People were also not all hospital-certificated nurses but a number had trained in Adelaide and Melbourne and had held responsible positions. Known by their given names only, they have been hard to trace. No charge was made for their services and they relied on the good offices of the people for their upkeep. Most of their efforts were directed to the nursing of the sick poor and each was required to make a report on the patients they had nursed, and to speak to these reports at the annual meetings of the organization held by the Wesley Church in Perth. The reports were printed and circulated in order to publicize the work among the more affluent members of the community and solicit their help. There were some members who refused to make public their 'case histories' as they considered it was unethical to give such information, and left the organization. However it is due to these printed reports, few of which have survived, that a picture of the conditions under which people lived in the closing years of the century and the need for social reform and responsibility for health care in the community is shown.

The *West Australian* of 2 November 1894 reports on a meeting in the Perth Town Hall on the occasion of the first anniversary of the mission, and states that it commenced with two Sisters but three more had been added and posted to Perth, Fremantle and Geraldton.

By 1897 the work had been extended to postings at Southern Cross, Kalgoorlie and beyond, York, Northam, and the timber mills of the south-west of the state.

In 1894, during the first session of the second parliament, legislation was passed by which the governor was given power to proclaim any place or places suitable, to be public hospitals, and also on advice to rescind these. This Hospitals' Act of 1894 also allowed for the administration of such hospitals by a board and for voluntary contributions from organizations and individuals.[36] A 'life' contribution of £10 gave the contributor some rights in the election of board members, two-thirds of whom was to consist of other than medical practitioners.

The first hospitals to be controlled by this act were Coolgardie, Perth Colonial, Kalgoorlie, and, later, Fremantle. However financial, staff and other difficulties resulted in Coolgardie and Kalgoorlie Hospitals reverting to the administration of the newly constituted Board of Health and the principal medical officer.[37]

In Western Australia there was no hospital acceptable as a training school for midwives. With the exception of the poorhouse, the only institution where a destitute mother could have her baby was the House of Mercy, founded in 1889 by a group of compassionate citizens.[38] This was the forerunner of today's Ngal-A which functions as a training school for nurses undertaking certificate courses in mothercraft and child health. Fortunately most of the records of this institution have been preserved and the nursing reports tell their own story.

This change in legislation and the demand for hospital beds by the ever-increasing number of indigent patients was the stimulus for the construction of new buildings and allowed in the case of Perth Public Hospital the appointment of medical practitioners to act as honorary staff, although the absence of a university precluded its use as a teaching hospital. It also meant the introduction of a nurse-training system, which commenced in 1896.[39] This probationer type of training was also started in the larger hospitals controlled by the Board of Health and in Fremantle Public Hospital in 1897.

There appear to be no guide lines set out for the above, the only uniformity being the appointment to each hospital of a matron who had gained experience through a nurse-training school. Miss A. H. Gordon from the Royal Adelaide Hospital was appointed to Perth Public Hospital in 1896;[40] Miss Bessie Steel of Addenbrook's Hospital, Cambridge, took the first group of probationer nurses from the Point Street Pensioner Hospital to the Knowle in Fremantle in 1897.[41] Miss Rosa Snodgrass of the Alfred Hospital, Melbourne, succeeded Miss B. Lee at Coolgardie in 1897 when the latter transferred to Kalgoorlie Hospital.[42] In spite of a personal tragedy,[43] Miss Snodgrass remained at Coolgardie to see the first group of nurses complete their course.

In 1896 Miss F. J. E. Way of the Royal Adelaide Hospital was appointed matron of Hannan's Hospital by the Kalgoorlie Progress Commiteee[44] but resigned to be married soon after the hospital was transferred to its present site and came under government control. Her successor, Miss C. Buckley, is officially listed as the first matron. In 1898 Miss Way, as Mrs Harvey, now widowed, was reappointed as matron of Kalgoorlie Hospital when it was officially recognized as a nurse-training school.[45]

In addition to other duties, the matron of a training school was responsible for giving theoretical and practical instruction in nursing. The number of young women accepted for training was very small and the wastage was high, which did little to alleviate the acute shortage of nursing help in the hospitals, so that in 1897 the P.M.O., Dr Lovegrove, visited the eastern states in an endeavour to recruit nurses.[46] The salary of £75 per annum with some amenities appeared very attractive, but dissatisfaction was felt when those recruited found that staff with less qualifications but with greater length of service were receiving higher salaries.

One of these recruits was the youthful Annie May-Steers, fresh from Sydney Hospital. Her expertise in nursing, especially in the surgical field, greatly impressed the matron and the medical officers, who gave her glowing references and a silver tea and coffee service when she resigned two years later to take up the position of matron of the hospital at Guildford. This hospital was made necessary by the casualties and sickness, especially typhoid fever, among the men constructing the Mundaring Weir, which was to provide a water supply for the goldfields, 640 kilometres away. Miss May-Steers subsequently became matron of Bunbury Hospital and was a foundation member of the Australasian Trained Nurses Association. She was the first nurse to become a member of the association in Western Australia.[47]

With her in Coolgardie and Guildford was her friend Ann Stafford Bird who, as Mrs Garnsey, has written the only book known to have been published by a nurse of those days, and titled *Scarlet Pillows*. However, many reminiscences of pioneer nurses have been published in various journals which reflect the attitudes people in the community held towards nurses. Roughly they divided them into two categories: the efficient, highly esteemed ministering angels, and the women who had taken refuge in drugs and alcohol. However, such is the sense of loyalty in nurses, the slightest hint of scandal or impropriety concerning their colleagues or members of the medical profession causes them immediately to close ranks.

Generally speaking, the professional nurse carried out treatment on the orders of a doctor if one was available, but this did not apply to the women who acted as midwives and undertook confinements in their own houses or in the patient's home. There was no legislation against such practice.

The common denominator of all nurses was the wearing of uniform, which in the strict sense of the word was never uniform as it was orientated towards the fashions of the day and the traditional cap of the wearer's school of nursing. The mark of authority was the chatelaine, with scissors, probe, thimble and keys. Except for the matron, all nurses wore aprons and starched collars and cuffs. Uniform was worn both on and off duty. There was nothing to prevent any woman from wearing the uniform if she so desired and instances are recorded of people masquerading as nurses in uniform for esteem, gain or protection. The question of entitlement to the wearing of a distinctive uniform and the use of the term 'nurse'[48] was a contentious issue and not confined to the local scene. Nurses were becoming increasingly conscious of their professional and social status and were realizing that they had no protection against piracy of their field by anyone who wished to call herself a nurse. This was a world trend, and in the United Kingdom efforts were being made to have nurses protected by an act of parliament, making it illegal for anyone who had not qualified by examination to take the title 'nurse'. This was an impossible dream, and did not eventuate.

The problem remains unsolved; people expect nurses to wear uniform of a traditional type even though it may serve no useful purpose. It may even be a danger to the environment as a vehicle of cross-infection.

> So may the outward shows be least themselves;
> The world is still deceived with ornament.

CHAPTER TWO

THE BEGINNING OF THE TWENTIETH CENTURY 1900-1914

The beginning of the twentieth century brought changes in the community which directly and indirectly influenced the role of the professional nurse. The entry of the Australian states into federation and the proclaiming of the Commonwealth gave rise to a new sense of nationhood, although the people of Western Australia were not wholeheartedly behind this merger as they feared the effects of being a minority in relation to population, in spite of having the largest land area, almost a third of the continent. The situation on the goldfields was becoming more stable but there was a great demand for nurses which had to be met by those trained outside the state. Many nurses married and settled down to undertake responsibility for husbands and families, and others returned to their home states, where contingents were being raised to go overseas to the Boer War.

The report of an interview with the newly appointed matron of Perth Public Hospital, Miss E. Wemyss, published in the *Western Mail* of 3 February 1900, describes the nursing situation and the inadvisability of sending nurses from Western Australia:

> Though there has been no question as to the patriotism and the humanity of the proposal to send a band of nurses from Western Australia to South Africa to tend the sick and wounded there, the question has been raised whether the colony, having regard to the requirements of the sickness of its own people, was not giving out of its own need rather than from its bounty in allowing any trained nurses to leave its shores.
>
> With the view to obtaining an expression of opinion on this point as well as upon other matters connected with the nursing of the Imperial troops, a representative of this journal sought an interview with Miss Wemyss, the matron of the Perth Public Hospital.
>
> Premising her remarks with an expression of diffidence in giving her opinions to a public amongst whom she had only

> lived some 12 months, Miss Wemyss said 'I really do think that the colony cannot afford to spare any of its trained nurses. There seems to me to be so much call for their services, apart from that I am delighted with the idea of sending out the nurses, because the experience thus gained will be of much value to them in their after life here. One cannot indeed over estimate the advantages it will be to them. It has been said that the nurses who are going are only to nurse Colonial and irregular troops, because they are not qualified to nurse the Imperial soldiers. They possess the requisite training, yet a difficulty stands in the way. By Act of Parliament the Imperial soldiers must be nursed by members of the Imperial Nursing Service. To belong to that corps it is necessary to have served 3 years in a public training hospital. Of course the members of that corps will nurse any sick or wounded who are brought to them, but the Imperial troops could demand to be attended by the Imperial service nurses. I thought there were only 300 or 400 of these nurses enrolled, but Dr White says that there are thousands, quite enough to meet all demands.
>
> 'Yes, I am leaving Western Australia' added Miss Wemyss . . . 'and I am truly sorry to go. I like the colony and the people here and I had hoped to remain amongst them at all events for some years. But you know I belong to the Imperial Nursing Corps and I have received a notification to present myself for service, and I must go. I am sorry to go in one way but you know I was born in the army. My father was the commander of a regiment of Hussars and all my family are soldiers. Major General Wauchope, who was killed at Magersfontein, was my cousin, and Colonel Stafford who was killed near the Modder River was also a relation of mine. You will understand then how gladly I accept the call for service and how anxious I am to be at work. I shall go away very soon, next month perhaps, but I shall always have pleasant recollections of Western Australia.'

However, Miss Wemyss's advice was not heeded and a group of nurses went to South Africa in charge of Miss Mary Nicolay. It was an independent unit, sponsored by Perth citizens and supported financially by a 'generous Public Appeal'.[1] The following excerpts from the *Albany Advertiser* 24 March 1900 outline some of their difficulties:

> The provision made by the Nurses Fund Committee for the West Australian nurses for their passage to South Africa, met with a good deal of adverse comment at Albany on Wednesday last. When the nurses first volunteered, it was understood that they were to be given first saloon passages to Cape Town. Later

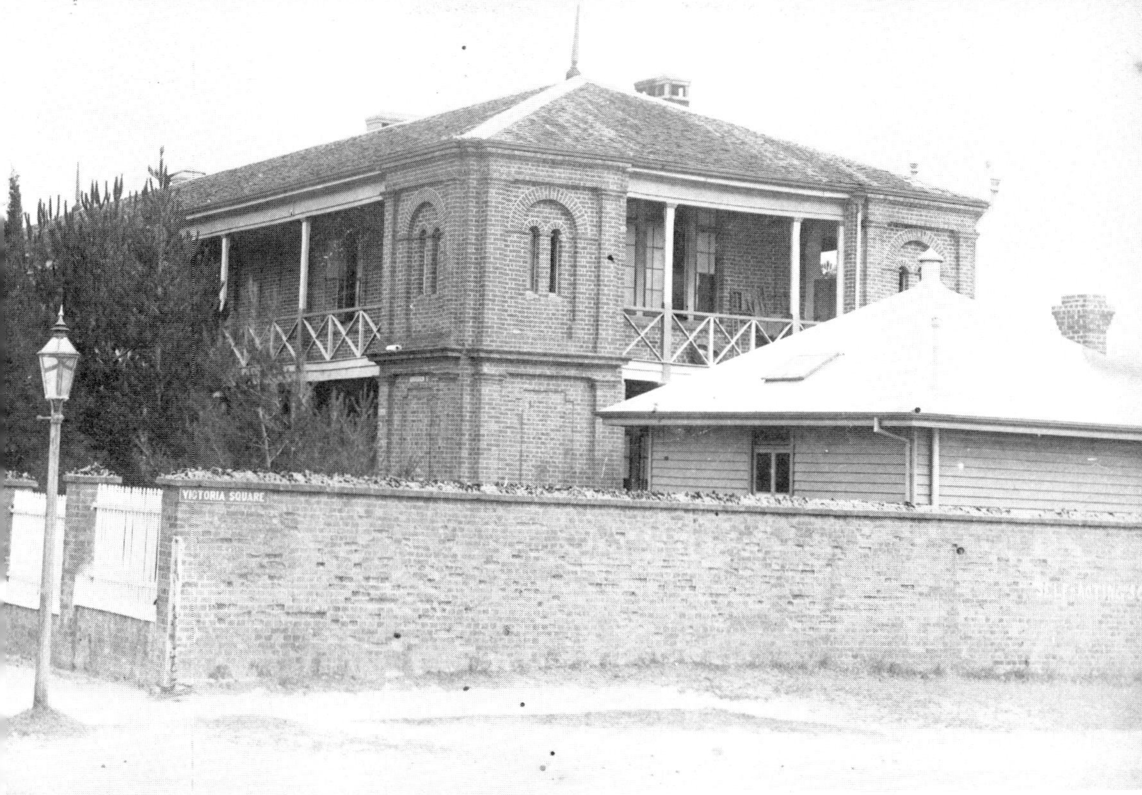

THE COLONIAL HOSPITAL, PERTH, C. 1894-95

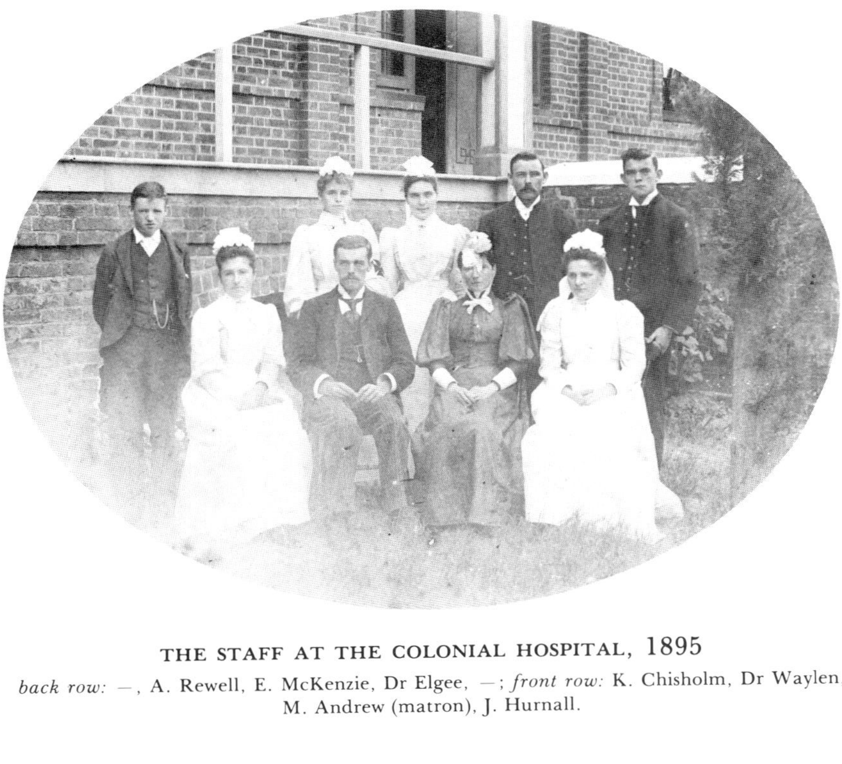

THE STAFF AT THE COLONIAL HOSPITAL, 1895

back row: —, A. Rewell, E. McKenzie, Dr Elgee, —; *front row:* K. Chisholm, Dr Waylen, M. Andrew (matron), J. Hurnall.

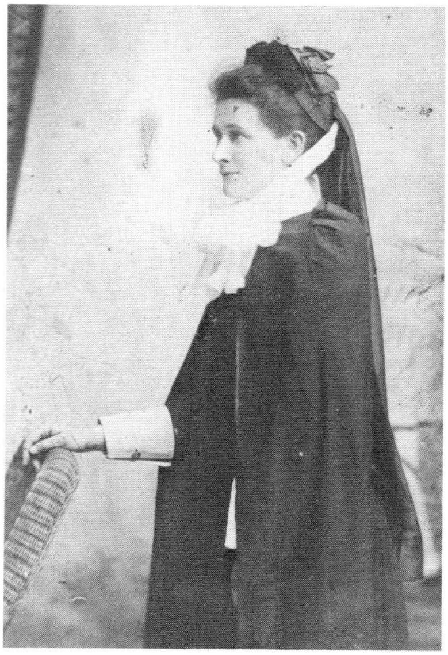

MARGARET O'BRIEN, 1895

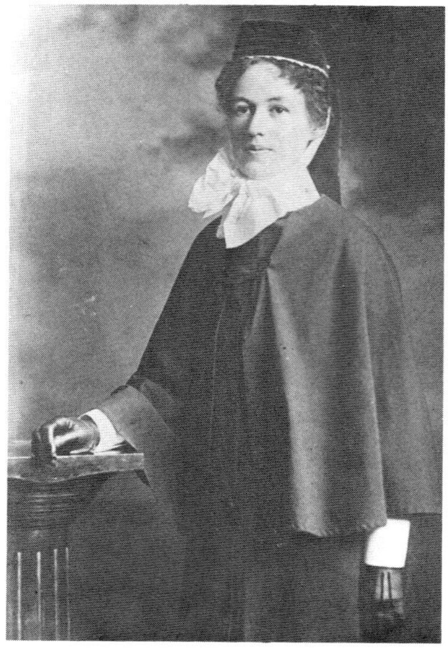

EMILY WHITE, 1901
outdoor uniform P.P.H.

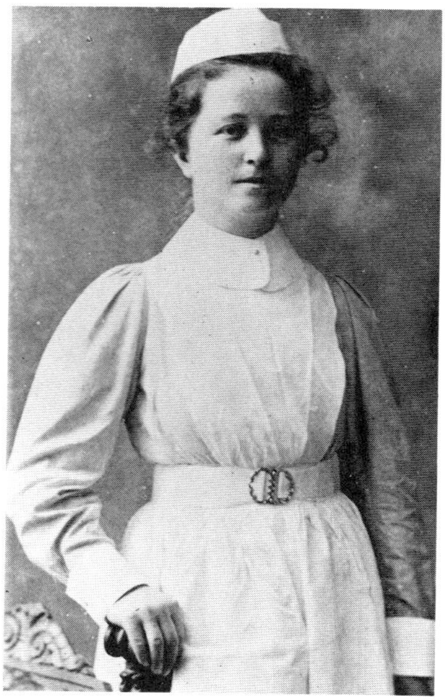

MAY ASHTON, C. 1903
probationer nurse P.P.H.

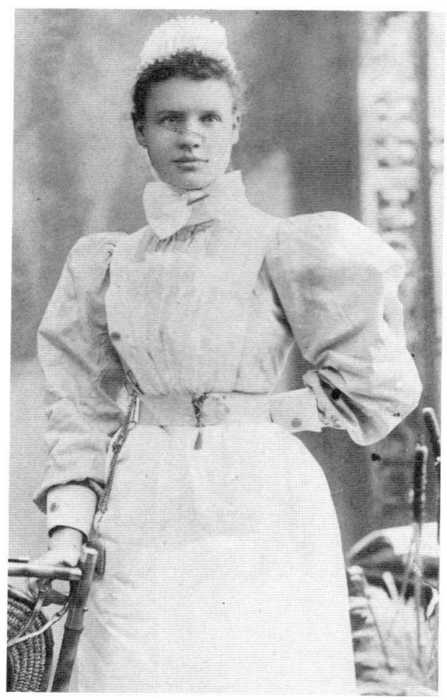

ANNIE MAY-STEERS, 1897

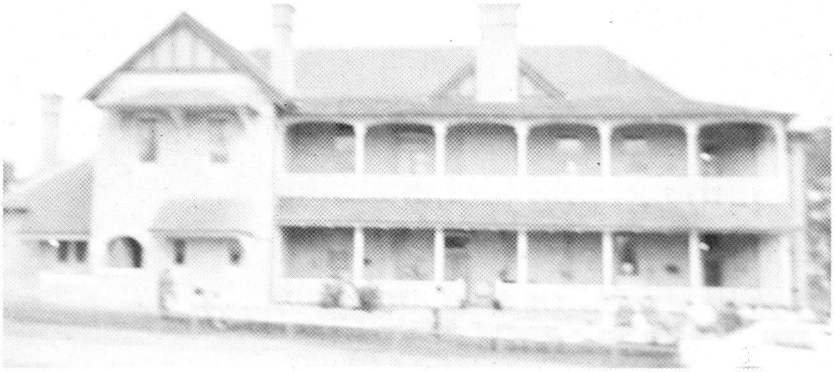

THE 'NEW' GOVERNMENT HOSPITAL, YORK, 1896
photo (1978) is of the restored building, now known as Mary Nicholas House.

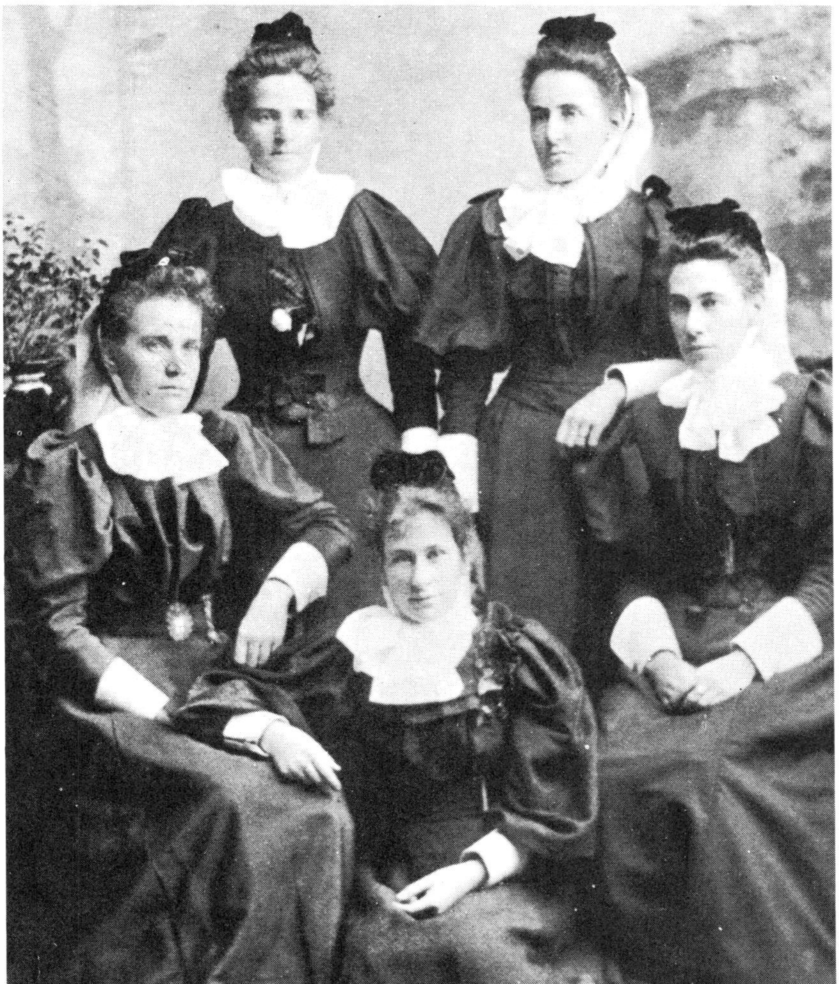

SISTERS OF THE PEOPLE, C. 1896

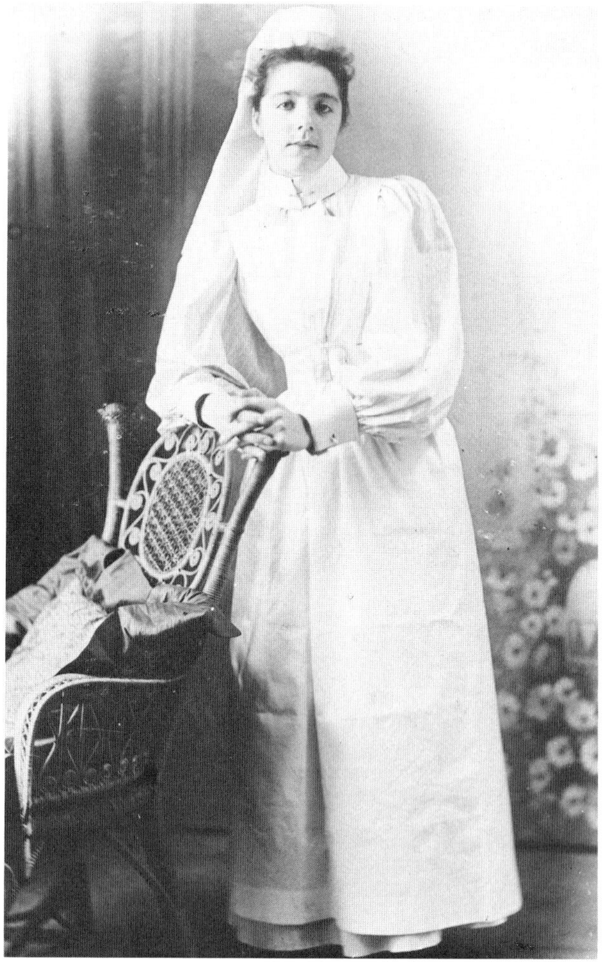

HELENA HUTTON, C. 1900

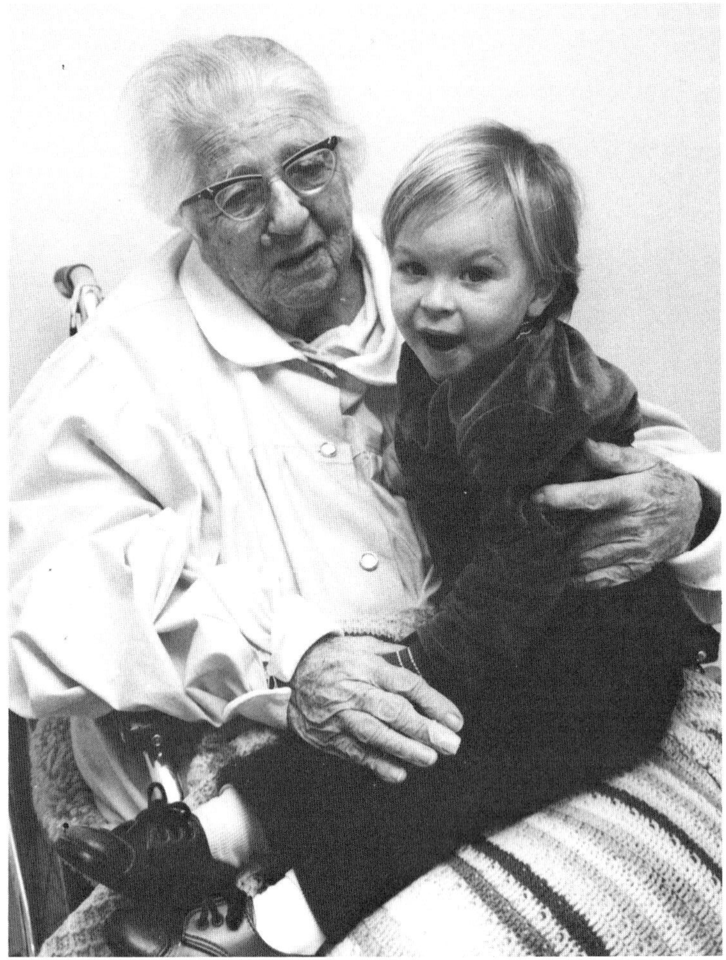

HELENA HUTTON, JULY 1978
with her great-greatnephew on her hundredth birthday.

on they were informed they would have to sleep in the steerage, but dine in the saloon. Immediately prior to leaving Perth in the train on Saturday afternoon they received the information that they would only be provided with steerage accommodation. As it was then too late to take any action the nurses decided to submit and inspect the accommodation before making any complaint. . . . The cabins were found to be ten-berth and the beds were minus sheets and pillow slips. . . .

[The nurses] were informed that for £70 more they could dine in the saloon. Telegrams were then sent to the secretary of the Nurses Fund Committee and also the Premier asking if they could be supplied with the necessary amount. The reply to the first telegram was that the money could not be sent, and no reply whatever came to hand from the Premier. The nurses decided that they would make the journey in the steerage. . . . They also had another cause for complaint. Before leaving Perth they were given to understand that £7 worth of luxuries had been put on the train for their use for the voyage but they never came to hand. On hearing the complaints made by the nurses several ladies made a collection in order to provide them with comforts during the voyage. Owing to the short notice only a limited number of people could be asked to contribute. In practically a few minutes the sum of £4.1s was subscribed. The following articles were then purchased and given to the matron; pillowslips 15s, 20 lbs biscuits, 20 pots Bovril, 20 meat extract, 2 doz unsweetened milk, 6 lbs prunes, 1 doz potted meat. Among those who knew the situation the nurses had been placed in there was an intense feeling of disgust at the treatment they had received.

As predicted, on reaching South Africa administrative difficulties arose and the group was disbanded. Some joined the Imperial Army Service and others, including Miss Nicolay, returned to Western Australia. A copy of the *Western Mail* of March 1900 gives pictures of the group prior to embarkation. Their names are given as Nurses Bole, Speers, Emmins, Armstrong, Rogers, Tchan, Naylor, Plover and Milne. Absence of initials makes it difficult to identify these women, but Miss Bole was one of the first graduate nurses of the Perth Public Hospital.[2]

It is also difficult to assess the impact on the local nursing situation caused by the withdrawal of trained nurses as no nursing registers were compiled, but the census figures throw some light on the situation, comparisons being given as follows:

Census of 1881

Nurses	7	female Aborigines [nursemaids?]
Midwives and sick nurses	22	

Census of 1891

Males: orderlies, hospital & poorhouse	10
Females: matrons, gaol hospital, lunatic asylum, etc.	10
Midwives	26

Census of 1901

Sick nurses:	male	1
	female	399
		400

Ages	*Distribution*
1 under 15 years	4 employed labour
20 ,, 25 ,,	4 assisting but not receiving wages
184 ,, 45 ,,	67 working on own behalf
178 ,, 65 ,,	271 receiving wages
16 over 65 ,,	11 unspecified
	42 unemployed

The above does not differentiate between trained and untrained, and it is possible that in the light of some of the current literature that some of the unemployed might have been unemployable. However, it was clearly time that both the graduate nurses and their patients had some type of organization to protect their interests and this was in part fulfilled by the founding of the Australasian Trained Nurses Association in New South Wales in 1899.[3]

The stimulus to form such an association seems to have stemmed from nurses domiciled in Australia who were members of the Matrons' Council of Great Britain and Ireland which had been organized by Miss Isla Stewart in 1894.[4] It was in 1899 at the second annual conference of this strong nursing body that Mrs Bedford-Fenwick proposed that steps be taken to organize an international council of nurses, along similar lines to the International Council of Women of which she was a member and staunch supporter. Miss S. McGahey, lady superintendent, Prince Alfred Hospital, Sydney, representing New South Wales, and Miss M. Farquharson, lady superintendent, Melbourne Hospital, representing Victoria, were both members of the Provisional Council of I.C.N. in 1900 and Miss McGahey was subsequently elected president at the first Quinquennial Congress held in Berlin in 1904.

At this stage Australian nurses did not have a national association. The A.T.N.A. mainly represented nurses in New South Wales but provision was made for the formation of state branches, with New South Wales becoming the parent association. Subsequently branches were formed in Queensland in 1904, South Australia in 1905, Western Australia in 1907 and Tasmania in 1908.

The position of New Zealand nurses is not quite clear, but it seems that they were affiliated with the A.T.N.A. until about 1906.

A strong nursing body, the Victorian Trained Nurses' Association, had been formed in Victoria in 1901 and an early basis for reciprocity was established with the A.T.N.A. However the two associations did not amalgamate and remained autonomous for nearly a quarter of a century.

In its first publication in 1900 the A.T.N.A. set out its rules and constitution (see Appendix III). Membership of the A.T.N.A. conferred upon its recipient the hallmark of being a professional nurse of the highest standard, and the badge of the association—a Maltese Cross in bright blue enamel outlined in silver, with the stars of the Southern Cross emblazoned in silver[5]—and the right to place the letters 'A.T.N.A.' after the person's name became status symbols. Association membership was not restricted to nurses and under its rules and constitution provision was made for the acceptance of members of the medical profession with full voting rights, auxiliary branch members—midwives—with limited voting, and honorary members without voting power. It was, as nominated, a *trained* nurses association, and its activities were directed to the protection and well being of the trained nurse practitioner who was self-employed in the private nursing field, which at this time was the greatest avenue of employment, the number of trained nurses employed as hospital staff being comparatively minimal.

Although the nurse in training did not qualify for membership, hospitals were invited to apply to the A.T.N.A. for recognition of their training programmes and the acceptance of their training certificates for the holder's subsequent membership acceptance. The value of the probationer nurse could not be overestimated in relation to the efficient functioning of the hospital both as a means of maintaining the standards of nursing care and also as an essential workforce, and therefore in this competitive field the hospitals accepted the directive of the A.T.N.A. in regard to their training syllabus. In so doing they virtually handed over the control of nursing training to the association.

Even though there was no branch of the A.T.N.A. in Western Australia until 1907, three hospitals applied for early recognition as A.T.N.A. training schools in 1900. They were Coolgardie, Kalgoorlie and Perth Public. Fremantle Public Hospital was not accepted at this stage but the trainees of this period were later admitted as full members.[6] A description of conditions in the hospitals of this period is given in an interview with two former probationer nurses when well into their nineties, Mrs de Moulin and Miss Helena Hutton,[7] and a report of the members of the select committee on the affairs of the Perth Public Hospital gives further enlightenment.[8]

As Miss Woodhead, Mrs de Moulin was one of the first group of five nurses selected as probationers at Fremantle Hospital in 1896-97. They were all interviewed by the principal medical officer of the Board of Health, Dr Thomas Lovegrove, at his office in Perth. Fremantle Hospital was then functioning in a building at the corner of Point and Cantonment streets near the port. Most of the patients were men of the older age group, but there was a six-bed women's ward, and a cottage at the rear for patients with grossly infected wounds. The nurses all shared one large room, with facilities for washing in one corner behind a screen, there being no bathrooms. There was a strict rule that uniform, which was silver gray, was worn off duty since the vicinity of the hospital was a 'red-light' area and this was a protective measure, the nurses being referred to as 'silver tails'.

The matron, Miss Bessie Steel, was a strict disciplinarian, but fair. She insisted that the nurses had time off duty, two hours in the morning or afternoon on alternate days, but would not allow them to go to their rooms to lie down, maintaining that they needed fresh air, so they had to go for long walks. She instructed them in their basic nursing skills of bandaging, dressing of wounds with the use of foot and hand baths, poultice making, and sponging, and bed making. Many of the patients admitted were from the ships and had been ill in their bunks for some time without hygiene, as a consequence the hospital had its fair share of bugs. Pneumonia was frequent in the older men, and the ever-present typhoid fever. Some surgery was performed, the senior surgeon, Dr White, always presented immaculately dressed in full morning dress. There was little antisepsis, the main agents used being corrosive sublimate, or a few drops of iodine added to the water for the bathing of wounds.

After a few months the hospital and staff transferred to the Knowle, which is still part of the Fremantle Hospital. After Point Street, the nurses thought it was 'heaven'.

The hospital was for people without means and the courses of most illnesses were lengthy so that nurses came to know their patients well and it was often distressing to find that after weeks of careful care, patients were discharged without means of rehabilitation. Mrs de Moulin quotes the case of a young man with typhoid fever who had been desperately ill, and within a few days of discharge from hospital was recognized working with a gang of prisoners in cleaning up the hospital grounds. Without a job, money or a place to live, he had smashed a street lamp in order to get arrested and assured of a meal.

Miss Helena Hutton was not quite eighteen when sent to Geraldton Hospital in 1897 as a lone 'probationer', and the long train journey of over 480 kilometres was somewhat of an ordeal. The hospital was the Victoria Hospital, an imposing two-storeyed building opened on the occasion of the Diamond Jubilee of Queen Victoria. A newer, larger block was in the course of completion in anticipation of a gold rush which did not eventuate, so it was not occupied for a long time. There was a reasonably good staff and the young probationer was instructed by the more senior members in nursing care of patients, which included temperature taking, urine testing, giving of enemas and the application of cold wet packs to reduce fever. Medications were given orally in mixture form, there being no tablets. A number of the patients were Lascars from the ships, and these were housed in a forbidding stone building removed from the hospital wards; the disease to be feared was typhus, which at that time was considered highly contagious.

After almost two years Miss Hutton became ill with typhoid, and on recovery was transferred to Kalgoorlie Hospital to complete her nursing training. During her time in Geraldton there was a minimum amount of ward cleaning done by the nursing staff, and the staff at Kalgoorlie were surprised that she was so well informed about nursing.

At Kalgoorlie she received her first lectures from the matron, Mrs Harvey, and the visiting doctors: anatomy and physiology, with emphasis on the Peyers patches and dietary care of patients with typhoid fever. The old adage of 'feed a cold and starve a fever' was strictly adhered to, and Baccus Marsh condensed milk was the only additive to boiled water allowed. In all patients with protracted high temperatures it was the practice to shave their heads as a measure of cooling, and on recovery from illness they would present literally as shadows of their former selves.

Miss Hutton's nursing certificate, gained in 1902, was accepted for membership of the A.T.N.A. when she registered with that body in 1906.

Building extensions to Perth Public Hospital did not result in improved nursing care, so that arising out of a series of inquests on patients who had died by misadventure, a select committee of the Legislative Assembly was convened to inquire into conditions at that hospital. During the hearing, members of both the medical and nursing staff were called to give evidence. Although the nursing staff consisted of mainly young probationers, their dignity, honesty and clarity of expression did them credit. The report, published after its presentation in November 1900, shows that the hierarchical order of nurse training had been introduced, matron, senior sister,

sister, staff nurse, third, second and first year probationers. There was no ancillary staff, and even junior probationers were questioned as to their knowledge of patients' social conditions and whether there was a place for them to go to on discharge from hospital, although the nurses could in no way have controlled this. No mention is made of lectures or time allowed for attending these, but hours of duty and conditions are shown in the evidence of Miss Annie Anderson, the matron, and a first and a third year probationer nurse. Miss Anderson said that conditions at Perth Public Hospital compared well with those of training hospitals in other parts of Australia and abroad. They compared very favourably with Melbourne Hospital, which was her own training school (1895-98), where a £10 premium was required and nurses received a very low salary.

> Here we give them print for their uniforms and caps every year Jessie Hurnall is the superintendent and Ella Techow is the night superintendent, they get £70 a year each, the other charge nurses get £52. The third year probationers get £30 a year, the second £20 and the first £12 . . . my own is £120 a year.

The duties and salaries of nurses were compared with those paid to wards-maids:

> There is more gentility in one department and more salary in the other—Nurses go there and receive training to fit them to earn their living.
>
> How many night superintendents are there? Only one.
>
> But is she not there every night? Yes every night.
>
> On duty continuously? On duty continuously. That is one of the drawbacks to our institution. That is the night superintendent. I cannot remedy it; she gets a salary of £70, while charge nurses get £52. It means a great deal to her because she is supporting a sister in Switzerland. I would willingly put her on but I should have to pay her only £52. She gets one night per month and two late nights a week. It is a great mental strain on her but I cannot remedy it for the reason that the salaries are different. We have a uniform salary of £52 a year for charge nurses and the night superintendent gets £70. It is desirable from a point of discipline to have one lady all the year round at this work.

Ann Bennett Hicks, examined.

> You are a nurse at the Perth Hospital? I am a probationer of the third year.
>
> You are working 10 hours a day? Ten hours a night. At

present I am on night duty. We go on at 9 o'clock and come off at 7 in the morning.

In your opinion do you think 10 hours too long a stretch? for continuous duty?— I would not mind the 10 hours if we could have a night off duty in the month. Before the rules were altered we went on at 8 and came off at 8 in the morning but we had a whole night off once a month and a 10 o'clock evening once a week. That was something to look forward to in the week; and it also gave us a rest because a great number of the night nurses slept badly in the day time owing to the noises. That is why we so much appreciated the night off and the ten o'clock evening.

You think 70 hours a week are rather too much especially for night duty? —Especially when we are three months on at a stretch, and we practically have only 9 hours off duty the whole three months.

May I ask what salary you receive? Thirty pounds a year but of course we have our training.

Ruby Frances Fry was a first year probationer, and out of her evidence arises the fact that the majority of staff in the hospital were probationers and that there must have been a great deal of wastage as the number of graduating nurses was very few. The responsibility for patient care was often beyond their clinical experience and the long hours on duty with little respite left them less inclination to go out in the meagre time they were off duty.

The records show that all the nurses who gave evidence went on to complete the three year training. Two of these became influential figures in nursing: Miss Maida Balding was matron of Fremantle Hospital for twenty-five years, and Mrs Florence Weller, née Shapcott, was a foundation member of the Florence Nightingale Club, and supporter of several nursing organizations.

The 1900 report is in itself a monument to the 'short but simple annals of the poor'. One of the findings was that the committee considered that the hours of labour imposed on nursing staff were too long, that the time allowed for recreation was too limited and the salaries paid insufficient. However, one recommendation did eventually bear fruit, and that was 'that a home for incurables and for the reception of patients suffering from mental or physical weakness should be established as it had come to the notice of the Committee that the Hospital was burdened with several incurables and also that patients had been discharged who were not mentally fitted to take care of themselves'.

The Home of Peace for the Dying and Incurable was formally opened in Hamersley Road, Subiaco, in 1902.[9] Sponsored by prominent citizens and supported by public subscription, its delay was due to the fact that the original site was not acceptable to the people in what was then considered a prestige area.

It is interesting to note that before the founding of the Home of Peace, the government was approached by the Anglican Order of the Good Shepherd for assistance in building an institution for the chronically ill, and that such assistance was refused on the grounds that it would have church control.

Although the Home of Peace was not acceptable as a training school, the matron, Miss Kate Anderson, treated her nurses as probationers, and taught them well. It was an unwritten law that when they were eligible to commence training they were sent to Fremantle Hospital. This practice continued for several years and among the many well-known nurses who commenced their careers in this way were Mary Carson, Ruth Bottle and others.

The years from 1901 to 1905 could almost be considered as the hidden years of nursing as little information is available. Although the recognition of their training schools by the A.T.N.A. gave them eligibility to join the association, it would seem that few of the Western Australian trained nurses did this, although they called themselves A.T.N.A. nurses. Reasons for this can only be conjecture, but it is possible that they were not sufficiently informed and also by not having a branch of the association in the state lengthy correspondence would have been needed to contact the head office in New South Wales.

The rules of the A.T.N.A. were also a deterrent, as members who had received their experience in the field of general nursing were forbidden to undertake the management of midwifery patients except in emergency, and there was no hospital in Western Australia deemed to come up to the standard as an A.T.N.A. midwifery training school. Failure to conform with the above rule meant deregistration. It is known that practically all Western Australian nurses practised in the above field.[10] Trained nurses usually worked with a medical practitioner who was responsible for the management of the actual delivery, but delay often meant that the nurse attendant had to officiate and the birth was complete before the doctor arrived on the scene. Analgesia, practically non-existent, was limited to chloroform, which was carried by the obstetrician and administered by the nurse.

The attitude of both doctors and members of the public towards midwifery patients is reflected in a paragraph in the *Western Argus*, Kalgoorlie, 24 January 1905:

Maternity Ward for Kalgoorlie

A letter was received from the Under Secretary at the meeting

> of the Kalgoorlie Municipal Council, Monday with reference to the subject of the establishment of a maternity ward at Kalgoorlie. The writer stated by direction that all medical opinions were against its establishment in the hospital grounds. To provide a separate building in a different locality would require a special vote by parliament. Cr Erson spoke against a maternity ward on hospital grounds. A maternity home should not be near a surgical ward . . . . It was the voice of all of the medical profession throughout the world that was against the building of a maternity hospital beside a surgical one. He thought that a separate piece of ground should be obtained and the medical profession would be pleased.

By 1904 a basis of reciprocity was reached between the Australasian Trained Nurses Association and the Victorian Trained Nurses' Association which allowed members registered with one association to transfer to the other without further assessment. It was also agreed that all hospitals already recognized as training schools for nurses by the Australasian association would be recognized by the Victorian association. However it was agreed that hospitals in Victoria would come under the jursidiction of the Victorian association, while in New South Wales and other Australian states the control would be by the Australasian association.

This historic document was signed by the presidents of both associations, who were both doctors, F. North Manning, M.D., for the A.T.N.A. and J. W. Springthorpe, M.D., for the V.T.N.A.[11] In the same publication, the A.T.N.A. set out its policies with regard to the recognition and registration of training schools for nurses; the schedule of study to be accepted as the minimum course for registration by the A.T.N.A.; and the Midwifery Nurses' Auxiliary Branch rules.

In Western Australia this paved the way for the formation of a branch of the A.T.N.A. in this state, which was still heavily dependent on nurses from other states for its matrons and senior nursing staff. Both the matrons of Perth and Fremantle Public Hospitals were from the state of Victoria.[12]

In 1905 the A.T.N.A. parent body issued what could be termed an ultimatum:

> In the case of all Nurses completing their training after June 30th 1906, it will be necessary to pass the examination for membership of the Association, except in the case of candidates presenting certificates from those other States or countries with which the Australasian Trained Nurses' Association has a reciprocal agreement.[13]

In the face of this it was imperative that a state branch of the association be formed which could appoint its own examiners and supervise the implementation of the rules and schedule for study. Without this, nurses from Western Australia would have had no opportunity within their own state of taking the examination and becoming members.

On 31 October 1907 a meeting was called to inaugurate a state branch of the Australasian Trained Nurses Association. Held in the board room of Perth Public Hospital, it was chaired by Dr Martin and attended by members of both the medical and nursing professions.[14] In the election of officers which followed it is interesting to note that there were country as well as metropolitan representatives and some of those elected were not present at the meeting, including the president, Dr Athelstone Saw. Miss K. Ryan and Dr Officer were elected vice presidents, and Miss McNamara and Dr Tymms, honorary secretaries. Members of the council included eight medical men and fourteen nurses. In deciding a quorum of eight, there was no mention that there should be an equal number of medical and nursing members. The medical men were accepted as members without further qualifications but nurse members had to be eligible under the rules of the association. However, over the subsequent years the medical members stood firmly behind the nurses. It was probably due to their influence as honorary doctors of Perth Public Hospital that the association was provided over the next fifteen years with a meeting place free of charge.

The minutes of the inaugural meeting of the West Australian Branch of the A.T.N.A. as recorded in the original minutes book of the association show that there were only twenty-five persons present, five medical men and twenty nurses, most of whom were non-members. The twenty nurses represented were matrons of Perth Hospital, House of Mercy, private hospitals and nurses' homes (employment bureaux), charge sisters and nurses engaged in private duty. Absence of initials has made recognition difficult but they have been identified as follows.

Miss Kate Power-Ryan: matron of Perth Public Hospital. Succeeded Miss Annie Anderson in 1906. Trained at Ballarat Base Hospital, Victoria, 1890-92. Charge sister and matron of Victorian country hospitals until coming to Western Australia in 1906. Member of R.V.T.N.A.

Miss J. McKimmie: matron of a private hospital, Perth, subsequently admitted to membership under Rule XXI.

Miss Eva McNamara: One of three sisters who owned and conducted the Waverley Private Hospital for general and midwifery patients. She was subsequently admitted to membership under Rule XXI.

Miss M. Anderson: matron, private nursing home. Trained at Ballarat Hospital, Victoria, 1897-1900.
Mrs Antoinette Harris, née Grafe: matron, House of Mercy, Perth. Trained Adelaide Hospital, 1895-98; Women's Hospital, Melbourne, 1905-06.
Miss Stronach: no training background. Matron of a nurses' home. Accepted as an honorary member.
Miss Susan Rose Lee: third-year nurse, Perth Public Hospital. First nurse to qualify by taking A.T.N.A. examination in this state, 1908.
Miss (? Frances Annie) Phillips: sister, Perth Public Hospital. Trained Perth Public Hospital, 1900-03. Member of the A.T.N.A. 1904.
Miss Mary Isabel Peile: sister, Perth Public Hospital. Trained Perth Public Hospital, 1903-06. Member of A.T.N.A. 1906.
Miss Maida Florence Balding: sister, Perth Public Hospital. After completing her training at Perth Public Hospital in 1902 Miss Balding joined the Medical Department and nursed in Geraldton and Coolgardie. She rejoined the staff of Perth Public Hospital in 1906. Subsequently she became matron of Fremantle Hospital, retiring after twenty-five years service. She joined the A.T.N.A. in 1906.
Miss Frances Elizabeth Potten: trained at Perth Public Hospital, 1904-07.
Miss Isabel Tait Borwick: sister, Perth Public Hospital. Trained Ballarat Public Hospital 1899-1903. Subsequently had a long and interesting association with nursing, both military and civil, and was awarded an associateship of the Order of the Royal Red Cross (A.R.R.C.).
Miss (? Marian Glenfield) Johnstone: sister, Perth Public Hospital. Trained Perth Public Hospital 1902-05. Member of A.T.N.A. 1906.
Miss Mary Francis Kelliher: recently completed training at Fremantle Hospital, staff nurse.
Miss Elsie Begg: nurse, Perth Public Hospital. Trained 1904-07.
Misses McClosky, McKenzie, Krugher and McCulloch: unidentified. They do not appear to have applied to join the association.
Mrs Helen May Dunn, née Monkhouse: completed training, Perth Public Hospital 1904-07.

Those who tendered apologies but were elected to office were:
Miss Alice T. Dixon: matron from 1900 of Fremantle Hospital. Certificate from Melbourne Hospital 1888-90. Member R.V.T.N.A.
Mrs Christian Shackell, née Nickoll: matron of a trained nurses' home. Widow of Dr Shackell. Trained Wakefield Street Private Hospital, Adelaide.

Miss Kate Anderson: matron, Home of Peace, Subiaco. Admitted to membership under Rule XXI.
Miss Jean Fyfe: matron, Bunbury Hospital. Trained Adelaide Hospital 1892-95. Came to Western Australia during the gold rush and nursed in many country centres. Senior matron with Medical Department (Served in World War I, awarded associateship of the Royal Red Cross).
Miss Miriam Plover: matron, Topsham Private Hospital. Trained Brisbane Hospital 1893-97. One of a contingent of nurses to accompany Miss Nicolay to the Boer War.
Miss Hannah Maria Gilbert: staff, Old Women's Home, Perth, formerly known as the Poorhouse. Cert. of Obstetrics from London Obst. Society.

Those elected to office but not present were:
Mrs Florence J. E. Harvey, née Way: matron, Kalgoorlie Hospital. Trained Adelaide Hospital 1891-95. As Miss Way she had been appointed to Hannan's Hospital in 1895-96 and returned as matron of the Government Hospital, Kalgoorlie, 1898.
Miss Frances Cully: private nurse. Cert. Women's Hospital, Sydney. Accepted for General and Obstetric Register, Rule XXIa.
Miss McLeod (? Lorn Edith Campbell McLeod): private nursing home, Perth. Cert. two years Hoemopathic Hospital, Melbourne Women's Hospital. Member of R.V.T.N.A.
Because of the duplication of names it is possible that there may be some mistaken identities. There were several Andersons, three McNamaras, two McLeods, three Dunns, two Phillipses, two Johnstones on the registers.[15]

The minutes of the inaugural meeting were signed by the president, Dr Athelstone Saw, and dated 10 January 1908, indicating that meetings were held at three monthly intervals.

At the first meeting of the council of the association it was agreed that the financial year would be from 1 January to 31 December, and the treasurer, Dr Martin, was authorized to open an account in the Bank of Australasia in the name of the Australasian Trained Nurses Association, West Australian Branch. Cheques were to be signed by the president and the honorary treasurer, both members of the medical profession. A telegram was received from the parent association, with congratulations and provisional ratification of the appointed council.

The first decision was the approval of membership, and it was agreed to elect all applicants who came under rules XVIII and XIX as laid down by the association, but to refer all other applicants to the parent association for approval. The thirteen medical applicants were approved, but of the forty-two nurse applicants, it would appear that a few did not meet the requirements. Many practising as nurses in Western Australia would have been ineligible to join the association unless the concessional clauses were extended. Arising out of this, a request was forwarded asking for amendments to rules XXI and XXIa which had become obsolete. The amendments to these rules were as follows:

> Rule XXI. That the rule be altered to read:—'to December 31st 1908' instead of March 31st 1900, and in line four after the word 'nursing', shall be inserted 'in Western Australia'.
> That rule XXIa shall be altered to read 'prior to 31st December 1908 has been engaged for a period of three years nursing in a hospital or hospitals recognized by or deemed worthy of recognition by the Council of the Australasian Trained Nurses Association and who has resided in Western Australia since 31st December 1905 and who can produce etc.'

The important matter of fees was introduced by the matrons of registered homes. These homes, which were employment agencies and hostels for trained nurses, supplied nurses for private patients and private hospitals, and there were many of them around Perth. If registered with the A.T.N.A. they had to conform to the rules, employing only A.T.N.A. members and charging fees laid down by the association; furthermore they could only supply nurses on the recommendation of a doctor. A subcommittee was formed to resolve the matter, and its recommendations subsequently adopted as follows:

> Ordinary Cases £3-3-0d weekly
> Day or night (12 hours) 10/6d
> Operation cases £1-1-0d
> These fees are inclusive of suburban travelling expenses.
> In the event of a case occurring where a nurse accepts a case at a reduced fee, she must report to the Council of having done so.

For those nurses engaged in private practice there was always an element of uncertainty. In some cases it meant nursing the patient in a large home, well equipped, and with adequate domestic staff, while in cases of the less affluent members of the community the nurse often found herself looking after both the patient and the family. Her salary, too, was not always forthcoming, and although the association rules required her to report unsatisfactory conditions, she was often reluctant to do this in view of the fact that the employing agents, medical men and matrons, were often members of the A.T.N.A. Council and there could be discrimination against her future employment. Nevertheless a nurse gained a lot of satisfaction in having the sole care of patients, and often formed a lifetime friendship with them and their families, returning to care for them when future nursing was required.[16]

A most important function of the Council of the A.T.N.A. was the organization of nursing education, for under the new ruling all nurses accepted for training had to be educationally assessed by a committee appointed from people in that specific field.[17] Whether they received payment from the hospital concerned, the association or the applicant is not known. It is possible that the service was honorary. Among the first personnel suggested were Mr Faulkner, High School, St Georges Terrace, Perth; Mrs Gouly, headmistress of Sisters of the Church, Cathedral Avenue; Reverend Brother Newman, Christian Brothers School; Miss Walker, principal, Bedford College; Mr Anderson, Scotch College. A ballot resulted in the election of Faulkner, Newman and Anderson. However the two latter subsequently declined to accept.

There was also the introduction of a curriculum, which was quite extensive (see Appendix III) and the appointment of instructors in invalid cookery.

A board of examiners was appointed for the association, consisting of Miss Power-Ryan, matron, Perth Hospital; Miss Dixon, matron, Fremantle Hospital; Miss K. Anderson, matron, Home of Peace; Drs Officer, Clealand and Anderson.[18] The first state examination was deferred until December 1908.

Although there was no interference with the domestic running of hospitals registered with the A.T.N.A. as training schools or the deployment of trainee nurses, nevertheless the management was required to furnish a yearly report, and list of attendances at lectures, etc. Furthermore the matrons had to be members of the A.T.N.A. as did also members of the trained staff. For those hospitals administered by the Medical Department this proved to be almost impossible, but the association was adamant, and could and did deregister any hospital which did not comply, thereby penalizing the trainees by ruling them ineligible to sit the A.T.N.A. examination.

Matrons were responsible for giving the lectures in nursing, setting and marking the examination papers as well as sitting in on the lectures given by the doctors in anatomy and physiology, surgery, medicine and hygiene. Students had to compile their own lecture notes from material given by the dictation method of delivery. Textbooks used were Foster and Shore's *Physiology for Beginners*, which was also the textbook used for the subject when taught in the schools; and *General Nursing* by Eva Luckes, first written when she was appointed matron of London Hospital in 1884, but rewritten and updated in 1898 with further editions in 1905. Evaluated against the knowledge of the day and age in which it was written this book is truly remarkable for its detail and insight of the patient as a person, the nurse's role as an observer and the very first requirement of a hospital as enunciated by Florence Nightingale, 'that it should do the sick no harm'.

A Handbook for Nurses by J. K. Watson, M.D., which was also used, makes reference to the fact that in 1908 it had been updated to include notes on X rays, the administration of oxygen, and enlargement of the prostate gland, although in the section of anatomy there is no mention of either male or female organs of reproduction. These are also omitted from the curriculum laid down by the A.T.N.A.

The training schools did not provide lecture rooms for nurses, the board rooms of Perth and Fremantle Hospitals being used for this purpose. Even the 'new' nurses quarters of Perth Hospital, now known as Kirkman House, did not provide facilities for study. Teaching aids were limited to a skeleton and blackboard and all practical instruction was given on the wards. With the emphasis on economy it would have been considered extravagant to use materials for practice only. Lint—which was used extensively for foments, padding for splints, and bandages—was washed and re-used. The few textbooks and nursing journals which comprised the library were kept under lock and key and available on application only. Invalid cookery was taught in the hospital kitchens, and of necessity had to be in the evening after the kitchen staff had finished.

The method of accepting probationer nurses for training was on a replacement basis; as one nurse completed her training or dropped out, another was called up to take her place. As soon as there was a sufficient number to form a class, lectures were initiated. It is not possible to give the exact number of nurses in training, but judging by the number put forward as acceptable by the Education Committee and those who completed training, the wastage was considerable. It is doubtful if there would have been an average of twelve per year graduating from all three training schools.[19]

In 1907 Perth Hospital accepted responsibility for the administration and staffing of Victoria Hospital (the Infectious Diseases Branch), and this could possibly account for the slight increase in nursing staff, noted at that time.

The pressure of business made it imperative for the A.T.N.A. Council to meet monthly instead of three monthly as originally planned, and even so there was a considerable delay in receiving correspondence from the parent body, which also issued all certificates. Difficulties of communication gave rise to problems regarding acceptance for membership and conduct of examinations. Under the rules, all nurses who wished to qualify for membership after June 1906 were required to take the membership examination, but at the first meeting of the West Australian Branch Council, 10 January 1908, it was decided to accept all those who qualified under Rules XVIII and XIX and refer all others to the parent body. However, at the next meeting a directive from headquarters refused membership to four nurses who had completed their training at Perth, Fremantle and government hospitals, requiring them to take the membership examination. Dr Haynes, a somewhat controversial member of the Branch Council, spoke up in defence of these nurses, saying that they would have had no opportunity of sitting for the examination, and asked that concession be made in their case. This was granted but an interim type of examination was introduced pending the setting up of a full examination board in this state. Sealed papers were sent from the eastern states and the written papers returned for marking and assessment. The two nurses to take this examination were Susan Lee and Alice Maud James, both from Perth Hospital, and both passed. The date of this is not known but a further examination held in June 1908 extended the pattern to include an oral assessment in addition to the written papers. The three nurses taking this also passed. They were Beatrice (Bridgit) Victoria Anderson, Alice Hilda Scharer and Alice Maud Newnham, all of Perth Hospital.

The first examination conducted by the West Australian Branch of the association was held at Perth Hospital on 8 and 9 December 1908, written, practical and oral. Questions had been forwarded to Sydney for selection, and the sealed papers sent back to Perth. Nurses taking this examination were from Perth and Fremantle hospitals, none from the government hospitals. Names of the nurses are listed below as they could be considered the first to take the Western Australian examination, which they all passed: Phyllis Bromley, Jessie Cassell, Annie Donnell, Dora Ellis, Martha Palfreyman and Effie Yelland, of Perth Hospital; and Florence Anderson, Olive Grace Davey, Isabelle Main, and May Isabella Waller, of Fremantle Hospital.[20]

It was the strict adherence to its rules in granting selective membership that gave the A.T.N.A., together with the Victorian association, control of professional nurses throughout Australia. A register was published every two years and in it was given all the members' nursing backgrounds and the terms of their admission to membership. As the rules were reprinted in each issue, it was a

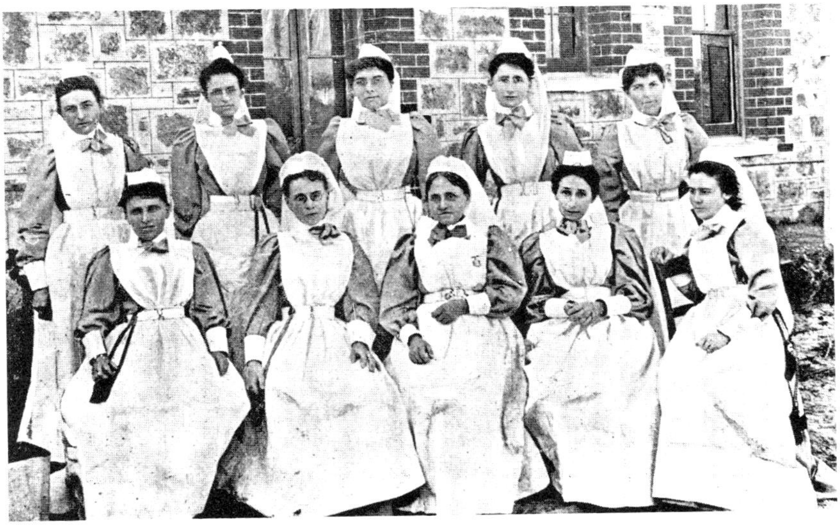

BOER WAR NURSES, 1900

back row: Speers, Emmins, Armstrong, Bole, Rogers; *front row:* Tchan, Naylor, Nicolay, Plover, Milne.

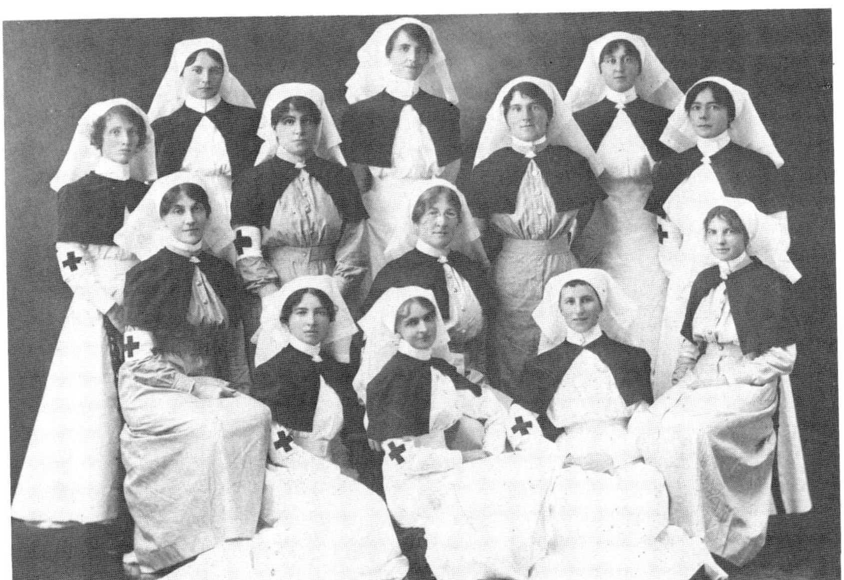

WORLD WAR I NURSES, 1915

back row: M. Scanlon, M. Hayes, E. Doherty; *second row:* R. Bottle, I. Lovell, H. Homan, M. Lightbody; *seated:* E. Crohan (?), J. Crosby (matron), D. Smith; *front row:* E. Hamersley, E. Phipps, N. Walsh.

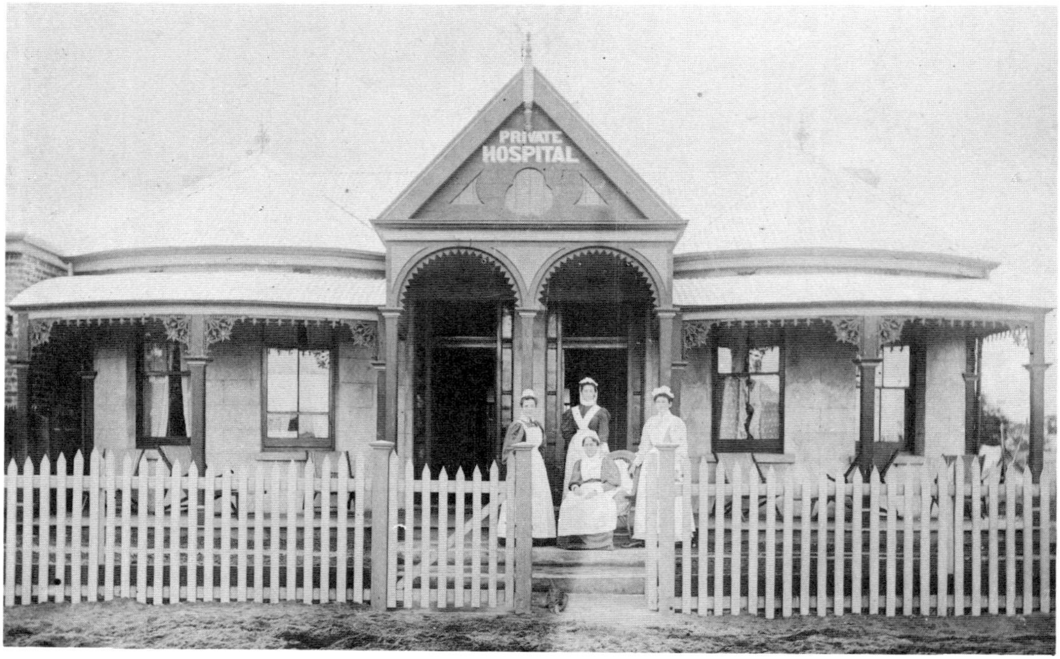

SISTER NICOLAY'S PRIVATE HOSPITAL, BRISBANE STREET, PERTH, 1897

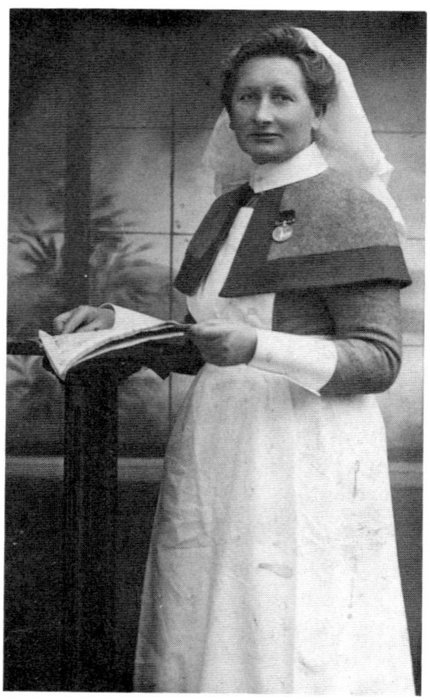

ELIZABETH BOLE, IMPERIAL ARMY NURSING RESERVE, 1901

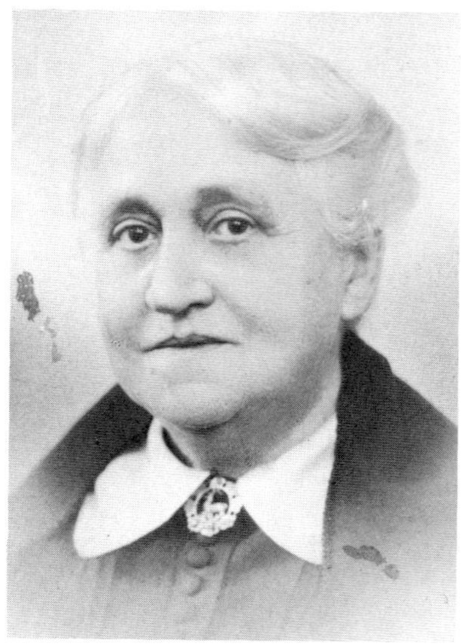

MARY NICOLAY, C. 1920

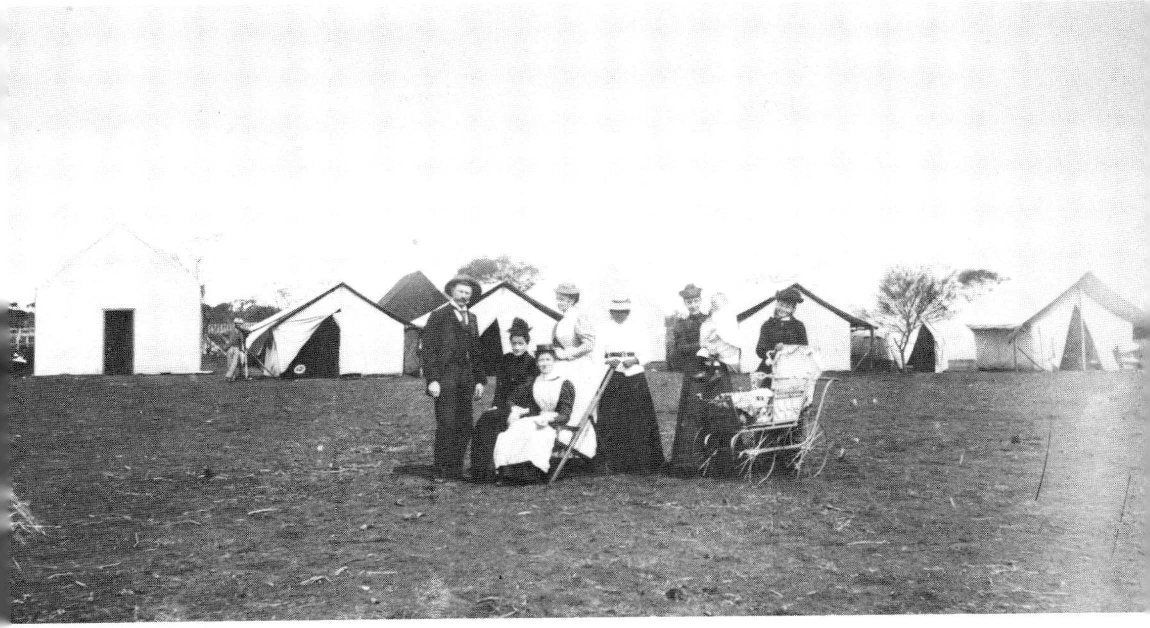

THE EARLY COOLGARDIE HOSPITAL, 1894

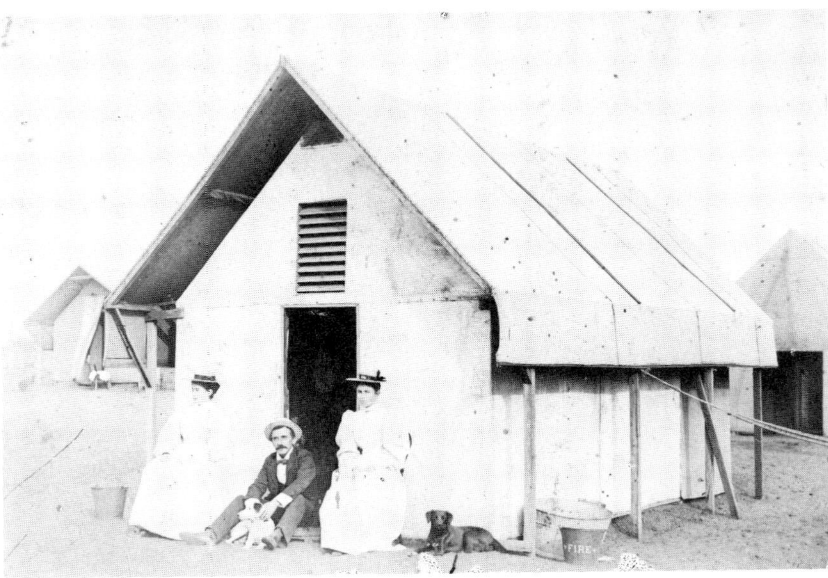

NURSES' QUARTERS, COOLGARDIE, 1898

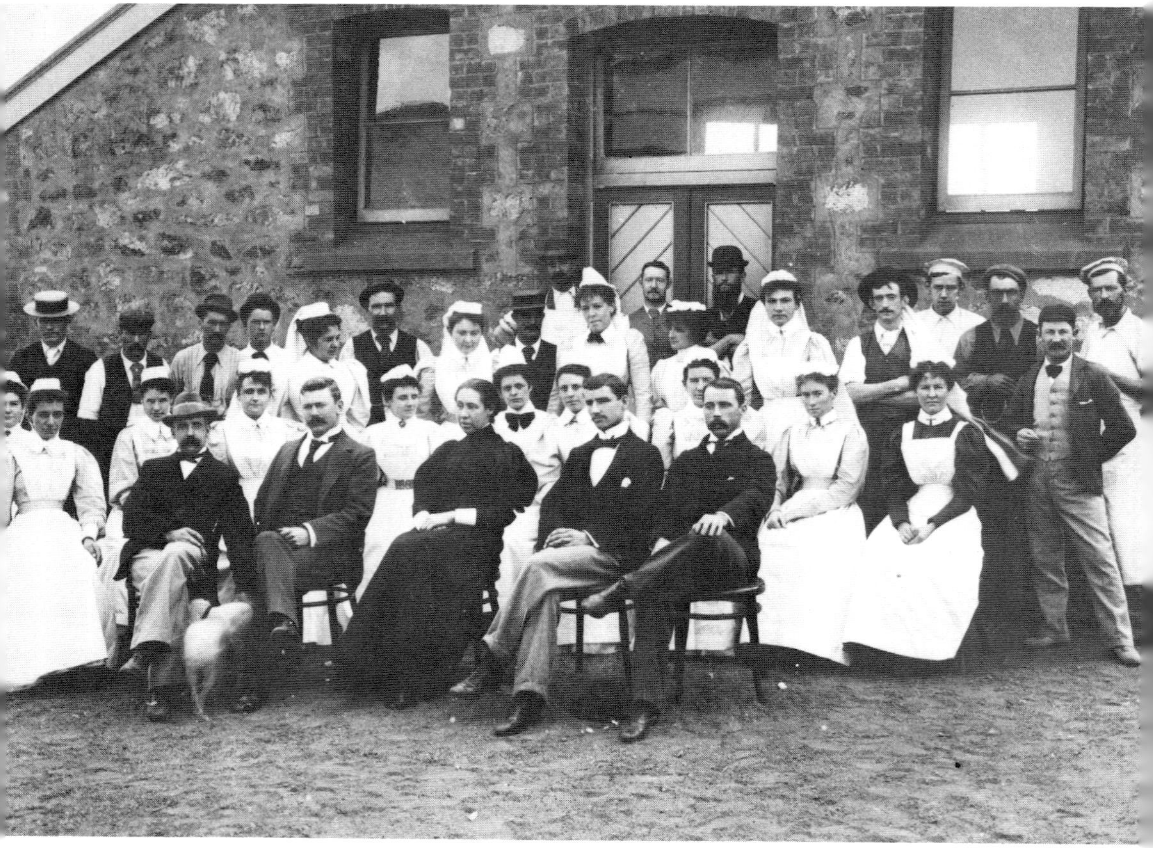

COOLGARDIE HOSPITAL STAFF, 1897

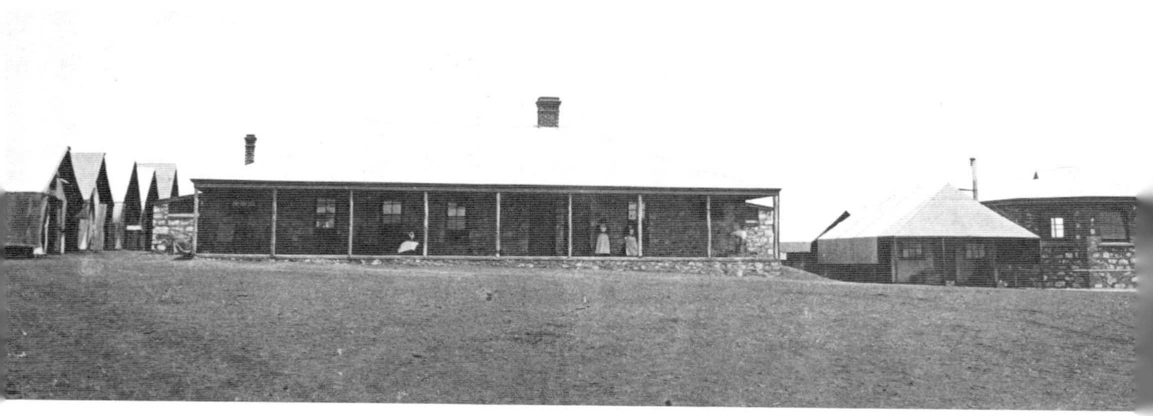

COOLGARDIE HOSPITAL, 1897

simple matter to look up the members' qualifications. There was evidently some feeling about this for as the years went on, those who had been accepted under concessional clauses tended to be looked on by some of their nursing colleagues as second-class (nursing) citizens. A copy of the register together with the A.T.N.A. journal, published monthly, was sent to every financial member and the former was available to the public. The cost of this was offset by the membership fees, half of which were sent to the parent body for this purpose. Joining fee was £1 1s 0d, life membership £5 5s 0d (with a limit of twelve years for free journals and registers) and annual membership 10s 6d. Medical members paid £2 2s 0d life membership but it is not known whether or not they received copies of the journal and the register. It is not known whether the registered nurses' homes and training schools contributed financially to the association. However arising from a resolution at the first annual meeting of the West Australian Branch, a request to have the fees reduced was acceded to.

The acceptance of the A.T.N.A. is shown by the applications of five nurses' homes for registration. They were from Mrs Shackell, 194 Stirling Street; Miss Stronach, 237 Beaufort Street; Mrs Strickland, née Byrne, Forrest Avenue; Miss Alice Moore, St Georges Terrace; and the Misses McNamara, Adelaide Terrace. These were accepted although it is known that the last two applicants were combining the nurses' homes with private hospitals. This often involved the employment of the nurse as hospital staff during the patient's stay in hospital, and on discharge accompanying him to continue caring for him during convalescence in his own home. The A.T.N.A. did not normally approve of this practice, which brought the private hospitals into competition with the nurses' homes.

There were also two applications from hospitals for registration as nurse-training schools. The first was 'Topsham', a private hospital conducted by Miss Plover and owned by Dr Haynes, and where the daily average number of occupied beds over the past two years had been twelve. It was duly registered as a five year training school for nurses. The second application came from the matron of St John of God Hospital, Kalgoorlie, asking for a special concession to allow four nurses who were in training to sit for the examination in twelve months to two years time. It was stated that they had already been nursing for nine, six, seven and four years respectively. The daily average number of occupied beds was shown to have been seven and a half during the past two years. This application was deferred as the average was too low.

It would seem that the matrons of nurses' homes were very much aware of the restrictions placed on them by being registered with the A.T.N.A. and one of them, Miss Stronach, asked if the medical men in private practice would pledge themselves to support A.T.N.A. members and nurses' homes. The reply to this was that all medical men who were members would endeavour to further the interests of registered A.T.N.A. nurses and homes.

The progress of the West Australian Branch of the A.T.N.A. is reflected in the report of the first general meeting, which took the form of a social evening for members and guests.[21] It was held in the Hibernian Hall, Murray Street, on 24 July 1908, and was given coverage in the press. Over one hundred attended, including a representative of state parliament and many members of the medical profession. The social aspect of the gathering was enhanced by items from people prominent in Perth's musical circles, and the serving of refreshments. Business was kept to a minimum, Dr Saw giving a short presidential address in which he outlined the objects of the A.T.N.A. and made a strong appeal for the establishment of a maternity hospital in Perth which could function within the rules laid down by the association, and become a recognized A.T.N.A. maternity training school for nurses. Dr Saw concluded his address with the following:

> They had had the Premier's policy speech at Bunbury, but he noticed that the Premier had not in his speech referred to something they considered of vital need in this State, viz the establishment of a Maternity Hospital where the poor might receive proper treatment and whereby also that nurses in this State might derive that experience and training essential to them in their calling. It was distinct hardship to the nurses in Western Australia that they had to go to the other States in order to get proper training in midwifery. There was no doubt that there was a very great need for a Maternity Hospital in the State and he hoped that the Government would shortly undertake to supply that much needed institution.

This was reported in the *West Australian* of 25 July 1908 under the headings: 'Trained Nurses' Association, Address by the President, Establishment of Maternity Hospital advocated.' At the subsequent council meeting maternity nursing continued to be a key issue. An approach was made to the House of Mercy by Dr Lovegrove and Mr Longmore of the Medical Department (Board of Health) regarding the use of possible extensions to their buildings for opportunities for the training of midwives but this did not come to fruition.[22] It was thought that until a training school for obstetric nurses was established, some concession should be made towards acceptance of those members of the association who had been in midwifery practice for some time.[23] Arising from this the following was forwarded to the parent association.

> That in the case of nurses in Western Australia on the general register who can produce proof of having attended under medical supervision, twenty cases of labour and who shall have passed an examination to be conducted by examiners approved by the Branch Council, such nurses shall be eligible for the Obstetric Register up to 30th June 1909. Nurses so registered shall be entered on the Register as admitted under Rule 1(d).

This was agreed to, but it is not known how many availed themselves of the concession.

Another matter of vital importance was the subject of state legislation to be introduced for the registration of all nurses, and although the association was of the opinion that this was desirable in Western Australia, it was felt that it would be more beneficial if a uniform act was passed to become operative in all states.[24] Concern was also felt at the manner in which the above legislation was to be controlled in Western Australia since it was mentioned that clauses were to be introduced into the proposed Health Act to provide for the registration of midwifery nurses under a Central Board of Health, and the possibility of including all nurses. Action on this matter resulted in the secretary being directed to forward the following to the colonial secretary: 'that this council would not consider it advisable that the State registration of nurses be vested in the Central Board of Health, but strongly urges that a Bill be introduced for a Board to control general, obstetric and mental nurses.'[25]

The first annual meeting of the A.T.N.A. held in the Hibernian Hall, Murray Street, on 15 January 1909 saw the election of a new council by ballot and a change of president, Dr E. A. Officer succeeding Dr A. Saw.[26] A new member of the council was Miss Cherry, a member of the newly formed Silver Chain Association. Miss Cherry had previously been refused registration of a nursing home, but no reason was given.

The control of nursing by an organization like the A.T.N.A. was not wholly acceptable to some members of the medical and nursing professions, hospitals and the Board of Health as it was felt that the rules were too restrictive, especially in the area of standardized fees and the field of midwifery. Dr Lovegrove, the retiring principal medical officer, had earlier sought reassurance that the fees laid down for the private practice nurse would not be expected by nurses employed as staff in the public hospitals. Disagreement with the

A.T.N.A. policies in both the above matters had early led to the resignation of Dr Haynes, who was conducting a course of lectures in midwifery in a private hospital, a procedure totally unacceptable to the association. Topsham Hospital had also withdrawn its registration as an A.T.N.A. training school.[27]

Following the resignation of Dr Haynes, which was accepted without regret, a letter appeared in the *West Australian* of 15 January 1909 over his signature and was to have the effect of bringing about a division in nursing in Western Australia.

> I wish to take a very strong exception to the report supplied to you and published in today's issue. For such a report is certainly misleading and against the Constitution of the Australasian Trained Nurses' Association, which centre is in Sydney. I was a member of this Association when it first started and I resigned because I found it an association founded for the grandisment of its members without any benefit to the sick poor. One of the by-laws was that no nurse of the association should take duty under three guineas in one case of illness and four guineas in another. In case of necessity she may take a lesser fee but must forthwith report her action to the committee or if no urgency she can attend at lower rate if receiving permission to do so. Is this not Trade Unionism? Not that I condemn Trade Unionism in other circles but such an association is scouted[?] in the Medical Profession because there are higher and more noble ends in the Medical Profession to serve than those for filthy lucre. However, this by law was passed at the last meeting I attended and I strongly protested against it, and I felt the Association was no place for me.
>
> From my experience among the sick for nearly thirty years I know too well that if nurses were to charge that amount, very few indeed, and especially in this State would pay the amount and as I pointed out, where are the butcher, the baker the landlord and the doctor to come in?
>
> The last straw referred to a nurse, I think in Bridgetown who was threatened with expulsion if she did not conform to the constitution of the association. In this writing I do not by any means wish to condemn the society for they have many excellent nurses and for those who can pay the wage no better nurses can be obtained, but my experience in this state and it is no small one, is that few indeed will be able to pay such a fee and therefore they will be compelled to engage Sairey Gamps. When I resigned I placed my views before Dr Lovegrove and Mr Connolly and pointed out how necessary it was . . .

This letter, which was answered publicly by the secretary of the A.T.N.A., gave rise to considerable correspondence, lengthy and wordy, from both the supporters of Dr Haynes and those of the association. The two examples given below serve to show the trend of opinion in the matter.

> Sir, I was pleased to note that the secretaries of the Trained Nurses' Association have replied to Dr Haynes letter. . . . The A.T.N.A. is a nurses' association and I fail to see why it should be linked even in name with the State or Central Board of Health. With this association nurses who are qualified, that is those nurses who have had three years in a training school are placed on a basis of equality. They are entitled, if it so please them to charge a fee of three guineas per week. By employing one of these nurses the general public is assured that it is procuring the services of a nurse who is considered certificated and holds a certificate recognized as worthy by those who are capable of deciding, that is the Council of the A.T.N.A. Surely it can be nothing but an advantage for such an association to exist? People who have been resident in Western Australia for long can tell many tales of so called trained nurses, who even though they have received their three guineas per week were no more fitted to be placed in the responsible position of a nurse than a child would be. Many of these nurses are imported from the other States and have received a few months training experience may be in some private hospital even in Perth. The decision to train nurses in a hospital of forty beds is a wise one. A nurse buys her experience and it costs a large amount of energy if not money and when she is competent to enter upon her career and may charge her fee, she does not always receive payment for what she has done, and so in like manner just as a doctor may reduce his forty guineas from one patient for a surgical operation, he may receive no fee at all for a similar one. I have never heard of a nurse who made her fortune with nursing. It is to be regretted that Dr Haynes should think that the standard set by the A.T.N.A. too high for nurses of Western Australia to climb to. The Association has done good work in the other States and there is every reason that it will do likewise in Western Australia.
>
> M/A.T.N.A. Perth January, 23rd. (1909)

> I do not profess thoroughly to understand the purport of the correspondence in your columns between Dr Haynes and the A.T.N.A., but I do hope that those connected with the organization named are not aiming at anything which may tend to bring about the discontinuance of the worthy doctor's praiseworthy efforts to ensure a good supply of fully qualified midwifery nurses in this State. The letter of Mother of three in your issue of this morning shows only too plainly how badly a larger supply of obstetric nurses is needed in this State and the emi-

> nent position that Dr Haynes holds in his profession should be sufficient guarantee that candidates who undergo his course of training and satisfactorily pass examinations prescribed by himself and his colleagues are quite as proficient as any who may be imported from the Eastern States, while the system inaugurated and carried out by him places it within the means of poor widows and wives of worthless or invalid husbands to qualify themselves of earning a living for themselves and young children who may be dependent on them. I do not for a moment wish to imply that the unqualified person should be allowed to register or practice, but there always seems to be a tendency on the part of the Foundation members of an association like the A.T.N.A. to impose restrictions on new aspirants which they themselves were never required to comply with and could not have complied with had they been called on to do so, the object no doubt being to bring about legislation calculated to make registration so difficult that those already on the roll may have less competition and thereby being enabled to fix their fees so high as to be [?] on the poorer classes. I think any proposed legislation on this subject requires careful watching so that while the public interest is preserved, there will be no playing into the hands of a particular association in a way that might assist its members in the establishment of a close cooperation for themselves.
>
> Candidate. North Fremantle
> ?26th January, 1909.

Resulting from the substance of Dr Haynes's letter and public reaction shown in subsequent letters to the press, it was agreed that the A.T.N.A. secretary should write to the colonial secretary requesting an interview by representatives of the Branch Council of the association to explain its objectives and the necessity for a maternity hospital. Members of the deputation nominated were all medical members—Doctors Saw, Officer (president), Montgomery, Anderson and Tymms. At the April meeting it was reported that there had been no acknowledgement of the letter, but at the May meeting the principal medical officer, Dr Hope, was quoted as having written to the association stating that it was proposed to establish a maternity home in Perth where women would be taught practical midwifery and attend a course of lectures on hygiene in particular reference to this branch of work. The course of training was to be six months only. He further stated that it was desired 'to be on all fours with the Association' and asked that the rules be so far liberalized as to embrace those trained for the term of six months to enable them to be registered with the association. After considerable discussion it was moved that Dr Hope be informed that 'this Branch does not see its way clear to recommend to the parent association any reduction in the time of training for obstetric nurses'.

At this period the Branch Council was heavily involved with other activities: arranging examinations, assessing people for membership, forwarding names for the roll and preparing items for discussion at the forthcoming conference of branch councils in Sydney to which it was hoped to send representation. Although the parent body offered to pay the fare of delegates and to offer them hospitality while in Sydney, the cost of such a venture had to be measured in time and availability of personnel. Sydney was a ten-day journey by sea. Delegates selected were Dr J. M. Y. Stewart and Mrs Scott, née McKimmie, matron of a private hospital in West Perth.[28]

Apart from the midwifery issue, the association was well aware of the difficulties facing Western Australian hospitals in regard to the A.T.N.A. rules of membership, and among the items sent for discussion were the reduction of life membership fees from £5 to £3 3s 0d; the abolition of private hospitals as training schools; the need strongly to urge a uniform registration act in all states under a nursing board rather than under the Central Boards of Health; in view of the fact that the majority of hospitals in this state were administered by the Medical Department and that probationers were often moved to smaller hospitals during their training, to urge that a concession be granted under approved conditions to permit these nurses to continue training under the association; and as there was still no maternity hospital in Western Australia Rule 1d was requested to be extended a further year.[29]

Although the number of nurses trained within the state was still comparatively small, there continued to be an influx from the eastern states and overseas and the question of employment was a matter of some concern. For those who preferred to nurse in hospitals rather than in private nursing the field was still limited, especially in the private hospitals in the city. Hospitals administered by the Medical Department did offer some stability in employment although it was feared that the introduction of probationer nurses would reduce the employment of the trained nurse as there was no clear-cut legislation to control the number of probationer nurses in proportion to those who had completed their training. However control of approval hospitals by the A.T.N.A., through its training programme, would have offered some safeguards against exploitation of the nurse, who would not have to meet the needs of the hospital to the detriment of her own needs in nursing experience.

A summary of the classes of hospital services within the state but outside the private sector in 1909 is as follows:

1. Under Hospitals Act 1904: Perth and Fremantle Public Hospitals.
2. Government and departmental: Kalgoorlie, Coolgardie, Geraldton, Albany, Bunbury, Roebourne and larger country towns.
3. Those controlled by local committees: board hospitals.
4. Hospitals at timber mills.
5. Consumptive Sanitorium, Coolgardie.
6. Children's Hospital, Perth (opened 1909), received a grant of £1250 per annum.[30]

In June 1909 it is recorded that the Children's Hospital, Perth, the foundation stone of which had been laid by the governor, Admiral Sir Alfred Bedford, G.C.B., on 27 June 1908,[31] was registered as a three-year training school for nurses subject to A.T.N.A. rules, and much publicity was given to this venture. The newly appointed matron was Miss Annie Anderson, who had previously been matron of Perth Public Hospital, 1900-06.

Discussion on the state registration of nurses dragged on. In June 1909 the colonial secretary wrote to the association stating that provision was being made in the 'new' Health Bill for registration of all nurses and that the principal medical officer had expressed the undesirability of this matter coming under the jurisdiction of an outside body since it might impose restrictions on the registration of midwives. Replying to this, the A.T.N.A. secretary pointed out the desirability of vesting registration of nurses in a board on the lines of dental and medical boards, and asked for a deputation to the minister from members of the council on the subject of registration. The P.M.O, Dr Hope, also wrote asking for more consideration for the registration of midwives, and in reply was told that the association had to abide by rules.

The upshot of this was that a deputation was received by the minister, the members being Drs E. A. Officer, Trethowan and Tymms, Miss K. Power-Ryan, Miss Stronach and Mrs Shackell. Their request was for an autonomous board for the registration of nurses, outside the Board of Health (Medical Department). In reply they were told that the amendment to the proposed act was to register midwives and that the period of training required would not be more than six months. A few medical men might be appointed to the board but no hope was given for the representation of nurses on this board.[32] Following the deputation there had been a further interview with the P.M.O. who stated that in framing the amendment to the act, training for obstetric nurses would be six months and for general nurses three years. There was no specification of what time should be spent in each area of experience.

A month later, in August 1909, the association members were shocked to read in the press that a second nurses' association had been formed and was to be known as the 'Western Australian Nurses' Association'. This is an extract from the report in the *West Australian*:

> A meeting of citizens interested in the formation of a Nurses' Association for Western Australia was held at the Town Hall last evening. The Mayoress (Mrs T. G. Molloy) presided.
>
> Dr Haynes explained that the meeting had been called to consider the 'advisableness' of forming the Western Australian Nurses' Association, the object of which would be to give practical education in medical, surgical and midwifery nursing.
>
> It would not by any means be in opposition to any other nursing association, but he was convinced that there was urgent need for the formation of such an organization as was now proposed. He pointed out that the nurses here did not have the same facilities as those enjoyed by those in other States, and if the same standards were applied to them in the matter of qualifications the local nurses would not be able to compete with those from the East. They had to make a start and receive their training in accordance with the opportunities that presented themselves. When those opportunities were increased the standard could be raised.
>
> In Western Australia, the country districts were sparsely populated, but there were many women in the bush, and it would be unfair to expect nurses to go outback who had all the qualifications at present required of city nurses. It would be better to have a half trained nurse in the bush than a woman who had had no training at all. The principal thing required of nurses in the country was surgical cleanliness which was as much removed from domestic cleanliness as domestic cleanliness was removed from dirt.
>
> It was proposed that nurses be allowed to attend at the different private hospitals in the city and as long as they had attended an average of six to eight patients they should be able after three years to present themselves for an examination which it was hoped would be conducted by the Government. In the meantime the Government might appoint lecturers to the nurses on various subjects such as medical, surgical and midwifery nursing and the care of infant life. If a woman could not learn nursing in three years she never would learn it. As a later stage when the association was in full working order, they should take into consideration the question of appointing an organizing secretary to establish branches in the country districts.
>
> Resolutions were carried that in the opinion of the meeting it was desirable that a Western Australian Nurses' Association

> should be formed and that a provisional committee should be appointed to draw up the Constitution. Officers of the new association were elected as follows. Patrons, Lady Edeline Strickland and Lady Forrest. President, Mrs T. G. Molloy. Vice presidents Lady Stone, Lady Parker, Lady Lee Steere. Committee, Mesdames J. W. Hackett, F. Wilson, W. T. Loton, Connolly, Gregory, S. Burt, J. M. Ferguson, Daglish, Lefroy, Haynes, Hill, Cowan, Foulkes, Rischbieth, Gover, Bird and Miss McLean; provisional committee Mesdames Symons, Ferguson, Rankinson [?], Johnson, Knight, Miller and Ross. Misses McKimmie, O'Connor, McDonough. Nurses Lloyd, Slattery, Mortlock, Ryan, Wiltshire, Knight, Loveland, McCallum, Wheeler, White and Chinnery. Joint hon. secretaries Mesdames Philpott and Booth. Treasurer Nurse Farquharson.
>
> It was decided that as an inaugural Ball should be held at an early date a committee was appointed to make the necessary arrangements.
>
> The meeting adjourned till Monday week, when the conditions as drafted by the provisional committee will be submitted for adoption.[33]

Although Dr Haynes was obviously one of the prime movers, there is no record as to the convenors of the above meeting. Absence of initials makes identification difficult, but quite a number of these ladies had affiliations with the newly formed Women's Service Guild which supported a lower grade of midwifery training than was acceptable to the A.T.N.A. The nurses' names in the list above approximate with those practising as midwives who were not acceptable for A.T.N.A. membership. One or two others were actually members of the A.T.N.A., having been accepted under concessional rules.

At the special meeting of the A.T.N.A. Council called for August to discuss the formation of the 'new' association, members were unanimously of the opinion that this was most undesirable.[34] Women in the bush needed trained nurses with the highest qualifications, nor was there any guarantee that those who received certificates from the new association would remain in the bush and not inundate the more populous areas, resulting in competition between two groups of nurses. There was a call for all medical men to support the A.T.N.A. nurses and not those of the proposed rival association. Finally there was a resolution that a reply to the article appearing in the press should be drafted and copies should be sent to office bearers of the new association drawing attention to the facilities which already existed in this state for the training of nurses. The response to this action was immediate and the secretary was inundated with letters and phone calls in reply to letters received.

This first W.A.N.A. apparently ceased to function quite early, as no records of any activity have been found.

A means of bypassing the A.T.N.A. regulations in relation to nurse training in hospitals controlled by the Board of Health was introduced by the P.M.O., Dr Hope. Under his scheme, nurses were to be imported from the United Kingdom. No details of this are available, but it would seem that some inducement was offered in return for satisfactory service. This the A.T.N.A. was opposed to, and suggested that the local supply be explored before taking this step.

Another matter suggested by the medical members, which received favourable attention, was the cooperation of nurses' homes in a scheme for supplying visiting nurses for those families who could not afford a full-time resident nurse, and were therefore inclined to employ the untrained nurse. Although approved, the venture seems not to have been a success. Transport, or lack of it, could possibly have been a factor, for people were beginning to move to the outskirts of the city area, and the day of the motor vehicle had not arrived.

Nevertheless the establishment of a maternity hospital in Perth was of paramount importance and in September 1909 Dr Officer reported an interview with Lady Strickland concerning the starting of a midwifery training school for nurses.[35] Following this, Lady Strickland called a public meeting to be held in Government House Ballroom at 4.30 p.m. on November 8 to discuss the organization of a women's hospital for maternity cases. Notice of this appeared in the Saturday issue of the *West Australian*, dated November 6, and on the following Monday the leading article gave prominence to the meeting called by Lady Strickland and in the same issue, under 'Social Notes' by 'Adrienne', Lady Strickland's view was stated. It was also stated that she hoped that the hospital would be self-supporting.

It is possible that impetus was given to the matter by an unfortunate happening in which a woman died after giving birth to a baby in a vehicle, having been refused admission to the House of Mercy and the Salvation Army Home in Maylands. In fairness to both these institutions, it would seem that their situation made it impossible to do otherwise. Mrs Harris, matron of the House of Mercy, did render aid, but was fearful of the introduction of infection and the risk to other women in the home, while the Salvation Army Home was full to overcrowding and was not geared to deal with maternity patients. The patient was subsequently taken to the

Women's Home (poorhouse) in Perth. This was in the process of being re-located in Fremantle, in the building formerly used as a lunatic asylum. Although the consensus of opinion was that the Women's Home should be relocated, many were appalled by the prison-like construction and atmosphere of this building. It could have been that the publicity given to the fate of the unfortunate woman brought home the fact that Perth was to be bereft of an institution which over the years had been the only refuge for destitute women, unmarried mothers and deserted wives.

Strangely enough there is no record of the meeting called by Lady Strickland in the A.T.N.A. minutes, but it is known that the association was well represented by the president, members of the council and other members. According to the report of proceedings given in the *West Australian* of 9 November 1909:

> Lady Edeline Strickland presided over a representative attendance of ladies and gentlemen, numbering about 400,— amongst those present were The Lieut Governor, Sir Edward Stone, Bishop Riley, Sir Edward Wittenoom, the Speaker of the Legislative Assembly (Mr T. F. Quinlan), Dr Hackett M.L.C., Messrs H. Daglish and W. D. Johnson, M's L.A. and many representatives of the medical profession and the different churches . . .
>
> A letter from the Premier was read in which he stated that he was prepared to recommend to Parliament to set aside an area of land for the proposed hospital in the neighbourhood of the Children's Hospital. . . . The secretary of the Eastern Goldfields Women's Labour League, wrote suggesting that the hospital should not be limited to maternity cases but should also be established for the treatment of women's complaints. Bishop Riley moved:— That the time had arrived when maternity hospital shall be established. . . .

The motion was seconded by Dr Saw. He brought up the problem of financing the institution as the government was only prepared to give the land, but it was stated that when the institution was established they could go to the government like any other charitable body, for a pound for pound subsidy up to a certain amount.

Unfortunately it was at this point that dissent arose between representatives of certain factions at the meeting. An amendment was moved and seconded by representatives of the Women's Service Guild that 'The hospital shall be for both married and single women'. This was opposed by a group led by Dr Ellis who, amongst other arguments, said 'that if they tried to provide a maternity hospital for both married and single women, the one class would not use it'. He urged that the matter be carefully thought out by people who had the necessary experience to deal with it. After much heated debate during which attempts were made both to persuade the mover of the amendment to withdraw it, and to have it ruled out on a point of order, the amendment was put to the meeting and passed overwhelmingly. The Reverend W. T. Kench moved that a provisional committee be appointed to make preliminary arrangements and report to the next meeting. He wished, he said, to refer to the good work being done by the House of Mercy amongst single women and he thought that they should confer with the principals of that home in regard to the proposed maternity hospital.

The following committee was chosen: Mrs Antoinette Harris (matron of the House of Mercy, A.T.N.A. delegate), Mrs Edith Cowan, Dr Haynes, Mrs Ruffy Hill (Women's Service Guild), Mrs H. Gregory, Dr Mead (A.T.N.A. delegate), Mrs Molloy (mayoress of Perth), Miss Anderson (matron of Children's Hospital, A.T.N.A. delegate), Mrs Scott, Mrs Hackett, Miss Ryan (matron of Perth Public Hospital, vice-president of A.T.N.A. Council), Dr Trethowan (A.T.N.A. vice-president), Mrs Butler, Mrs O'Grady, Mrs Lefroy, Dr Officer (president, A.T.N.A. Council), Dr Harvey, Mrs Harvey, Mrs J. B. Holman, Mrs Wheeler, Mrs Ross Harwood, J. S. Battye. Mr Battye was appointed convenor. The meeting terminated with a vote of thanks to Lady Edeline Strickland.

It will be noted that in fact many of the committee were council members of the A.T.N.A. Records of a 'follow on' from this meeting have not been located so the result is inconclusive. It is known that a fund was launched in 1910 by which people were asked to donate one shilling towards the establishment of a maternity hospital and it is possible it was a memorial fund to King Edward VII who died in May 1910. Miss K. Anderson, matron of the Home of Peace, urged members of her staff to contribute. Miss Ruth Bottle, then a young nursing assistant waiting to commence her training at Fremantle Hospital, remembers that the shilling was very hard to come by and that the contribution was no small sacrifice.

In 1910 an invitation to members of the A.T.N.A. to join the Women's Service Guild was flatly refused.[36] The guild was told that the Western Australian council could not take any part in their movement. It is presumed that the invitation was to the female members of the association only.

At the end of 1909 the former Lunatic Asylum in Fremantle became vacant when patients were transferred to the new establishment at Claremont and the former building was reconstituted as the Women's Home. The following was promulgated in the *Government Gazette* of 24 December 1909: 'His Excellency the Governor in Council has been pleased to declare the building known as the

Women's home, situated in Finnerty Street Fremantle to be a Poor House within the meaning of the Public Health Discipline Act 1882.'

In his annual report the principal medical officer, Dr Hope, expressed his views as follows:

> There is a lack of maternity nurses in this country, which has been felt for some time, and the public mind has been exercised as to how to remedy this defect. Committees who are managing some of the Homes in connection with both 'lying-in' women and the care of children have been impressed by this want of skilled assistance, and efforts have been made to overcome the difficulty.
>
> Lack of means has been somewhat the cause of failure to this end, but it is hoped that the near future will prove that this is not an unsurmountable difficulty.
>
> There is, and has been for a considerable time the material for training a fair number of women year by year, but the trouble has been in utilising it.
>
> Now an attempt is on foot by the Government to induce women to come forward and be trained with the means at disposal, and classes have been inaugurated in Fremantle, where with two institutions which receive maternity cases, and number about eighty (80) per year, practical instruction at the bedside coupled with lectures, both extending over at least a six months course will, if successful enable the want to be partly met.
>
> The idea is that when these women receive this instruction, and have passed an examination to prove their knowledge of the work, their training in hygiene, and care of the patient, they will be assisted by the Government in the way of subsidy to take up their living in different parts of the State where they will be able to give the necessary assistance, in the back country, to women requiring their services, but who may be too far from a medical man to secure his attendance, or may have an objection to leave their homes for some weeks, to come to a town for this event, and further may not have the means to face such expense.
>
> It is well known that most women view the on coming trial with equanimity, although not without some anxiety, but would not for a moment entertain the idea of going from their family, for they are able while there to feel that they are supervising the children, are in close touch with that in their life with which they are so intimately connected and which forms their chief interest.
>
> The presence of a trained woman in this respect will enable such events to be undertaken with the minimum interference of home life and the saving of expense.

> In some quarters it is thought that only thoroughly qualified and trained nurses should be entrusted with maternity cases, but the practice in many parts of the world has been in the direction of giving special women training for this work without requiring them to be thoroughly certificated trained nurses; the result is that it has been eminently satisfactory as regards the shorter time necessary for women to be trained, giving an opportunity to certain women who are well fitted to carry on this work, and the very happy results which are evidenced by the low mortality where this practice is in vogue . . .
>
> Coupled with the plan above referred to, in larger centres can very well be initiated a system of rendering assistance to poorer women in their homes at a nominal charge, where under ordinary circumstances the attendance they receive is only such as can be given by a friendly neighbour.
>
> Maternity nurses who receive the training in this State to make them efficient for the work required should be protected and have their positions secured for them.[37]

(The second institution mentioned in the foregoing has not been definitely identified but it is known that the Salvation Army conducted a home for women in North Fremantle, called 'Hopetoun'. This was later relocated as a maternity hospital at 'Hillcrest' which in 1920 became a recognized training school for midwives.)[38]

The Fremantle Midwifery Training Centre commenced sometime in 1910. There is some confusion as to its organization and it is referred to as a 'school', a 'centre', 'a course of instruction' and a 'midwifery training class'. It was inaugurated by Dr David Ernest Williams, who combined the duties of resident medical officer and secretary at the Women's Home in Fremantle. He was also quarantine officer and assistant to the principal medical officer in the field of health.

There are few details available of the first courses and their content. When compulsory registration of midwives was introduced in 1911 twenty-six women from the Fremantle Midwifery Training School were granted full recognition as certificated midwives and Mary O'Grady was given Certificate No. 1. Among the twenty-six is noted the name of Mary Fraser, matron of the home, and at least one staff member, who evidently had undertaken the course.[39] Mary Fraser had been with the medical services for a very long time and had worked at Coolgardie and Kalgoorlie Hospitals, and although uncertificated was gazetted a 'matron' in the Public Service, having qualified for the position by seniority.

Hannah Maria Gilbert, an early member of the A.T.N.A. Council, representing obstetric nurses, who had been in charge of the maternity section of the Women's Home in Perth, had transferred to the Fremantle establishment, but whether she played any part in the instruction of midwives or supervised their clinical experience is not known.

In his annual report of 1910 the P.M.O. makes the following statement, under the heading of 'Maternity'.

> A school for training women is being conducted at Fremantle and women who have thus qualified and are willing to reside in the agricultural and goldfields areas will be subsidised by the Government so to do. Their services will thus be available to women who with their husbands are opening up the country and who being remote from medical men would review this event in their lives with considerable anxiety. By the aid of these midwives, these women will be enabled to remain in the midst of their families where they can supervise their domestic concerns to the last moment and where during the critical period they can receive such skilled assistance as will relieve both them and their husbands from any mental distress.

However there is no mention as to whether the women undertaking the midwifery course received remuneration or if they paid a fee for their instruction.

The part of the Women's Home reserved for expectant mothers was the east wing facing Ord Street. It also contained offices and nurses' quarters. However not all of the midwifery students resided at the home, many of them being mature women with considerable experience with their homes and families. They were 'on call' for cases. Those who did live in were used in caring for the other inmates of the home in the geriatric section.

When the Midwives Board was constituted in 1911, the training school had to conform to the regulations and the schedule of instruction laid down by the board. These were based on the regulations of the Central Midwives' Board of Great Britain. The period of training was stipulated as six months but was later extended to twelve months, during which time the pupil midwife was required to attend no fewer than twenty labours and nurse twenty women and their infants during the ten days following labour. That the experience was hard to come by is demonstrated by the case book of Mrs Frances Appleton, née Moore, who had to wait eighteen months to get the required experience. Although no addresses are given, it suggests that the practical aspect of midwifery was not confined to the Women's Home. Mrs Appleton's certificate, dated December 1913, is headed 'Fremantle: Midwifery Training Class', and is signed by the lecturers, the examiners, the secretary and the P.M.O., but there is no signature of a matron or supervising midwife.

The lecturers were W. T. Dermer, M.B., M.R.C.S., L.R.C.P. Lond., and A. H. Gibson, M.B.B.S. The examiners are designated Arthur T. White and Owen Paget, M.D. All of these were well-known medical men in the Fremantle area. The textbook used was the *Rotunda Midwifery for Nurses* by G. T. Wrench, M.D., assistant master of the Rotunda Hospital in Dublin. Its choice could have been dictated by the fact that both Drs Williams and White received their qualifications there. The text is sophisticated and extensive, but it is not known at what stage in training it was introduced. Mrs Appleton's copy shows that it was certainly valued and well read. Of special interest is the appendix, which sets out the regulations for the issue of certificates and conditions of admission to the Roll of Midwives as acceptable to the Central Midwives' Board. These were adopted in full by the Midwives Board of Western Australia.

It could be said that the years 1907 to 1912 were vital to the survival of professional nursing in Western Australia and of the A.T.N.A. as so many changes took place. New nurses' quarters erected by Perth Public Hospital in Murray Street—now Kirkman House—meant that the space occupied by nurses in the hospital itself could now be used to accommodate patients and be converted into a ward—the old Ward VI. Perhaps it would be fair to say that the move from the nurses' quarters was precipitated by unwelcome publicity in the press owing to complaints from patients in the wards above Ward VI—Wards VII and VIII— about being disturbed by music and singing from the nurses' sitting-room, which was under the main operating theatre.[40]

The opening of the Perth Children's Hospital in 1909 meant that the transfer of children to that institution provided more beds for female patients at Perth Public Hospital. There was either a dramatic increase of sick children at this time, or perhaps a greater acceptance of hospital care, for the Children's Hospital had to guarantee a daily bed average of forty occupied beds to conform with A.T.N.A. registration. This excluded those with infectious diseases, who were nursed at the Infectious Diseases Branch. Typhoid fever was still prevalent and patients with this disease were still nursed in the wards of the general hospitals.[41] The use of departmental hospitals increased as people migrated from the goldfields to the rural areas and the expansion of the timber industry meant the birth of small hospitals in isolated areas. These were supported by the timber mills and in some areas such as Jarrahdale, the hospital was quite large. Nevertheless the daily occupied bed average of some of the departmental hospitals was still too small to allow their registration as nurse-training schools.

In November 1909 St John of God Hospital in Kalgoorlie was granted permission to operate as an A.T.N.A. training school (five years), presumably within its own order.[42] However Sister Mary Gleeson was refused acceptance as a matron because she had been admitted to membership under a concessional clause. Eventually the matter was resolved by acceptance of those admitted under concessional clauses as 'nominal' matrons providing that a nurse with the qualifications required of a matron was on the staff. On their return, delegates to the A.T.N.A. Sydney conference reported that requests from the local branch had been agreed to. In particular, the clause allowing the movement of probationers to the smaller country hospitals paved the way to better relationships with the hospitals which provided the main agencies for employment. Another important conference decision was the setting of the educational standard for entry to nursing to be the completion of the fifth standard of primary school in New South Wales, which had a dramatic effect in reducing numbers.[43]

As early as 1910 arrangements were made for lectures on a post-basic level to be given to A.T.N.A. members by doctors and nurses. The timing of these lectures was at 9 p.m. after the monthly meetings of the council. A publications committee was also formed to prepare material for the A.T.N.A. journal, which was issued monthly by the parent association. Those who had life membership were required to pay for their copies of the journal although this was included in the annual subscriptions of members. Lady Edeline Strickland asked that a copy of the journal be sent to her, but it is not known if any other people outside the profession were able to obtain copies either by courtesy or subscription. Unfortunately no early copies of the journal have been found to exist in this state.

It seems strange that the death of Florence Nightingale on 30 August 1910 is not mentioned in the A.T.N.A. minutes, although her obituary was given full page coverage in the *West Australian*. However there was a lot of concern about the employment of the trained nurse, and her status. Objection was raised to the signing on of nurses as stewardesses with the Orient Line[44] and it was urged that they sign on as nurses and come under the authority of the medical officer. It was also stated that A.T.N.A. members of the Bush Nursing Association should receive the recognized salary paid to other members. Furthermore it was resolved that a member of the Bush Nursing Association be a member of the A.T.N.A. Council. There was a problem too with the A.T.N.A. registered nurses' homes, in that there were nurses residing there who were not members of the association but who were gaining employment on the assumption that they were.

In 1911 there is reference to an infectious hospital in Kalgoorlie being refused recognition as a training school unless controlled by the parent hospital.[45]

Following the refusal of a request for sustenance by a member because a benevolent fund was not functional, steps were taken to commence such a venture and on 20 January 1911 a benevolent fund was commenced, the interest on the £150 in the bank to form the nucleus. This was to be added to by grants from the council and voluntary subscriptions. The incoming council was authorized to frame the rules.

There was a great deal of correspondence between Dr Hope and the association regarding the position of matrons of country hospitals with the ultimatum that they sit for membership examination or have the hospitals under their control deregistered as A.T.N.A. training schools; particularly named were Northam and Bunbury Hospitals.

In February 1911 St John of God Hospital in Subiaco was accepted for registration as an A.T.N.A. training school within the order.[46] The period of training was for five years. It is understood that previously the Sisters of the Order of St John of God were offered Topsham Hospital by Dr Haynes as he thought that the Subiaco site was too far out and surrounded by bush.

In March 1911 there was a move to register mental nurses with the A.T.N.A.[47] in this state and a subcommittee was formed to meet Dr Montgomery (of Mental Health Services) to discuss the syllabus. There was also a change in the Educational Assessment Committee; following the resignation of Mr Faulkner, Miss A. E. Walton was appointed. Miss Walton was headmistress of one of the colleges in the metropolitan area.

In August 1911 the association was asked for a contribution to the Nightingale Memorial Fund. Five guineas was given by the council, and nurses were to be circularized for subscriptions to the fund. However there are no more details available of the nature of the fund or the response.

The bill pertaining to the Health Act was introduced in parliament on 3 August 1910 by the minister for mines, Henry Gregory, during the Moore government (Liberal). The act was assented to on 16 February 1911. By the end of 1911 there was a change of government to Labor, and W. C. Angwin is stated as being in charge of the Health Act. The section of the act which dealt with nurses and was designated under 'Protection of Life', caused a great deal of debate from both sides of the house which reflected the attitude and knowledge of the role of the nurse. While they were generally agreed that it was urgent to recognize midwives and raise the standard, the nurse with the General Certificate presented a problem, because they were unable to define either the term 'nurse' or the scope of her activity. They felt that it was going too far to say that no person should practice unless she was registered. As far as midwives were concerned it was a different matter: their role could be clearly defined, they could be controlled by compulsory registration and become answerable to a board set up for that purpose. There was also some dispute as to who should qualify for the term 'matron', and after a petition from a number of doctors and deputations from nurses, the whole of the clause pertaining to the registration of the nurse with the General Certificate was struck out.

During the debate, tribute was paid to the late Dr Haynes and his part in maternity nursing, the doctor having died earlier in the year.

Provisions under the act, which finally became law in 1911, can be summarized as follows:

252 Setting up of the Midwives Registration Board. Restriction of the name or title 'Midwife' or 'Midwifery' to registered midwives only.

253 Prohibiting any but midwifery nurses from conducting a hospital where maternity cases were being nursed or to act as an assistant nurse unless registered under the act—special concessions to apply in emergencies.

254 A register to be styled the 'Midwifery Nurses' Register' was to be kept by the clerk to the Midwives Registration Board and to contain the names of all midwives registered under the act together with their qualifications and places of residence.

255 Provision for existing midwives allowing them to register if they had been in practice for two years or more prior to the commencement of the act. The examination of such persons' qualifications was to be at the discretion of the board.

256 Appointment of examiners and regulations prescribing the qualifying examinations. Candidates for examination required to provide evidence of having undergone at least twelve months training in an approved institution and having conducted a prescribed number of cases.

257 Production of a certificate from the examiners. Yearly re-registration. Notification of change of address. Failure to comply resulting in removal of name from register.

258 A copy of the register certified by the clerk to the Midwives Board to be published annually in the *Government Gazette*.

259-60 Circumstances under which names might be removed from the register and penalties for wilful falsification.

261 The acceptance for registration of midwives registered else-

where in British Dominions. (The first amendments to this section were No. 3 of 1912 and No. 28 of 1912 which provided that women holding acceptable diplomas need not take a board examination. The main purpose was to ensure the acceptance of midwives from the Fremantle Training School who were not recognized by the A.T.N.A. or the Central Midwives' Board of Great Britain.)

262 Empowering the Midwives Board to make regulations for the supervision and within due limits the restriction of practice of midwives, and also for any purpose tending to protect the lives of mothers and infants.

263 Furnishing reports on patients, stating where they have been attended.

The introduction of legislation to control midwives had a profound effect on the whole of nursing in this state, for it forced the nurse with the General Certificate who had gained her midwifery experience before 1909 to register as an uncertificated midwife or undertake a further course of training at the Fremantle Training Centre, which would of course have resulted in her being disaffiliated from the A.T.N.A. For those nurses who completed training after 1909 there was no choice but to go outside the state to further their obstetric training, or to restrict their nursing to the field of general nursing. Conversely there was nothing to prevent the registered midwife from entering the sphere of general nursing providing she carried out the rules of hygiene between patients. In those hospitals which catered for both general and obstetric patients, she was often employed in preference to the single certificated nurse as being more useful and economical.

However, compulsory registration did bring control of midwifery practice with the inauguration of a Midwives Registration Board under the chairmanship of the principal medical officer and consisting of two medical men and two midwives.[48] Members of the board were Dr Hope, chairman; Drs A. T. White and O. S. Hicks, M.L.A., Matrons M. Tate and A. Harris. The first meeting was held on 1 July 1911 and dealt with the implementation of the act. The secretary of the board was a departmental member of the Public Service. At the second meeting held on 9 August the board gave notice that it was prepared to accept applicants for registration. It also decided which institutions would be recognized. Those approved by the A.T.N.A., R.V.T.N.A.[49] and Central Midwives' Board of England and Wales were among those approved. It is interesting to note that these are listed on the front page of the original minutes book and include Fremantle Training School, with the date 20 December 1913, and King Edward Memorial Hospital, Subiaco, with the date 23 October 1914. The latter is rather strange as K.E.M.H. did not come into being until 1916.

Another provision under the Health Act was the compulsory registration of maternity homes—as apart from hospitals—and the issuing of licences to the proprietors, who had to be registered midwives. The rules concerning these homes were strictly enforced. A number of double certificated nurses were employed by the Department of Public Health as inspectresses and they made constant visits to detect any breaches of the rules.[50] Maternal or infant mortality arising from proved neglect or infection could result in prosecution and closure of the premises, and deregistration. Well-known names among those appointed were Misses N. U. Lynch, A. Broomhall and E. Bole, and Mrs McClemans.

This employment of nurses in the field of public health was not new but there are few details available. In 1910 a nurse, Ethel Pengelly, gives her address as Bernier Island, off Carnarvon, care of Dr Lovegrove.[51] At this time, Bernier and Dorre islands were used for the isolation of Aborigines suspected of having syphilis.[52]

The annual meeting of the A.T.N.A., which was held on 19 January 1912, was significant in that there was a change of office bearers and both the president and vice-presidents were medical men. Dr Deakin was elected as president. The honorary secretaries were Miss K. Anderson and Dr H. B. Gill. The main business discussed was the attitude of the association towards the Midwives Registration Bill and concern at the outcome. The move in Queensland for the introduction of a State Nurses' Registration Bill which would include all nurses was viewed with some trepidation, and as posing a threat both to the structure of the A.T.N.A. as a national nurses' body and to its proposed affiliation with the International Council of Nurses. Although it was agreed that the W.A. branch of the A.T.N.A. would abide by the decision of the parent body in the above matter, it is difficult to know how affiliation with the I.C.N. was to be achieved in view of the fact that there were two very strong nursing associations, the R.V.T.N.A. and the A.T.N.A., functioning in the one country, and both were dominated by medical members.

At this time, also, a move was being made to include members of the mental health field in membership of the A.T.N.A. in this state. The matron of the Hospital for the Insane at Claremont asked for a special register for mental nurses but there were insurmountable difficulties, mostly due to the unacceptable educational standards both of the students wanting to enter this field and of those already trained, which would preclude them from taking examinations.

It is interesting to note that the June A.T.N.A. examination of 1912 was held at the Children's Hospital for the first time[53] and was taken by the first trainees of that institution, who all passed. They were Eulalie Margaret Hamersley, Mona Miller, Olive Waterhouse and Alice Williams. It is also noted that Mary Josepha O'Brien was appointed matron of St John of God Hospital, Subiaco, this being the first appointment of a matron within the order.[54] The previous matron, Miss Carpenter, had left to return to the eastern states, and for some two months the hospital had been without a matron.

It is obvious that at this time pressure was being put on the matron of Perth Public Hospital, Miss Kate Power-Ryan. In a letter to the A.T.N.A. Council she refers to a communication from the Board of Management of the hospital objecting to the test examinations of the A.T.N.A. This resulted in a special meeting of the council and a deputation to the board of Perth Hospital.[55] The report of this was received but there is no indication of its contents. However, it is interesting to note that only three candidates from Perth Hospital and none from the government hospitals sat for the June examination as the A.T.N.A. had refused others permission to sit because of irregularities in their training. In due course Perth Public Hospital wrote accepting the conditions of the A.T.N.A.

In December 1912 the affairs of Perth Public Hospital received wide publicity when the matron resigned and both the chief resident medical officer and the hospital secretary were dismissed by the board.[56] The result was that the acting Public Service commissioner, acting with the powers of a royal commission, was appointed to hold an inquiry into the affairs of Perth Public Hospital and the allegations concerning the dismissal of the two officers.[57] The hearing continued over several days and was reported at length in the press, but the exact nature of the matter is very difficult to follow and the report of the commission seems to have been suppressed. The main issues appear to be concerned with 'sectarian bigotry' in the administration of the hospital and staff. Strangely there is no mention of this in the A.T.N.A. records nor of Miss Power-Ryan's resignation either from her position at Perth Hospital or as a member of the council, and it is interesting to note that she was asked to represent the W.A. Branch of the association at the forthcoming conference to be held in Sydney.

Of particular interest at this time was the discussion of fees for the trained nurse engaged in private duty. Should a nurse who was caring for more than one patient in a private home be entitled to extra salary? Ten shillings and sixpence per week was suggested but this was left to the discretion of the doctor.[58] The other question was the position of the nurse who was ill and her entitlement to salary during her illness (this applied to those on the staff of hospitals). It was decided that nurses should be treated at hospital expense, but not receive salaries during illness and convalescence. However, apart from the fees of the private duty nurse, there was a great reluctance on the part of the association to become involved in the salary arrangements and the domestic affairs of board and departmental hospitals. This is evidenced in an inquiry from the matron of a board hospital as to what action could be taken regarding holidays, as she had had none for four years. She was told that this was a matter between herself and the board.

A matter of concern to the A.T.N.A. was the admission of 'paying' patients to public hospitals, which particularly applied to the Children's Hospital. At a special meeting convened for the above purpose the following resolution was framed:

> The Australasian Trained Nurses Association, W.A. Branch strongly protests against the action of the Children's Hospital Board in admitting private paying patients to a public institution built and supported by public subscription and subsidised by the Government. Such a step seriously affects private hospitals and also tends to deprive the fully trained nurse of her means of livelihood.[59]

At this time there was still no treatment carried out in hospitals which could not be carried out in the patient's home. Even patients with infectious diseases were successfully isolated, an accepted barrier being a blanket inpregnated with carbolic being hung across the door of the sick person's room.

At the annual meeting of the W.A. Branch of the association held on 17 January 1913 the first paid secretary of the association was appointed, salary £20 per annum.[60] She was Miss Ruby Anderson, who was not a trained nurse, and one of the three Anderson sisters who conducted a private hospital in West Perth.

In 1913 the University of Western Australia was founded. It commenced in a complex of wood and iron buildings in Irwin Street, Perth, and became familiarly known as 'Tin pot alley'. The effect of this was not immediate as far as nursing was concerned but the eventual introduction of the Junior Certificate examination gave some guidelines to the assessment of probationers for nursing. Prior to this they were obliged to sit as external students for the examination conducted by the University of Adelaide. Because of the close links between the eastern states and the Eastern Goldfields, children being educated in these areas had greater opportunities of secondary education than those living in the agricultural areas and other parts of the state.

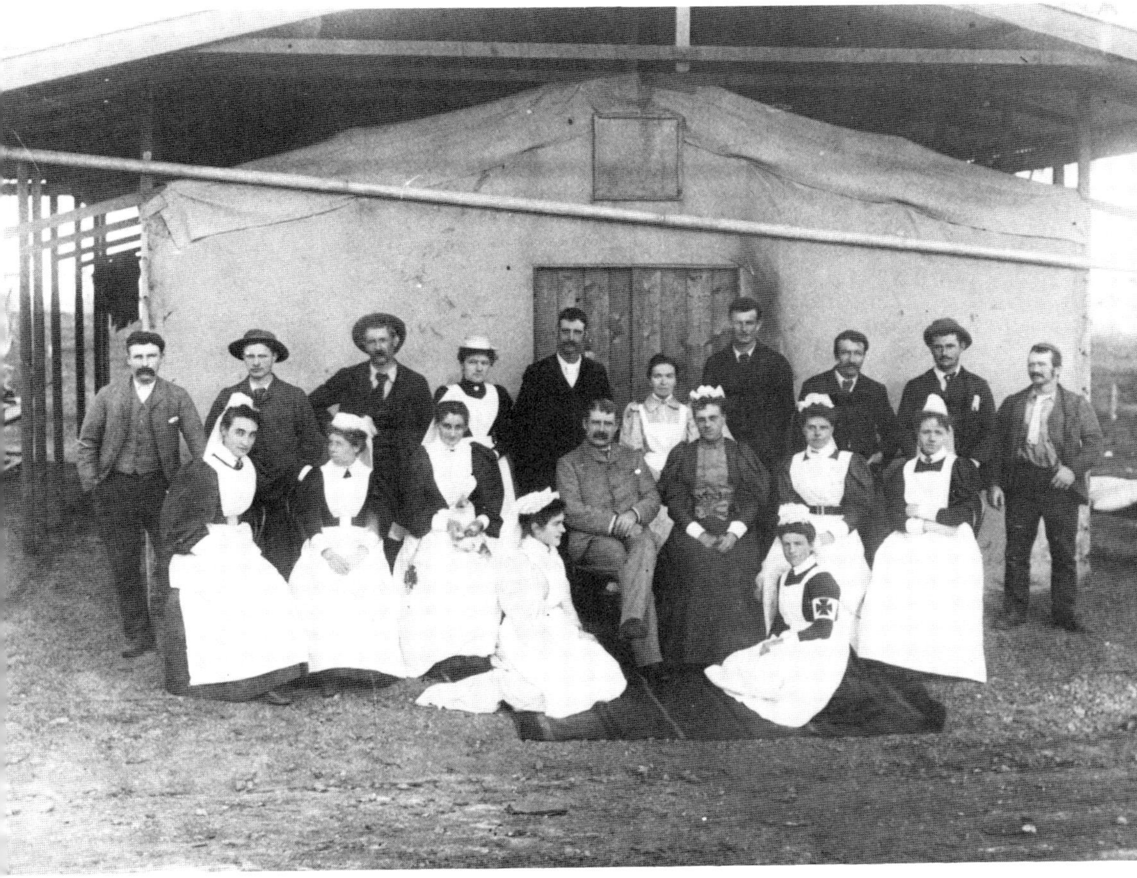

KALGOORLIE HOSPITAL STAFF, 1896 (ABOVE) AND 1930 (BELOW)

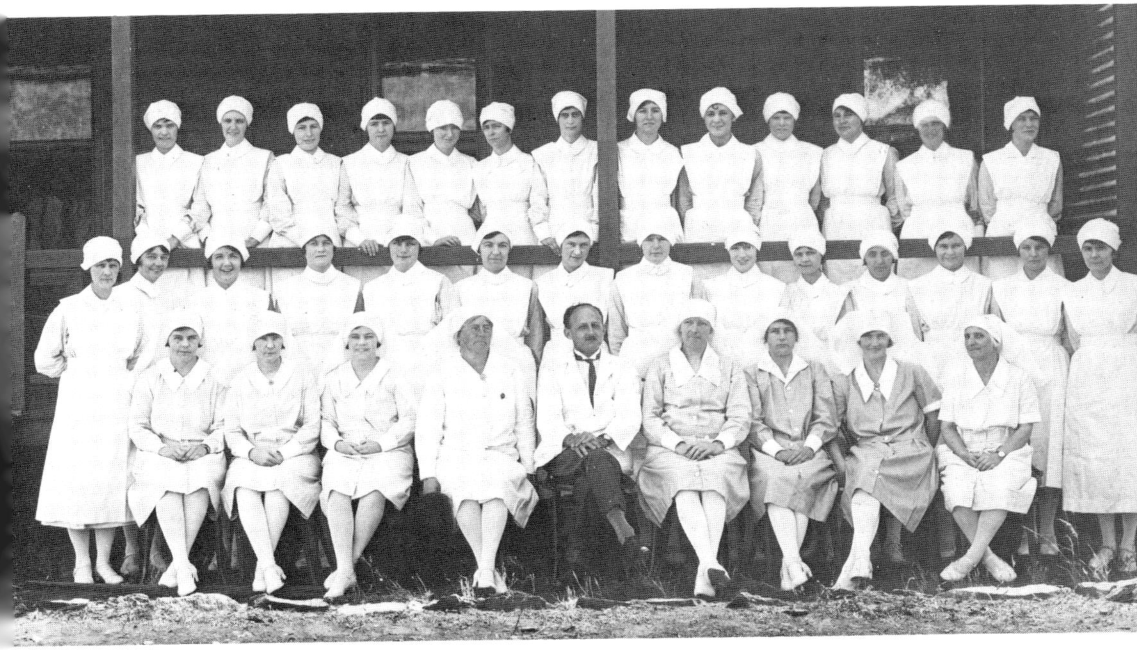

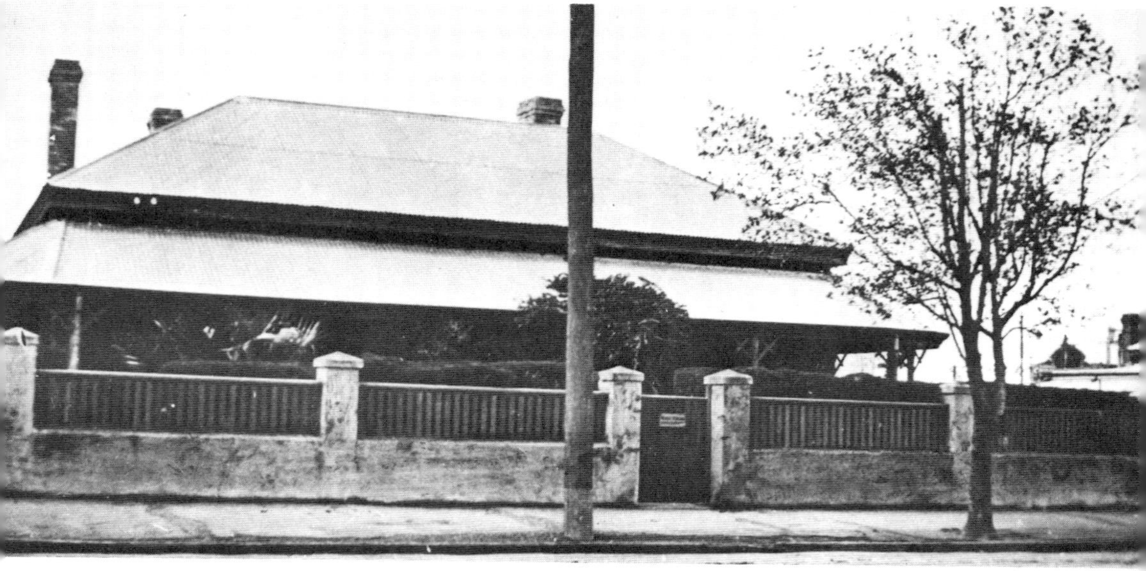

NURSE O'GRADY'S PRIVATE HOSPITAL, FREMANTLE, C. 1915

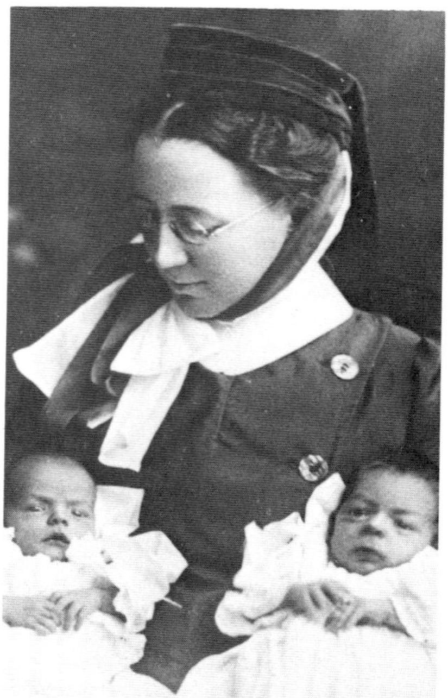

MARY O'GRADY
first midwife registered in W.A.

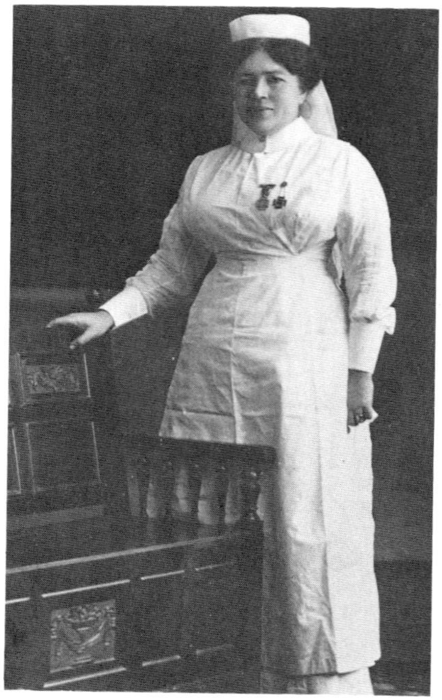

FRANCES CHERRY, C. 1910
early superintendent of the Silver Chain Domiciliary Service.

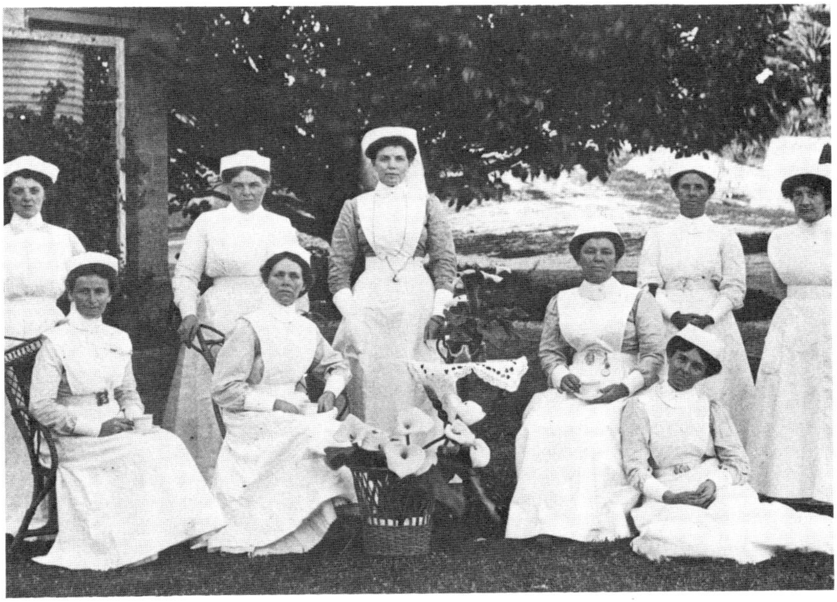

GRADUATES OF FREMANTLE MIDWIFERY CENTRE, 1913

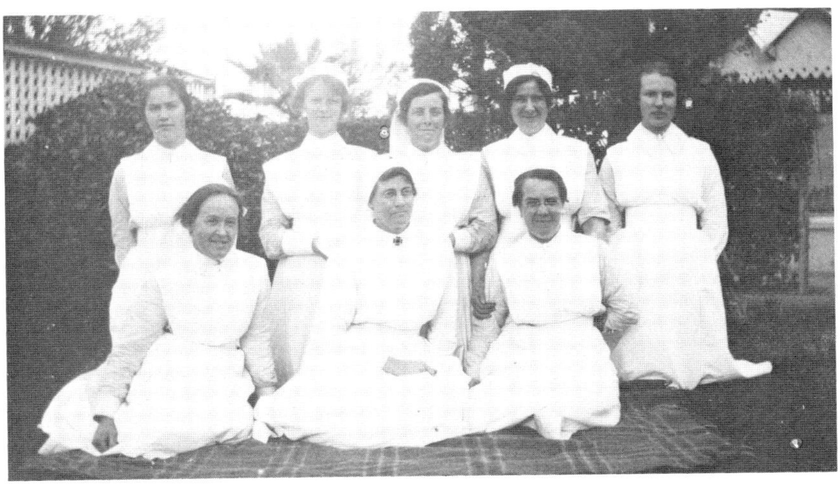

HILLCREST MATERNITY HOSPITAL, 1922-23

Miss A. Sutherland (matron) and first graduates.

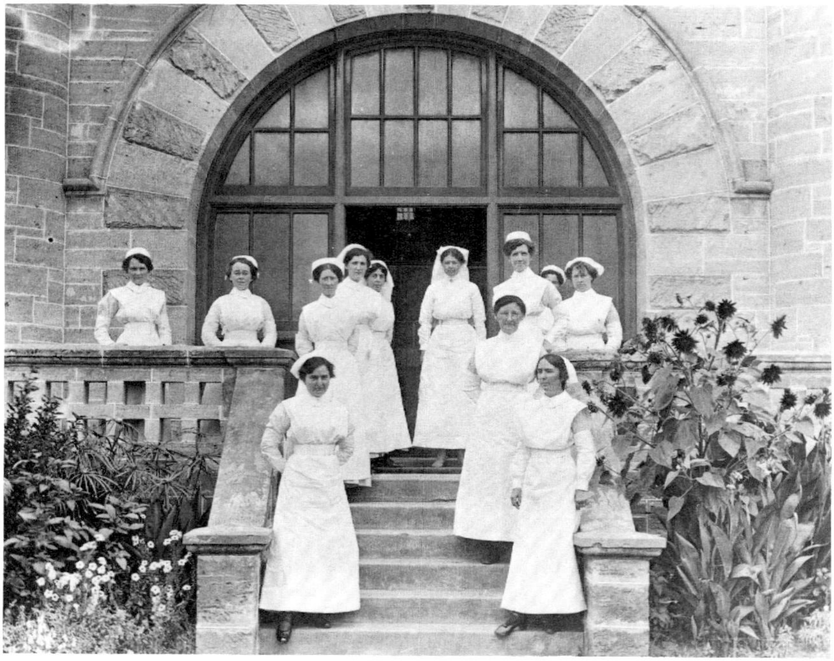

KING EDWARD MEMORIAL HOSPITAL
Miss Harvey and early graduates, 1917-18.

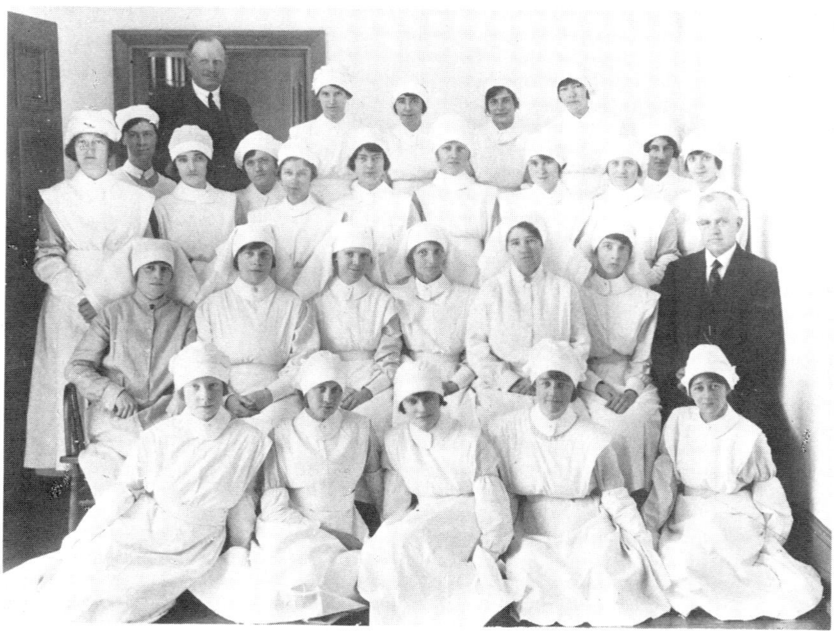

K.E.M.H. TRAINEES, 1926

back row: Dr Clement, Hitchen, Lawson, Waite, Banks; *second row:* —, Milne Robinson, Nelson, Smith, Lindsay, Boneham, Groves, —, Buzza, Griggs, Weston; *seated:* Lloyd, Lukin, Grant, Bottle, Walsh (matron), Carson, Dr Couch; *front row:* Waugh, Hitchings, Allen, Mettam, McLeod.

For many years there was no medical school attached to the university. This meant that tasks in public hospitals usually carried out by medical students were carried out by probationer nurses, which gave them a very wide experience, especially in the field of surgery, and stood them in good stead when working in isolated areas.

When it was agreed that examinations in arithmetic and English set by the members of the Education Committee of the association be introduced in lieu of individual assessment of the applicants' educational qualifications, there was a 50 per cent failure rate, especially in arithmetic. It was these 'test' examinations that were objected to by the authorities of Perth Hospital as they seriously restricted the numbers applying for entry.

In 1914 there was again a move towards the amalgamation of the two associations, A.T.N.A. and R.V.T.N.A., with the object of joining the International Council of Nurses. However this was held back because of the outbreak of war.

Another matter of concern was the industrial action taken by the matron and nurses of Perth Children's Hospital in protest against the unethical behaviour of the medical superintendent.[61] It was done quietly and discreetly. The sick children were transferred to Perth Hospital with their nurses and volunteers were brought in to care for the convalescents. The Hospital Board was divided on the matter, but the A.T.N.A. Council upheld the matron and nurses and the training school was deregistered to prevent the replacement of the dissenting nurses.

Three issues of the *Medical Journal of Australasia* gave coverage of the matter, referring to it as 'a mole-hill and a mountain', and upheld the medical superintendent.[62] The matter resolved itself when the medical superintendent left and the matron joined the Australian Army Nursing Service for which she was granted leave of absence, and the training status of the hospital was reintroduced.

The 1914-18 war had a profound effect on nursing for practically every trained nurse who was eligible rushed to join one of the army nursing services, either the Queen Alexandra's Imperial Medical Nursing Service, which was recruiting nurses in Australia, or the Australian Army Nursing Service, which had been preparing nurses as a reserve for some time. Service was on a part-time basis. The Australian Army Nursing Service had its beginnings when the federation of the Australian states was followed by the creation of the Australian Army Medical Service in 1902. An order to this effect was promulgated and July 1 of that year is taken as the birth date of the A.A.N.S. It is stated that 'An Army Nursing Reserve will be organized from those trained nurses who are qualified and willing to serve as such with stationary Field Hospitals and Base Hospitals when required upon national emergency.'[63]

The uniform was modelled on that of the Imperial British Nursing Service and a badge was issued to be worn with the uniform. In 1904 lady superintendents were appointed in New South Wales, Victoria, Queensland and South Australia, and in Tasmania in 1906. The service was not extended to Western Australia until 1909. Mrs Christian Shackell was appointed lady superintendent and fourteen sisters and staff nurses were foundation members. At this time an approach was made to the State Branch Council of the A.T.N.A. concerning the recruitment of nurses.

Miss May Ashton, who later became well known in nursing circles, states that she was No. 7 and at one period four of the members went into camp at Tammin with the troops for a week. During the winter months weekly lectures were given by Col. McWhae or Col. A. White and Certificates of Efficiency were awarded. A certificate gained by Miss E. A. Bole, dated June 1911, states that 'she has attended a course of lectures on the organization of military hospitals, hygiene and Military Surgery'. Miss Bole's number is twenty-three, which gives some indication of the large number of nurses drawn from civilian sources in 1914. Initially the number was calculated on a population basis, which did restrict Western Australian nurses and also affected their seniority. Subsequently the title lady superintendent was changed to that of principal matron. An interesting remark made by a contemporary historian of the nursing service is that no account was taken of the age of those who volunteered for overseas service and that some were veterans of the Boer War, and were 'past it'. Miss Ashton was among the first group of nurses who went overseas in the hospital ship *Kyama* leaving Fremantle on 14 December 1914. Miss Bole, impatient with the delay, went to England at her own expense and rejoined the Q.A.I.M.N.S.(R), having served with the British army during the Boer War.

In 1915 the war was very much a major issue. In addition to the newly qualified nurses joining the nursing service, the matrons of three of the major training schools, Miss E. Gray from Perth Hospital, Miss H. Homan from Perth Children's Hospital and Miss J. Fyfe from the government hospitals, all requested and were granted leave for army service. There was also a reminder from the office of the high commissioner in London warning that only fully qualified nurses were acceptable to the British Army.[64]

In matters nearer home, some action had to be taken to cope with the worsening situation in civilian hospitals and a measure to overcome this was the re-opening of the A.T.N.A. register to admit members qualifying by means of concessional clauses,[65] thereby allowing a number of matrons in the government hospitals who had been debarred from positions in training schools, to assume these positions.

CHAPTER THREE

FIRST WORLD WAR AND AFTERMATH 1915-1929

The war not only affected health care by reducing available nursing staff, but by depleting medical staff as well. The minutes of the A.T.N.A. Council meetings reflect this aspect in the number of resignations of medical men from the council because they were on active service. This shortage of medical practitioners resulted in extra responsibilities for nurses for which they were not adequately prepared. The technique of such procedures was usually demonstrated by another nurse who had gained her expertise by recent practice. No provision was made for extending the curriculum to cover the theoretical knowledge needed for safe practice nor was there any lessening of the domestic tasks performed by nurses to cover the extra time involved in medical procedures. No allowance was made for error. A mistake on the part of the nurse meant instant dismissal.

There were also outbreaks of sickness among troops in camps such as Blackboy Hill, especially respiratory cross-infection. Voluntary Aid Detachments were joined by many women of the civilian population who were an enormous help in army hospitals. A suggestion that some of these might replace the dwindling supply of probationer nurses was accepted but any suggestion that they might receive some recognition of training was opposed.[1]

The uniform and status of the V.A.D. was somewhat controversial as she wore a red cross on the bib of her apron and on her cap and was rightly called a red cross nurse, a term also applied to members of the A.A.N.S. by both service and civilian personnel. The popular song, 'The Rose of No Man's Land', is an example of such confusion, which was to lead to many post-war difficulties.

As the birth rate tends to rise during all wars, there was an increase in women needing maternity care in Perth which renewed the demand for a public maternity hospital. To this end, the Women's Service Guild approached the A.T.N.A. asking for representatives on a deputation to the premier regarding a women's hospital.[2] In reply to this, the association council agreed to send a representative, but stressed that the onus of organization was on the Women's Service Guild. The name of the representative is not given but it is presumed that it was Dr Gertrude Mead, who was both a trained nurse and a medical practitioner, and who was the obstetric representative on the A.T.N.A. Council. The outcome was that the government proposed to build a new maternity ward at Perth Public Hospital, a move that was not favoured by the council, and it was moved and carried unanimously that 'this council finds it expedient that the maternity ward should not be built in connection with the Perth Public Hospital'.[3]

The scheme involving Perth Public Hospital was shelved and in 1915 the Reformatory or Industrial School in Barker Road, Subiaco, was made available as a maternity hospital. It was a grim building with few amenities, but it was a beginning. However, the fate of the hospital as a midwifery nurse-training school was undecided. An Advisory Board was appointed by the government in April 1916, the chairman being Lady Hackett and the secretary Mrs Edith Cowan.[4] Miss Eleanor Harvey was appointed as the first matron. She was registered as a midwife in Western Australia on 14 June 1916. In order to comply with the A.T.N.A. ruling, she sat and passed the association's examination for acceptance to the Obstetric Register.

Miss Harvey had had an outstanding nursing career. The daughter of a doctor, she gained her General Certificate at Perth Public Hospital in 1911, where she joined the staff as theatre sister. She subsequently went overseas and undertook her obstetric training at the Rotunda in Dublin. Graduating with honours, she was appointed labor ward sister for the next twelve months. She then joined the staff of Kent Fever Hospital, but her stay in England was cut short by the illness of her father, which forced her to return home. When appointed to K.E.M.H. Miss Harvey was sister in charge of the Infectious Diseases Branch. Eleanor Harvey had a great feeling for her fellow nurses, and when a member of the A.T.N.A. Council, it was her great ambition to work towards a scheme which would provide for those who were no longer able to work. She deplored the fact that many were housed in small back rooms with little comfort, or had no alternative but to go to the Women's Home. It is a fitting tribute to her that the present Eleanor Harvey Home was named in her honour.

At K.E.M.H. Miss Harvey's task was difficult. The hospital opened on 6 July 1916 and the first patient was admitted. At a special meeting of the Midwives Board it was decided that the course be six months residence and lectures for women holding a three-year certificate of training in medical and surgical nursing, and for unqualified women twelve months residence and lectures. Pupil midwives were required to pay a training fee of ten guineas. They did not receive any salary during their course of training. It was also decided to register K.E.M.H. as an A.T.N.A. training school for obstetric nurses.[5]

The hospital was only available to those who could not afford other maternity care and the budget was very tight. The matron and staff were housed in a galvanized iron building with cubicles only. In common with other public institutions there was great reliance on the groups of women who formed auxiliaries and came regularly to mend and sew. Too much cannot be said for these women especially those who for years came to K.E.M.H. which had special problems related to both mother and baby. Napkins, baby gowns, shifts, binders and perineal pads were all made in the sewing room. Every bit of old linen was salvaged to make pads which were used, laundered (by the nursing staff), sterilized and re-used over and over again, a practice which continued for many years until the pupil midwives rebelled against it.[6]

Other areas, too, had their problems. In Kalgoorlie the work load was increased by casualties both medical and surgical among men working on the construction of the transcontinental railway. As with the gold-rush days, typhoid fever was a problem. The railway, which was commenced in 1913, was completed in 1917 when the construction workers who commenced at Port Augusta in South Australia linked up with those who had started from Kalgoorlie in Western Australia.[7]

In 1915 a sanatorium was built at Wooroloo in the country 65 kilometres or so outside the metropolitan area. This followed the world trend in the treatment of patients with tuberculosis by the so-called 'fresh air' method. On the goldfields the disease was prevalent amongst the miners, who were treated at Coolgardie Hospital, which had become almost specialized in this regard and as a result lost its status as an A.T.N.A. training school.[8] By 1916 the patients had all been transferred to Wooroloo as were those from the Infectious Diseases Branch. Along with this, many of the iron buildings at Coolgardie and at other redundant hospitals were removed and re-erected at I.D.B. and K.E.M.H. No doubt the heating of the iron to burning point by the hot sun had a deterrent effect on the pathogenic micro-organisms.

At Wooroloo, too, there was a small isolation section separate from the main building for patients with Hansen's disease, and this for many years was occupied by a matron who was said to have contracted the disease while working in Broome.

With Wooroloo there arose the usual question of staffing, and the position of the student nurses who were seconded to the institution during their term of training. Eventually the matter was resolved by an agreement that it could become part of the training programme providing that all nurses spent at least eighteen months at Kalgoorlie and another six months at an approved country hospital.

Naturally the A.T.N.A. centred a great deal of discussion and activity around those nurses who were on active service and what plans were being made for their future and readjustment to civil life. Together with other agencies, they set up a welfare committee and commenced a fund to provide a rest and recreation centre for them. This eventually resulted in a residence being provided in Wilson Street (Parliament Place), West Perth. By 1917 nurses were returning from overseas on hospital ships and troopships with the sick and wounded, and many went back for a second tour of duty. The A.T.N.A. and nurses generally expressed dissatisfaction that the proportion of Western Australian nurses selected for overseas service was much less than that from the eastern states.[9] The A.T.N.A. still continued to hold its council meetings at the Perth Public Hospital board room, and its larger meetings at the Hibernian Hall. There were no headquarters or rooms for extending hospitality to the nurses returning from overseas or the large number from the eastern states who arrived on the troopships en route to the war zone. At this stage the Karrakatta Club in Perth, which had been established for women, rendered invaluable service by making available their facilities to members of the nursing profession, as part of the war effort.[10] A centre was also provided in Fremantle at the Church of England rectory.

It is noted that in 1918 sixty-seven applicants sat for the entrance examination, and of these twenty-four passed in both subjects and eighteen failed in both subjects. The examiner asked if the standard required was too high, but the council did not consider that this was so.

A world problem at this time was the increase in venereal disease. The commissioner of public health suggested the forming of a branch council in the state with the National Council of Great Britain. Dr Gertrude Mead represented the association on the Western Australian committee convened for the purpose, and in a report drew attention to the fact that more education was needed on the subject. She emphasized that nurses were not adequately informed.[11] Miss Gill, matron of Perth Public Hospital, was appointed to augment the committee. However it was a very long time before the subject was discussed openly and methods of contact explained to the general public and members of the nursing profession.

War ended in 1918 but there was another enemy, the so-called 'Spanish' influenza, which did not differentiate between nations and was to become pandemic. Because of its isolation Australia was not as vulnerable as other countries, but the returning troops brought the infection back with them. The first two troopships to return had reached South Africa only but their personnel had come in contact with the disease and on the return voyage there were many sick and some deaths. In order to prevent the infection reaching the civilian population, the ships were placed in quarantine off Woodman Point, a few kilometres south of Fremantle, and the sick and their attendants, which included all the nursing staff, were transferred to the small quarantine hospital, which was not geared for such an influx. The staff was augmented by sisters from No. 8 Base Hospital and some civilians. Many contracted the disease and thirty men and four nurses died.

In spite of the strict security measures taken, it was not long before the infection was manifest in the civilian population and every available nurse was pressed into service.[12] In addition to the existing facilities, temporary hospitals were set up by the public health authorities. One of these was the isolation hospital in Victoria Park, formerly known as the Rotunda and now Edward Millen Home. The matron appointed was Mrs Annie Campbell, formerly Annie May-Steers of the Sydney Hospital, who had returned to nursing during the war years. Epidemics were not new to her as she had formerly nursed at Coolgardie in the 1890s and had been appointed matron of Guildford Hospital when typhoid fever became endemic among the men working on the Mundaring Weir at the turn of the century. A member of the A.T.N.A. since its inception she retained her interest in nursing affairs. Nursing care was still basically the same: it aimed at relieving the symptoms. There were no curative drugs.

The shortage of nursing staff to deal with the epidemic is reflected in the request from Dr Atkinson of the Health Department for nurses to be released from training at King Edward Memorial Hospital for nursing people with pneumonic influenza. This was granted without penalties for broken training. On the general side it was found that the facilities afforded at No. 8 Base Hospital were inadequate to cope with the number of returning sick and wounded and in addition there was need of accommodation of a temporary nature for those returning with their 'war brides' and awaiting discharge. A large pavilion-type hospital was built at Keane's Point and named 'Anzac'.[13] (This is now the Royal Freshwater Bay Yacht Club.) It was staffed by members of the Army Nursing Service, some of whom had not had the opportunity of serving overseas.

This was later to create a problem when it came to eligibility for membership of returned servicemen's institutions.

In 1920 the main avenue of employment for trained civilian nurses and those being discharged from army service was private nursing. In this the younger army nurses were at a disadvantage as many had not had experience in this field, and there were no services for rehabilitation. Most had single certificates and opportunities for gaining further qualifications in maternity nursing were limited as both K.E.M.H. and the newly opened Hillcrest Hospital in North Fremantle were restricted in accommodation.

Another problem was the closure of the well known nurses' homes or bureaux during the war years. To this end the A.T.N.A. held a special meeting on 30 June 1920 to consider the establishment of an A.T.N.A. club for trained nurses.[14] A special committee was formed and empowered to make decisions regarding the leasing or purchasing of a suitable property and to consult the solicitors Unmack and Unmack in the matter of forming a registered company. A deputation to the premier with a request for a block of land had met with a favourable response, but dissatisfaction arose with its situation. An acre of land in East Perth valued at $1100 was offered with the suggestion that a building be erected from funds raised by the nurses themselves.[15] This was rejected because of the proximity of the old East Perth cemetery and the locality. The offer was taken as an insult. Its inconvenience was stressed by the fact that people employing private nurses were moving north, south and west of the city. After much discussion and the investigation of many properties it was finally decided to purchase the lease of a property at No. 9 Mount St to be known as the A.T.N.A. Club.[16] The money was loaned by the association and members were encouraged to become shareholders. The club became the headquarters of the A.T.N.A. and from January 1921 all meetings were held there A letter of thanks was sent to Perth Public Hospital which had given the association a meeting place free of charge since its formation in this state in 1907. The first matron of the A.T.N.A. club to be appointed was Miss Henrietta Jarvis, formerly of Guy's Hospital, London. The idea of a club was well supported by the nurses themselves. When the venture was launched at a special meeting and welcome home to the returned sisters in April 1920, there were a hundred applications for shares, and arrangements for a fete and other fund-raising activities were enthusiastically supported.[17]

The wartime experience of all who served, combatant and non-combatant, had a marked effect on their attitude and so coloured their outlook that never again would they see things in the same light as before. They were a race apart. Before her death, a half century later, Elizabeth Grover (A.A.N.S.) spoke of her reactions when she nursed the men from the Gallipoli campaign and subsequently brought some of the first Anzacs back to Australia. These men with their badly battered bodies and indomitable spirit made a lasting impression on her, as did the quiet of the Australian countryside after the noise and intensity of war. On her return to the theatre of war she nursed in a prisoner of war hospital. The nurses were well liked by the Turkish soldiers, who never forgot their kindness.[18]

Ruth Bottle has also spoken of the impression made on her when, returning on a troopship, one of the chaplains, Bishop Riley, spoke to the men and told them that as they had stood together in war, so must they stand together in the difficult post-war period, and urged them to join the newly formed returned soldiers' associations being raised in each state to safeguard the interests and rights of ex-service men and women.[19] These associations later amalgamated to become a national association, the present-day Returned Services League. Returned nurses were accepted for membership on the same terms as the men, but because of their unique service in all being women and all trained nurses, they formed a Returned Sisters' Association, which was later to become a sub-branch of the R.S.L. In 1971 both Miss Grover and Miss Bottle were honoured in receiving certificates for fifty years' continuous membership.

In April 1920 representatives from the W.A. Branch of the A.T.N.A. were invited to join the Returned Sisters' Association of the Returned Soldiers Association to wait on the minister and present their request for the state registration of professional nurses.[20] Although the A.T.N.A. agreed in principle, the letter arrived too late for them to take any part in the discussion. The copy of the Returned Sisters' request to the minister tells its own story:

1. That the standard for State registration for General Nurses be that of the Australasian Trained Nurses Association, now general throughout Australasia.
2. That the Registered Board be composed of at least three parts trained nurses.
3. That it be made illegal for either Physician or Surgeon to allow any unregistered nurse to take charge of either operative or medical cases.
4. That it be made illegal for nurses registered only for Midwifery nursing to undertake general nursing.
5. That all nurses non-members of the A.T.N.A. must be registered within twelve months of the passing of the Act.
6. That all private hospitals be registered and compelled to employ at least one registered nurse to every six patients.

7. That only registered nurses be allowed to wear the Army Nurses cap which has been so largely copied by untrained women.

It would appear that the deputation was well received although a report is not available, the minutes of the Sisters' Association having been lost. There is also no record in parliamentary papers of the deputation being received, but on 12 October 1920 a bill was introduced into the Legislative Council — the Nurses Registration Bill — by the minister for education and health, H. P. Colebatch. After debate it was passed on to the Legislative Assembly and further debated, when it was found to be out of order on a technicality. Because expenditure would be involved in the setting up of a registration board and the payment of examiners, the bill should have rightfully been introduced into the Assembly first. It was therefore withdrawn on Thursday 25 November 1920 by the speaker.

Almost ten months elapsed before the bill was recommitted and introduced into the Assembly by the colonial secretary, F. T. Broun, on 20 September 1921. The debate resumed over the next two months and it was reintroduced into the Council on 15 November 1921. It was finally returned to the Assembly and received with Council's amendment and passed. It was assented to 31 January 1922 to become Nurses Registration No. 7 of 1922, to be cited as the Nurses Registration Act of 1921.

It should be noted that during the passage of the Nurses Registration Bill through parliament, between the first and second presentation, there were events of some importance to the parliamentary system throughout Australia. In 1920 a bill had been introduced and passed to allow women to nominate and be elected to parliament. In the 1921 state election the government was returned, with a difference. Mrs Edith Cowan was elected and became the first woman to sit in an Australian parliament. She was a strong supporter of the registration of trained nurses. From the outset she made it clear that in this and other matters she would, if she found it necessary, vote according to conscience and not along party lines. The effect of this on the final outcome on nurses' registration is difficult to know and assess.

No copies of the actual bill appear to be in existence but the measure received a mixed reaction by members of both houses, many of whom were ill informed on the role of the professional nurse. Their derogatory remarks deserve only contempt. Recorded in Hansard, they will go down in history as a testament to the ignorance and bigotry of their authors.

However, there were members who were sympathetic towards the nurses and endeavoured to meet their requests, even though some of the members' suggestions were outside the scope of the legislation. These included the establishment of a registered nurses' home for the purpose of domiciliary care for people unable to afford fees for full-time nursing; shorter hours and more pay for probationer nurses; less time to be spent at the Wooroloo Sanitorium during the training period and an interchange of trainees between the metropolitan hospitals, Perth Public and Fremantle, with those in the country training schools, in order to afford the latter a more systematic course of training.

The requests that preference be given to registered nurses in the government hospitals when vacancies became due and that nurses wear a distinctive uniform were opposed on the grounds, firstly, that it would deprive older women, unable to qualify by the passing of examinations, of employment; secondly, the need to wear uniform at all was queried as it was thought that a distinctive badge would suffice.

A contentious issue was the control of nurses by the A.T.N.A. and the latter's involvement, if any, with the registration board to be created under the proposed act. One member in particular stressed that the nominees for such a board should be from the nurses' organization and he doubted the wisdom in appointing a public servant as secretary and the principal medical officer as permanent chairman (ex officio).

There was also a suggestion that the register be opened to all those who had served as V.A.D.s during the war, especially overseas, on the basis that their experience in army establishments was equal to that gained by nurses in recognized training hospitals.

It is mentioned that the register would be divided into two sections, one for the registration of mental nurses and the other for general nurses. However it seems that the former did not eventuate. (An interesting point is that nurses are referred to in the feminine, possibly because there were at that time no facilities for the training of male nurses in Western Australia. The rules of the A.T.N.A. did not discriminate on the basis of sex.) Overall, the main concern seems to have been that the supply of probationer nurses, which was the mainstay in the cheap and efficient staffing of hospitals, would be inhibited if conditions for registration were made too difficult.

Under the act, the Nurses' Registration Board of five members was constituted and met for the first time on 13 July 1922 to draw up the rules and regulations. Members of the board were Dr E. Atkinson, principal medical officer (chairman); Mr F. Hadley, surgeon; Miss A. Broomhall, inspectress, Department of Health, and hon. secretary, A.T.N.A.; Miss I. J. Gill, matron of Perth Hospital; Miss H. M. Homan, matron, Perth Children's Hospital, and member of Returned Sisters' Section of Returned Services League.[21]

The regulations, under the provisions of the Nurses Registration Act 1921, were based on the rules which applied to the A.T.N.A. and had been reprinted in 1920.[22] It was agreed that the examination for registration would be that of membership of the A.T.N.A. and that for the time being the association would continue with this function. The first secretary to the board was D. Stewart, a clerk employed in the Medical Department. The board position was considered to be only part time. Miss Broomhall had hoped to have been appointed to the position as she was already employed in the Department of Public Health. This was largely a factor in her leaving the state to take up the position of secretary to the Victorian Trained Nurses' Association. Trained at Fremantle Hospital, she had gained most of her nursing experience in Victoria[23] and the Victorian home for retired nurses, Eadrie, contains a memorial plaque to her.

A comparison of the curriculum given in the N.R.B. regulations with that of the A.T.N.A. shows that the former gives guide lines only for general nursing, anatomy and physiology and does not extend it to the other subjects required, i.e. medical and surgical nursing, invalid cookery and hygiene. In both there is no alteration from the first curriculum of 1904.[24] The minimum number of lectures remains the same and organs of reproduction in male and female are omitted. However in the list of textbooks suggested, gynaecological nursing is mentioned.

In the association rules, under Rule 18, the following is of interest.

> The attention of Training Schools is drawn to the following definition of the duties of a Matron, drawn up at the suggestion of the Board of Health (N.S.W.) and approved by the Council:
>
> The MATRON shall have sole charge of the Nursing Housekeeping and Domestic Staffs, and shall be responsible to the Hospital Board of Directors or Committee, through the Medical Superintendent for the due and efficient performance of their duties. Where there is no Medical Superintendent the matron shall be responsible for the general superintendence of the whole Institution. The Matron shall select the candidates for admission to the Hospital Staff as pupil nurses, and shall submit their names to the Board or Committee, for approval. She shall see that the pupil nurses regularly attend the lectures arranged by the Medical staff and shall herself instruct them in the theory and practice of nursing.[25]

In August 1922 a Nurses Registration Act Amendment Bill was introduced in the Council by Minister for Education Colebatch, the subject of which was to extend the period of registration to July 1923 to allow those who were possibly not aware of the legislation and its implications extra time to register.

The second alteration was to specify nursing organizations, for example, the Australasian Trained Nurses Association, the Royal Victorian Trained Nurses' Association, the Royal British Nurses' Association, etc. whose certificates of membership would be recognized for registration. The bill was passed on 14 November 1922 without further amendment and assented to 30 November 1922, to become No. 25 of 1922. There were no further amendments to the act for another seventeen years.

The first register, published in the *Government Gazette* 1 February 1924, lists 645 names.[26] These include about two hundred who trained outside Western Australia, and many who had been accepted by the A.T.N.A. under concessional membership. There is no indication of how long these nurses had been nursing and if they were still in practice. Registration was not compulsory but it was a status symbol, although there was some confusion between A.T.N.A. membership and state registration.

Western Australia was the third Australian state to achieve registration of nurses. In 1912 Queensland registered midwives, nurses and physiotherapists under the Health Act. Both South Australia and Western Australia attempted legislation in 1920, but the delay in passing the act put Western Australia in third place. In New South Wales and Victoria registration was achieved in 1924, in Tasmania in 1927, and in the A.C.T. in 1933. Overseas, the General Nursing Council for England and Wales was established following the passing of the Nurses Registration Act 1919, designated 'An Act to provide for the Registration of Nurses for the Sick'. This body's acceptance of Australian nurses has fluctuated over the years. In Australia there is no national register and nurses are required to re-register in the state in which they are practising. The original Western Australian Register is divided into two parts, female and male nurses. Under the latter there is one name: Walter George W. Clark, Military Hospitals, England. The registration of midwives remained unchanged and they continued to be registered under the Health Act of 1911 by the Midwives Registration Board.

Regarding the Mental Health Services, certificates had been granted following examination as early as 1903 but refusal to comply with A.T.N.A. requirements re standard of entry etc. precluded these nurses from the A.T.N.A. register, and they were not included in the Nurses Registration Act of 1922. The certificates could be classified as evidence of competency within a particular field of custodial care.

Although general nurses practising under the state act did not receive preferential treatment for positions in government hospitals, trained ex-service nurses confidently thought that in the nursing of military and repatriation patients they would be given priority of employment. Unlike in New South Wales and Victoria, there were no large hospitals built for the above purpose in Western Australia where, except for Lemnos for the mentally ill which was built at West Subiaco (Shenton Park), the only new building was a block at Perth Hospital. This consisted of three wards, 9, 10 and 11, and an operating theatre. For many years it was referred to as the 'Military Block', although it was gradually taken over by the authorities of Perth Hospital. At this time, also, the old colonial building was extended to Murray Street to provide out-patient clinics for assessment of repatriation patients, and, later, to provide the hospital out-patient department. It is believed that at this time a lecture room and new living quarters were added to the Murray Street nurses' home (Kirkman House), thus completing a quadrangle. (The lecture room was converted into bedrooms when the new hospital was built in the 1940s.)

When the Military Block first opened, trained ex-army personnel were employed, but they were gradually phased out in favour of the probationer nurse. Many of the long-stay patients in the above category were eventually accommodated in the various private hospitals in their own areas. Those with tuberculoses were cared for at Wooroloo Sanitorium for a time and later at the Edward Millen Home in East Victoria Park. The hospital for the mentally ill, Lemnos, continued to employ trained staff. The repatriation hospitals were under Commonwealth government control and outside the jurisdiction of the state. At this stage the federal seat of government was in Melbourne, which meant that there was a large number of 'Commonwealth' nurses in Melbourne. An organization, the (Victorian) Trained Nurses' Guild,[27] affiliated with the Victorian Women Citizens' Movement, made application for registration as a union in the federal Court of Arbitration, and was accepted (1921). It is reported that the R.V.T.N.A. applied for deregistration of the organization, but the circumstances surrounding this are not clear, and the move did not succeed. There was also concern that in Queensland nurses had formed an association registered with the Trades Hall and had applied to arbitration re salaries and hours of work. Both the A.T.N.A. and the R.V.T.N.A. considered this so serious that a conference planned to discuss their amalgamation was postponed. Earlier discussions on this matter had been shelved for lack of unanimity. The W.A. Branch of the A.T.N.A. was represented at the conference, which was eventually held in Sydney in July 1921, by Misses Eleanor Harvey and A. Broomhall. Following their report on proposed unionism in other states, it was decided that legal advice on arbitration matters be obtained with a view to altering the constitution so that 'the nurse in training in recognised hospitals be brought immediately under the influence of the Association'.

The ruling on arbitration was reported by Miss Harvey:

> Nurses who are workers within the meaning of the Act can form a Union under the Industrial Arbitration Act 1912, the number applying to be not less than fifteen and only those 'employed' would be eligible for membership.[28]

This virtually ruled out the A.T.N.A. whose members were generally employers (private hospital matrons) and private nurse practitioners. There was a suggestion that trainee nurses be granted 'honorary' membership of the association and that some positive steps be taken to improve working conditions and remuneration for all grades of nurses.

An interesting note in the minutes of this time is the conferring of honorary life membership on Sister Mary Nicolay and her acceptance. Miss Nicolay had retired from active nursing but had become a well-known figure in Perth by virtue of the fact that she always wore an 'outdoor' uniform. Once a week she visited Perth Hospital as the guest of the matron for a midday meal, a custom which continued over many years.[29]

State registration of nurses in the separate states deprived the nursing organizations of much of their bargaining power, and clearly there was a need for unity if they were to survive. There was also the question of a national body to represent Australia in the International Council of Nurses. There was a great deal of confused thinking about the I.C.N. and there were some who thought and taught that national membership would confer on an A.T.N.A. member, through its affiliation with the I.C.N., acceptance as a trained nurse throughout the world. This was a misconception which persisted for a great many years both in the community and amongst the nurses themselves, and this 'world-wide' idea of nursing was even used as a draw card to induce young women to take up nursing as a career.

The sixteenth annual report of the W.A. Branch of the A.T.N.A. for the year ending 1923 gives the following statement by Miss Broomehall, the honorary secretary:

> one very important feature of the year's work was the interstate Conference held in Melbourne in June last. It was decided to meet in Melbourne so that the two Associations (the R.V.T.N.A. and the A.T.N.A.) could meet and discuss their points of difference, with the object of forming one body and although the way is not at present clear to a complete amalgamation of the two Ass. it was considered possible to form a governing council—composed of two delegates from each of the six States of the Commonwealth. It is proposed that this Federal body which would be called the Australian Nursing Federation, should meet at stated intervals (or in emergencies) Members of either Ass. would automatically become a member of the A.N.F. without payment of any further fee, an arrangement being made for the transference of a certain amount from either Ass. for the upkeep of the Federal body.
>
> Already a very beneficial result has taken place regarding the better understanding between the R.V.T.N.A. and the A.T.N.A. The Victorian Ass. has greatly appreciated the assistance which it has received from all States to fight a very unsatisfactory Bill which was introduced before the Victorian Parliament recently. Advice now comes to hand that a satisfactory finality has been reached and that the training decided upon is in accord with the suggestions made at Conference by the Federal Council.

The Western Australian delegates to the above conference were Misses F. Marrett and A. Broomhall.

In 1924 the Australian Nursing Federation became a reality, the first meeting of the council being held in Sydney on 27-30 May. The representatives of the branches were Miss Conyers, R.R.C., O.B.E. (Victoria), Dr Millard and Miss Kendal Davies (New South Wales), Dr Marks (Queensland), Miss Murray (South Australia), Misses Broomhall and Gill (Western Australia), and Miss Carpenter (Tasmania). The secretaries of the R.V.T.N.A. and the A.T.N.A. (Misses Crocker and Evans) were also present. The original report of this meeting, supplied by Miss Evans, is on file in the archives of the West Australian Branch of the R.A.N.F. and a first edition of the Constitution, 1 July 1924, is also available. Both these are lengthy documents. The preamble to the Constitution is quoted below:

> Whereas it is expedient that the Nurses' Associations of Australia should unite in a Federation in order to promote the best interests and protect the rights of the nursing profession in Australia now the Australasian Trained Nurses Association and the Royal Victorian Trained Nurses' Association have

> agreed to form a Federation called the Australian Nursing Federation and have adopted the following Constitution . . .

It is stated in the report that:

> Owing to the changed conditions in the various states each state must exercise more domestic autonomy and the A.N.F. now being an accomplished fact there is no longer any parental control and only matters of a Federal nature will be dealt with by the Federal Council. For the time being the Sydney Office will be the office of the A.N.F.

Although there was general acceptance of the A.N.F., the individual state branches still retained their former names, A.T.N.A. and R.V.T.N.A., which led to a lot of confusion among members, especially life members who, under the new constitution, would be phased out. One matter which met with the approval of the West Australian Branch was the matter of voting: it was decided that each state branch should have equal voting power of two votes instead of voting being proportionate to the number of members enrolled. Unfortunately there was some disagreement on the appointment of a federal secretary. The A.T.N.A. (N.S.W. Branch) wanted to retain the services of Miss Evans who, although not a trained nurse, had been an efficient officer over the years. The Victorians, however, thought the position should be beld by a nurse. Another condition of the Victorians entering the federation was that their branch retain the prefix 'Royal'.[30]

Following federation, the West Australian Branch settled down to sort out its domestic problems and there were many. Nurses were widening their horizons, and new opportunities of service were offering in the community outside the narrow limits of hospital-based practice. However, most of these activities required that the applicants be equipped with basic nursing training, but in turn a higher educational standard was demanded to qualify for many of these positions. Failure to recognize this need cost nursing dearly as it was by-passed and the opportunity for it to progress to the field of higher education was lost. Sadly, the reason for this was the fear that the source of labour for the hospitals might dry up if the demands on entrants became too severe.

In the twenties the hospitals were completely nurse orientated, and nurses were filling the positions of dieticians, social workers, radiographers, laboratory technicians, assistants and, in some cases physiotherapists. At Perth Hospital the chief resident medical officer always had a trained nurse in his office to keep the patients' medical records.

In the outback, nurses ran the mission hospitals almost single handed with an occasional visit from the doctor. The Australian Inland Mission, which began in 1912, did not envisage a flying doctor service, which was introduced in 1928 in eastern Australia. Some of the first mission hospitals were at Lake Grace, Esperance, Halls Creek, and Port Hedland.

Following the British pattern, the medical examination of school children was commenced in Western Australia in 1906 and continued spasmodically until 1913, when the 'visiting nurses' from the Health Department, whose duties were primarily the inspection of midwives, were also required to visit patients with tuberculosis, to follow up the school medical inspection to make sure corrective action was taken by parents, and also to give instruction to mothers regarding the feeding of infants. In 1917 Dr Roberta H. M. Jull was specifically appointed school medical officer and given the part-time service of the visiting nurses, but in 1921 two school nurses were appointed on a full-time basis. It is noted that when these appointments were being made, the A.T.N.A. urged that the positions be given to Western Australian rather than overseas nurses. In 1925 Dr E. M. Stang was appointed school medical officer to allow Dr Jull to spend half her time supervising the newly formed Infant Health Service. On the retirement of Dr Jull in 1928 Dr Stang took over both positions.

The Infant Health Service offered trained nurses another avenue of employment. This service evolved partly from the Silver Chain Visiting Nursing Service, and partly from the Children's Protection Society. It was also supported by the Red Cross Society. Administration was by the Infant Welfare Association, a body subsidized by the government but relying mainly on voluntary effort and help from local authority. Understandingly, the salaries were low. The sister who ran the North Perth Clinic, established by the Silver Chain, was paid £100 per annum. The Perth Clinic, which shared the premises occupied by the Children's Protection Society Day Nursery for working mothers, opened almost simultaneously with the North Perth Clinic in September 1922. The sister in charge of the Perth Clinic was Miss Cole, and in 1932 the building was extended to accommodate a 'correspondence' sister, Miss R. Nicholson, who had been with the service since its inception. Miss Nicholson spoke with affection of the mothers she met through her letters.

When it was first introduced, infant health training varied from state to state and the examination and certificates were those of an 'in service' nature; there was no state register provided for under the Nurses Registration Act. The two systems advocated for infant feeding were Karitane (Dr Truby King, New Zealand) and Tresillian (Sydney). Inevitably there was some disagreement as to the best method to be used in the local situation.

In 1926 a move was made to set up a training course in infant welfare in Western Australia, using the facilities of King Edward Memorial Hospital. This venture did not get complete support from medical men, who saw the infant health nurse as a threat to their practices, although the clinics dealt only with healthy babies and those who were considered in need of treatment or medical advice were referred to the doctor. Infant health sisters were not allowed to prescribe treatment or advise on medical preparations.[31]

Prior to this, in 1924, Mrs Walsh, matron of K.E.M.H., was granted leave of absence to undertake training at Tresillian in Sydney. On return she inaugurated a series of lectures in conjunction with Dr R. Crisp for members of her staff and midwifery trainees. In 1927, on the recommendation of the Infant Welfare Association in a report to the minister, an approved training centre was established at K.E.M.H. in one of the new buildings in Hensman Road (Ward 8) and incorporated the Infant Health Clinic for the Subiaco area.

The length of infant health training advocated was two months for trainee nurses at K.E.M.H. and three months for others. The requisite was a Midwifery Certificate. This was in conflict with the eastern states pattern of training which was four months, but it was pointed out that this was available to untrained nurses and included invalid cookery and other subjects which would account for the extra time. However the K.E.M.H. course was finally settled for four months. Because of numbers it was divided into two periods of two months, before and after midwifery training.

The course was inaugurated by Janet Chalmers, a friend of Mrs Walsh from their training days at the Royal Hospital in Paddington, Sydney.

Agnes Marion McLean Walsh had joined the staff at K.E.M.H. in 1920, on completion of her general training at Perth Hospital. A young widow, she had gained her Midwifery Certificate before coming to Western Australia.[32] Her appointment to K.E.M.H. followed the resignation of Kathleen McAleer, a senior sister, the matron being Mrs Charlotte Latta. At this time the hospital was Rotunda (Dublin) orientated, as Eleanor Harvey (the first matron), Kathleen McAleer and Charlotte Latta had all obtained their Obstetric Certificates from that institution. Dr Dixie Clement, the honorary obstetrician, was also a Rotunda graduate.

When Mrs Latta resigned in 1922, Agnes Walsh was appointed matron, a position she was to hold for the next thirty-four years, during which her association with nursing and midwifery was to become almost legendary. She had a dominant personality and was able to influence people at all levels of the community, businessmen, politicians and those in 'high places' as well as the 'mothers' who had sublime faith in her ability as a midwife. For many years she was the sole administrator of the hospital, answerable only to the commissioner of public health. The fact that the institution was able to operate within its budget was quoted as an example to other health services, but the economies practised were certainly not appreciated by the student nurses.

Agnes Walsh had an outstanding ability to assess the potential of people within their own field, and on this basis she chose her staff, and having done so, allowed them to 'get on with it' with a minimum of interference, which resulted in their unswerving and sometimes undeserving loyalty. This delegation of authority enabled her to enjoy and participate in activities outside the hospital. She was a keen racing enthusiast; she also had an interest in music, and had a fine contralto voice. She was indeed fortunate to staff the hospital with people of the calibre of her lifelong friend and assistant, Mary Carson, and Ruth Bottle, Agnes Tait and Dorothy Edis.

In 1927 there were changes in the administration of Perth Hospital which were reflected in a change of pattern in nursing practice, with the resignation of Miss Isabella Gill as matron and the subsequent appointment of Miss Ethel McNevin in 1928.

Isabella Jane Gill had been matron of Perth Hospital since 1916. She had come to Western Australia at the invitation of Miss Ethel Gray, with whom she had trained at Royal Melbourne Hospital, to take charge of the casualty department, which was the kind of work she enjoyed. On being persuaded to accept the matronship during the difficult war years, she introduced the pattern of the Royal Melbourne Hospital which gave nurses graded experience according to their seniority. A blackboard in her office showed the deployment of the nursing staff, and was the forerunner of what was to become later the 'manning chart'.

She had very definite views on the way nurses conducted themselves both on and off duty, and her strict religious beliefs did not allow her to accept the permissive society of the twenties. This led to a difference of opinion with the Perth Hospital Board on the matter of discipline so that her resignation was inevitable, to the distress of many members of the nursing staff. Her salary of £120 per annum was not found to be conducive to further applicants for the position and the amount was doubled. Within a year Miss Gill was appointed matron of Perth Children's Hospital, where she died of a heart condition on duty on 10 August 1929.[33] The following tribute in the Children's Hospital *Magazine* (1930) was written by one of the trainee nurses on the occasion of Miss Gill's death.

No more in spotless white you tread
The paths trod by our feet.
No more in passage, hall or ward
Your gracious form we meet
No longer in the midst of work
You stay and give us cheer
Your noble form has left us now
We weep and mourn you here.
No more your kindly words of praise
Will lift our spirits high
No more your wisdom ease the doubts
That in our hearts might lie
No longer with us gracious soul
You leave a memory fair
Of a noble heart and great
And a personality rare.

Following Miss Gill's resignation as matron of Perth Hospital there were two interim appointments to her position, Janet McDonald and Florence Stuart, but in 1928 Ethel McNevin was appointed. From the outset she made it clear to the board that she would not brook any interference in the matter of discipline. She was strict but she was just, and genuinely concerned for the welfare of the nurses under her charge who were very young and often immature, for the Nurses' Registration Board had reduced the age of entry into nursing from twenty-one to eighteen years.

Ethel McNevin was one of Perth Hospital's youngest matrons and came from New South Wales, where she had trained at the Coast (now Prince Henry) Hospital, obtaining her Obstetric Certificate in the same state. She introduced some changes in nursing techniques and hospital procedure, including the concentration of all ward staff, both day and night, on duty in the wards in the early hours of the morning so that all patients could be bathed and all beds made before breakfast. Miss McNevin also changed the uniform of the probationer nurses by introducing short sleeves and soft shirt collars in lieu of stiff collars and cuffs. The stiff collars and cuffs were at this stage a status symbol and the change was resisted in some quarters, even though it benefited the hospital by several hundred dollars in laundering and starch. Nevertheless it was ten years before long sleeves and cuffs were dispensed with in the uniform of trainee nurses at Fremantle and government hospitals. Perth Children's Hospital was more realistic and the nurses' smart coat-type frocks with fashionable, very low belts were the envy of their colleagues.

Miss McNevin was not insensitive to the fact that the nurses had to work very hard and fully realized that the A.T.N.A., because of its structure, had little control over hours worked and salaries paid. In response to a request from the association, the Medical Department and hospital boards agreed to reduce the working hours to fifty-four per week for day duty and sixty for night duty,[34] but there was no reduction in the work load, which was disproportionately loaded with domestic duties.

Miss Gill's replacement on the Nurses' Registration Board was Eileen Ivy Curwood, who had been a prominent member of the A.T.N.A. Council since completing her nurse training in 1918.[35] Miss Curwood had represented the West Australian Branch of the association at the two conferences which followed the formation of the Australian Nursing Federation in 1924. In 1923 she had been branch secretary during the absence of Miss Broomhall and had subsequently been appointed treasurer.[36] During her term of office in this capacity a committee was formed to investigate a proposal from Miss I. Bradshaw that a home be started for aged and otherwise incapacitated nurses. The committee thus formed consisted of Misses Bradshaw, Dunn and Jarvis, Mrs Watkins, Dr Anderson, and the president, Mr Hadley, and secretary ex officio.[37] As a preliminary investigation it was suggested that they should inquire into the possibility of accommodation in convalescent homes for 'immediate necessitous cases'. This was the precursor of the Society for the Care of Aged or Incapacitated Nurses (W.A.) Inc. which was formed in 1941, and eventually founded the Eleanor Harvey Home. Under the original scheme it was suggested that £1 per annum be contributed by association members. In 1925, with an economic depression already being felt, the idea was too ambitious, but the fund remained and was contributed to over the years.

In 1927 it was found that the accommodation for the private practising nurse as provided by the A.T.N.A. Club was at a premium, and with the lease expiring on No. 9 Mount Street, a new venue was purchased in 25 Richardson Street, West Perth, from Dr H. Gray and added to. Miss Jarvis, the previous matron, resigned to take up the position of matron of Kalgoorlie Hospital and the new club opened in March 1928 with Miss Curwood as matron.

Apart from providing a 'status symbol', there was at this stage little tangible incentive for nurses to become members of their professional body. The Nurses' Registration Board had relieved them of their examination function and furthermore had taken the step to appoint board members who did not necessarily have to be association members. Membership of the I.C.N. still demanded a reconstruction of the governing body of the A.N.F. and even so the cost of joining was prohibitive — an invitation to attend the Congress in Montreal as observers was ruled out because of lack of funds.[38]

Because of the economic conditions of the time, the trained nurse was being by-passed, especially by the private hospitals which were employing the less expensive nursing assistant and allowing her to wear the traditional uniform complete with veil. An appeal by the nurses in New South Wales to have the veil registered for the use of trained nurses only was disallowed on the count that it was not their property. To counter this, the Australian Nursing Federation introduced the woven cap badge and sold it to members along with the veil itself.[39] (Except for the addition of the prefix 'Royal', the badge has remained unchanged.) Nevertheless it was difficult to police and a satisfactory answer was not found until the cap itself was registered under the act in 1937.

Despite the fact that the Nurses' Registration Board had the power to register nurses, the Australian Nursing Federation still exerted control over the standards relating to the training of the probationer nurse and her eventual acceptance, on graduation, for membership. The worsening economic situation and lack of job opportunities was forcing more and more young women into the nursing field, and there were long waiting lists for entry into the nurse-training schools. This resulted in the age of entry being raised in 1929 from eighteen to twenty-one years. Furthermore, many had higher educational standards than those required by the board. Perhaps through necessity rather than vocation many joined the Mental Health Services to tide them over until they would be called up for entry into general nurse training. For a number of years the qualifications of the matron of Claremont Hospital had not been acceptable for membership of the A.T.N.A. In 1928, in view of her long service and the fact that she had qualified in 1904, she was deemed a matron of a training school and those undertaking the three year period of training were granted inclusion on the A.N.F. Mental Register.[40] Complications arose when it was found that although there was a surplus of female applicants with the required standards, male applicants had difficulty in coping with the educational entrance examination. As the male nurses were the backbone of the institution, because they alone staffed male wards and they tended to remain in their jobs as their area of employment was limited, the educational test was deemed unnecessary and the hospital lost its training-school status.

The centenary of Western Australia was celebrated in 1929, one of the years of the Great Depression, and the functions were rather

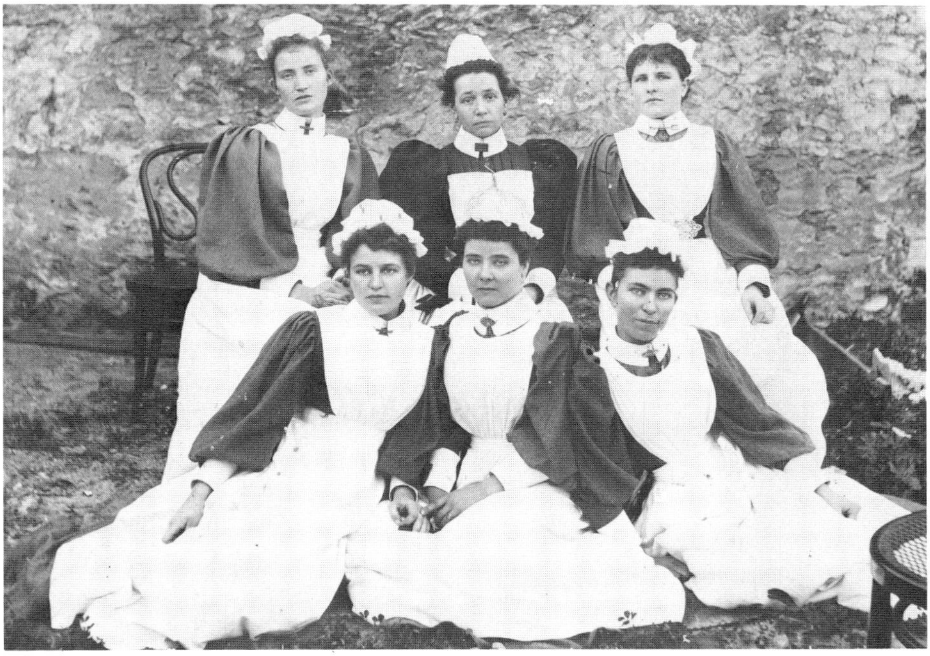

FIRST TRAINEES, FREMANTLE PUBLIC HOSPITAL, 1897

back row: —. Mortimer, B. Steel (matron), D. King; *front row:* E. Woodhead (later de Moulin), M. Price, M. Grover.

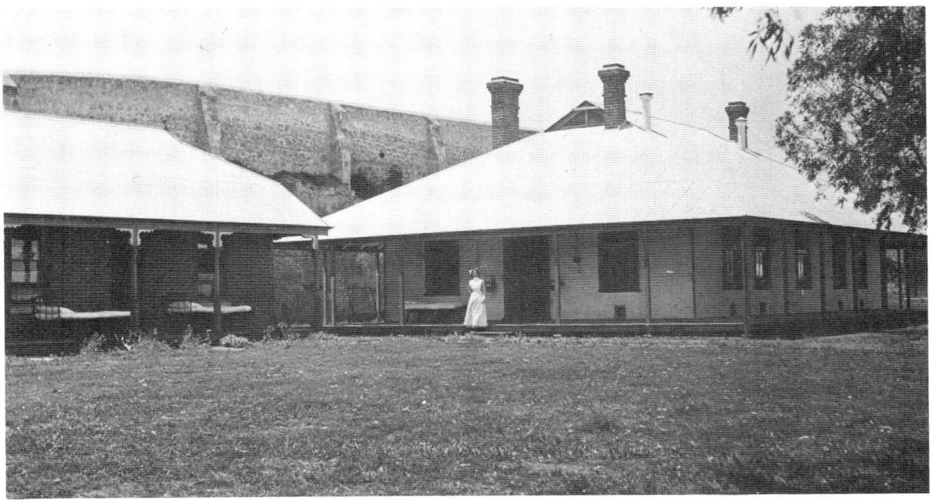

ISOLATION BLOCK, FREMANTLE PUBLIC HOSPITAL, 1910

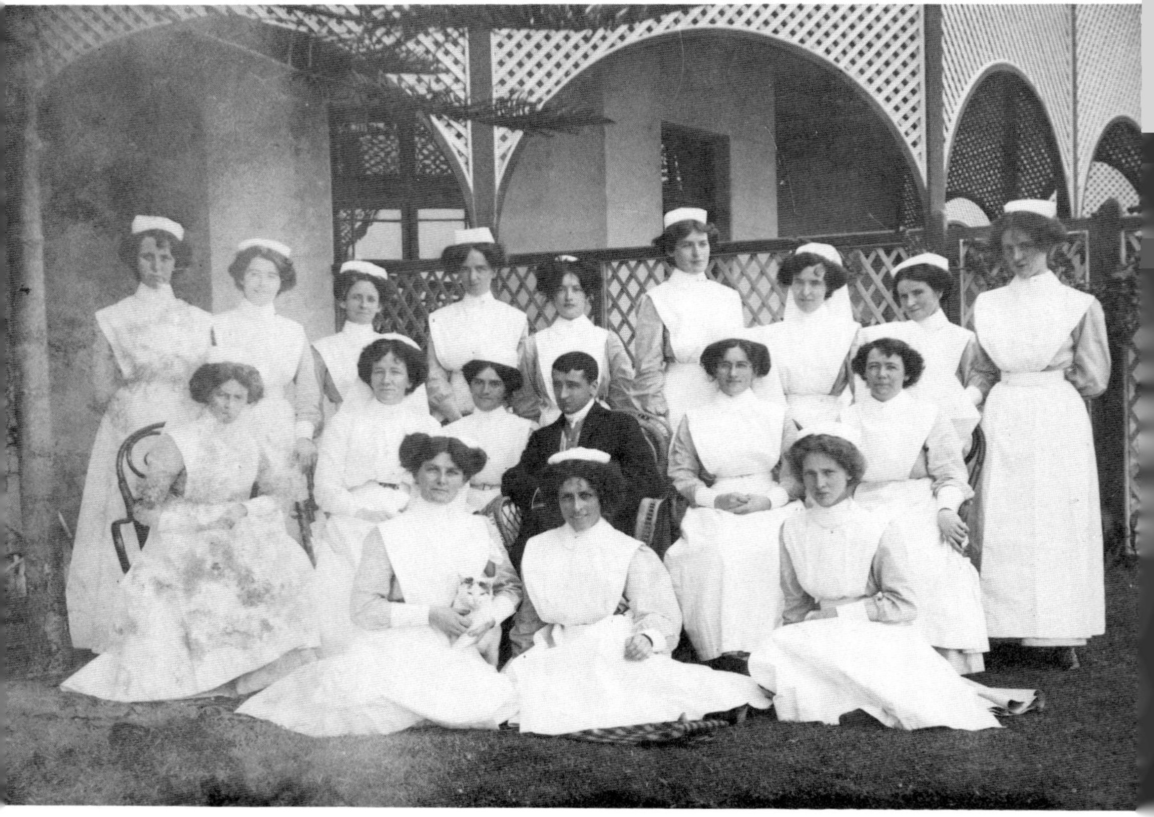

FREMANTLE PUBLIC HOSPITAL STAFF, 1910

back row: —. Baker, L. McGurk, L. Baillie, M. Hayes, M. H. Hicks, B. Giles, K. Davidson, L. Lyons, M. Carson; *second row:* F. Edsall, D. Cameron (matron), M. Haines, Dr G. Barker, E. Kerr, M. Grimley; *front row:* S. Kirkham, L. Cardew, R. Bottle.

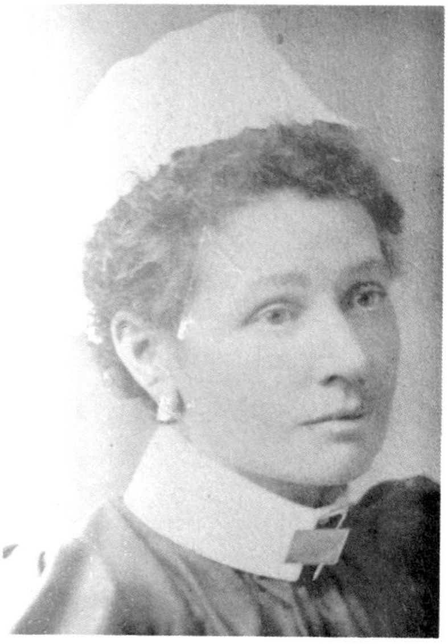

BESSIE STEEL

matron F.P.H. 1897-98.

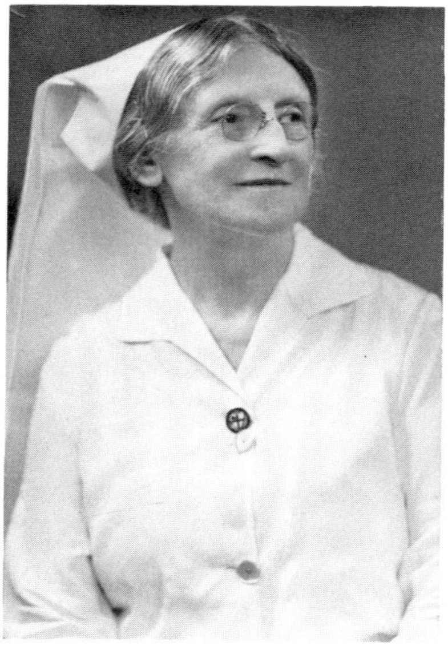

MAIDA BALDING

matron F.P.H. 1913-39.

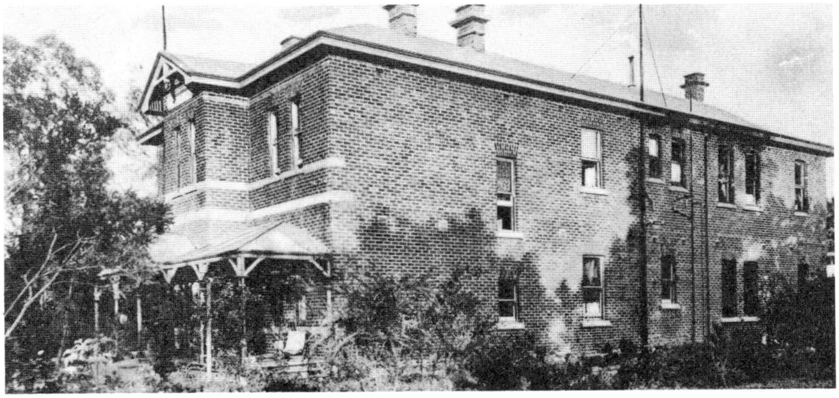

HOME OF PEACE, SUBIACO, 1913

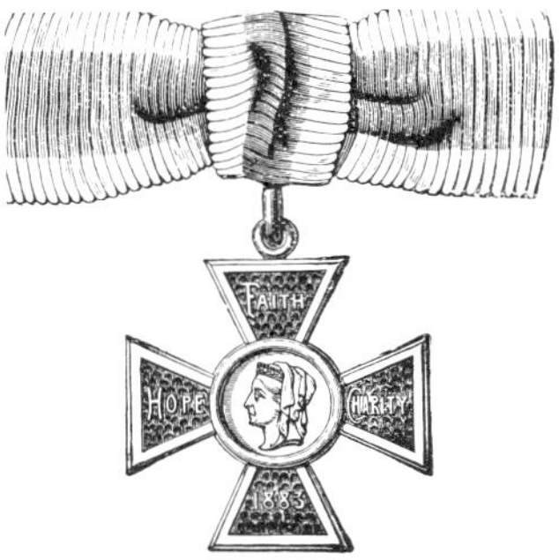

ROYAL RED CROSS

This decoration was instituted by Royal Warrant, 23 April 1883, to reward nurses for outstanding service in attending the sick and wounded of the army and navy. Later amended to include associates of the order (A.R.R.C.).

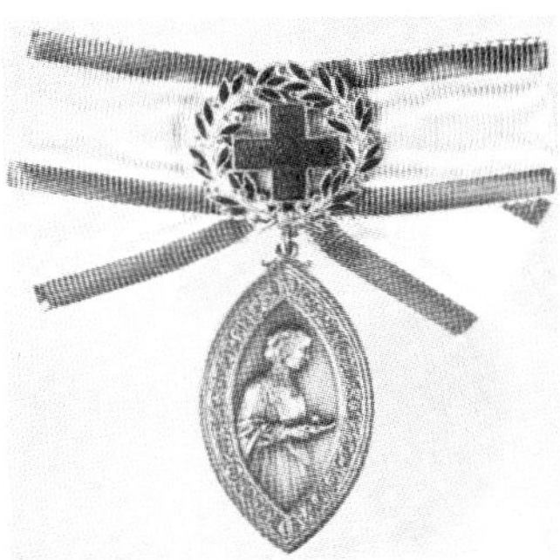

FLORENCE NIGHTINGALE MEDAL

Instituted in 1912 by the International Committee of the Red Cross in memory of Florence Nightingale, for meritorious service to nursing. The three Western Australians who hold this award are M. D. Edis, J. Ferguson and E. Harler.

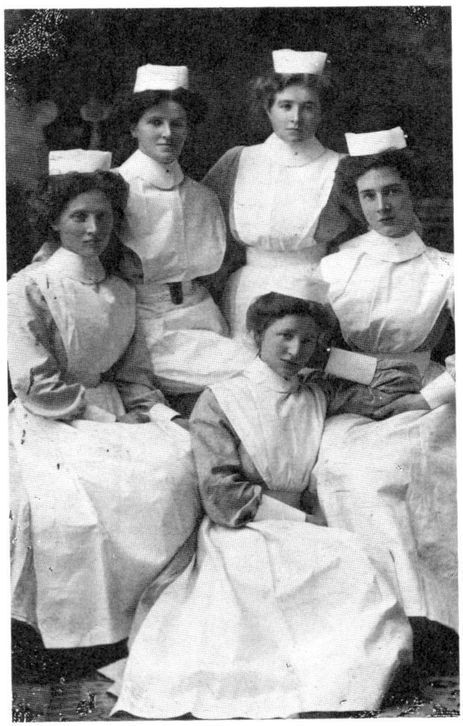

HOME OF PEACE NURSES, 1909

standing: Liddell, Lyons; *seated:* Carson, Brown, Bottle.

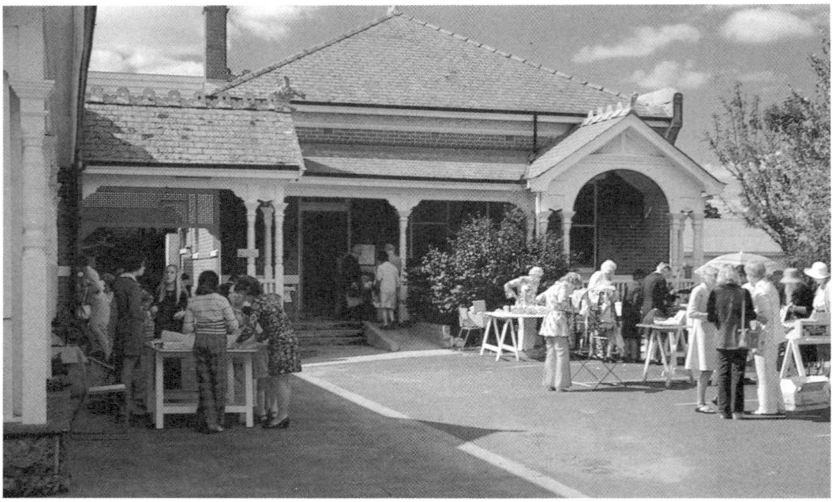

NURSES' MEMORIAL CENTRE
the photo was taken during a fete for Eleanor Harvey House, 1974.

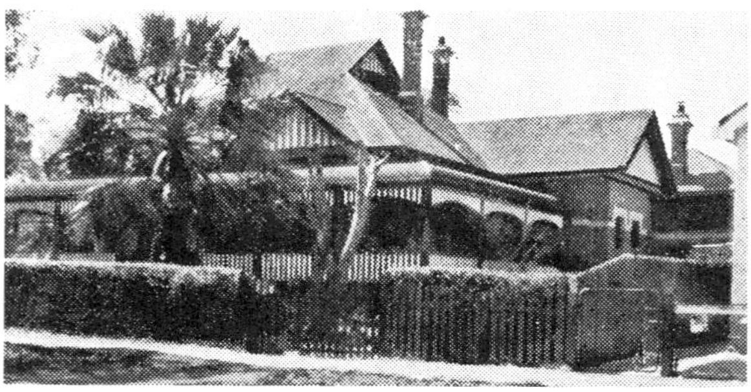

ELEANOR HARVEY HOUSE
home for aged and incapacitated nurses

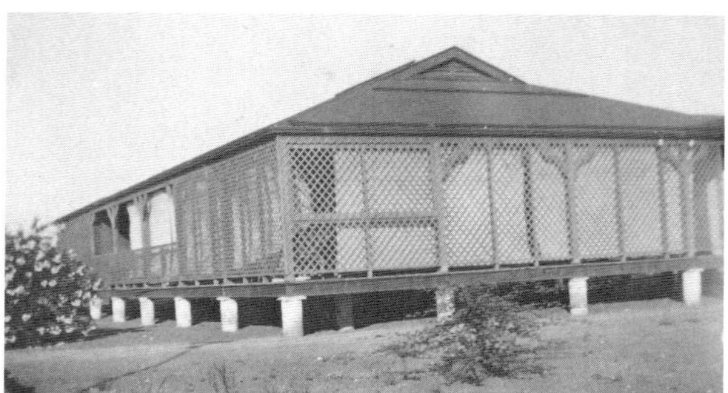

A.I.M. NURSING HOME, PORT HEDLAND, 1931

low key as funds were in short supply. There appears to be no evidence to show that nurses were in any way involved in the various social activities which marked the occasion. Neither the minutes nor the annual report of the W.A. Branch of the A.N.F. make mention of the event. However a fund was inaugurated for additions to King Edward Memorial Hospital. This resulted in the erection of the Centenary Ward, which was finally opened and the first private patients admitted in 1932.[41] In marking the centenary of the state the emphasis was on the 'practical' aspect and some of the country hospitals had additions at this time, but they have not been documented.

CHAPTER FOUR

THE THIRTIES

The effect of the depression on nursing was felt in a number of ways, and those most affected were the trained nurses in the private field, as people could no longer afford to employ them at the statutory fee. The doctors' surgeries were empty and pharmacists were forced to close, while the out-patient clinics and dispensaries of the public hospitals were full to overflowing as more and more people qualified for the means test. More than ever, the gynaecological wards of the Perth and Fremantle Hospitals told their own story of the 'backyard' abortionist, and self-induced abortion and the frightening thought of puerperal sepsis with its tragic results.

In 1928 the first patients had been treated with radium at Perth Hospital, and in 1930 the Radium Building was opened. Nurses who worked there were not informed of the danger to staff, nor of the measures they could take for their own protection. It was considered a light ward to work in, and no steps were taken to reduce the hours and limit the exposure.

Despite improved hygiene in sewerage and water supplies, typhoid fever was still a disease to be feared, although patients with this condition were nursed in the medical wards. The deaths of two nurses at Perth Hospital alerted the authorities to the need for staff immunization. In the realm of infectious diseases, children fared worse than others for they were usually nursed at home. Reluctance to call the doctor because of inability to pay often meant that help was left too late, especially in diphtheria, which in the thirties was in almost epidemic proportions. The Infectious Diseases Branch, staffed by nurses from Perth Hospital, was totally inadequate, and primitive conditions made nursing difficult and dangerous. There were still no curative drugs in general use, with the exception of mercury for syphilis and quinine for malaria. Conversely the nurses who received their basic training at Wooroloo Sanitorium, which was exclusive to patients with tuberculoses, rarely picked up the infection, possibly due to the very strict regimen.

The day of the motor car had not really arrived, but the motor cycle with or without sidecar certainly had. This was particularly so in the city and gave rise to surgical emergencies with head injuries and fractured limbs. A full-time operating theatre staff and a nurse for casualty were put on night duty at Perth Hospital, whereas, before, these departments had been staffed on night duty by nurses on call from the wards.

Treatment of surgical patients was still very conservative and patients were confined to bed and limited movement several days post-operatively, during which time they had to be lifted and moved with care as well as being fully sponged in bed. The post-operative nursing of patients who had had abdominal surgery involved sitting them up with anything from eight to ten pillows and an air cushion, and a bolster under the knees. Except for emergencies, pre-operative preparation of such patients was detailed and time consuming. The routine of painting the skin with a variety of antiseptics was repeated at least twice in the ward and once in the operating theatre. Even the normal midwifery patient was kept in hospital from twelve to fourteen days after delivery, for eight of which she was at bed rest.

In the early thirties there was an increase in the building of small country hospitals administered by local boards of management and subsidized to some extent by the government. There were usually from ten to fifteen beds available, including those for midwifery patients. The staff consisted of a matron, a sister, a cook-laundress, a wards-maid and a boy for odd jobs and messages. These hospitals were an incentive to doctors to take up residence locally. It also meant that people could be nursed in their own environment, usually within a radius of a hundred kilometres. The local practitioners did most of the surgery, and very few patients were sent to the city for specialist treatment. Hospital facilities left quite a lot to be desired. Instruments, gloves, bowls, etc. were sterilized by boiling on the large kitchen stove, and linen was treated in a pressure-cooker type sterilizer over a primus stove. Sometimes the doctor would get the doctor from the neighbouring town over to assist, but often he managed alone, with the matron administering the anaesthetic and the sister assisting the surgeon, and the wards-maid acted as nurse assistant in looking after the hospital patients. Many of the towns did not have electricity, so lighting was by Aladdin lamps and hurricane lanterns. There was no deep sewerage or septic tanks; the pan system operated with disposal by the local authority. A specially marked 'pan' was kept to receive the excreta from patients with typhoid, and after being mixed with saw-dust, its contents were disposed of by burning.

In the absence of a local pharmacist, the hospital supplied most of the medications, and the dispensary was managed by the matron. Most of the medications were in liquid form, there being very few tablets. There was no night staff; matron and sister took alternate nights of being 'on call'. Nevertheless it was an experience enjoyed by most nurses and they were well thought of by the people in the area. It was the custom for the Education Department to provide 'one-teacher' schools in the towns, and there was a high marriage rate among the teachers and nurses.

In December 1929 the Council of the A.T.N.A., W.A. Branch A.N.F., received a letter from the matron of Fremantle Public Hospital, Miss Balding, which read:

> Since consideration of an Insurance Scheme for Nurses is before the Council at the next meeting on the 10th December, I would be glad if you will bring up the following matter for discussion:- 'The advisability of forming a professional union for Nurses, and especially those attached to Public Hospitals in order to promote their interest and welfare'.
>
> Matters for consideration would be:- Salaries, holiday leave, sick leave, long-service leave, and retiring allowance etc.
>
> I think if these matters were discussed by the Council, they would probably have the support of all members of the Nursing profession.[1]

After discussion, it was decided that the matter would be given further consideration and that Miss Balding would be asked to attend the next council meeting and enlarge on the matter. However the reply received was that she would be unable to attend and requested that the matter be dropped. What prompted the letter is not known, but Fremantle Hospital was expanding. A children's ward, known as the Adelaide Samson Memorial Children's Ward, had been added in 1927, and a surgical block was functioning in 1928. Although patients with infectious diseases were still being transferred to I.D.B., trainee nurses from Fremantle Hospital were no longer required to spend part of their training period at that hospital, so that Fremantle Hospital became a self-contained unit, which of course would have meant an increase in trained staff. Miss Balding herself was getting towards retiring age and she must have had some feelings of insecurity in the face of the economic climate of the depression.

At this time, too, the council was receiving requests from members regarding terms of employment, on which, in view of their non-legal status in these matters, they were unable to advise. There was also a dropping off of interest, and with it membership of the association. At the annual meeting of 1929 there were no new nominations and the council was re-elected en bloc. The composition of the council is of interest, there being seven medical members, and the following matrons and nurses: Miss Ashton, industrial nurse and examining matron for N.R.B.; Miss Bruce, assistant matron, Perth Hospital; Miss Cox, private nurse from A.T.N.A. Club; Miss Curwood, matron of A.T.N.A. Club; Miss Dunne, matron of Wooroloo Sanitorium; Miss Harvey, matron of a private maternity hospital; Miss Homan, vice-president, matron of a private hospital and examiner for N.R.B.; Miss Marrett, Public Health Department (pathology section); Miss McNevin, matron of Perth Hospital; Miss Ryan, ex A.A.N.S., private hospital matron (?); Miss Salmon, Infant Health Clinic, Fremantle; Misses Sandilands and Thompson, positions unknown; Miss Ward, sister in charge of X ray department, Perth Hospital; Mrs Walsh, matron of K.E.M.H.; Mrs Watkins, matron of a private hospital. The president was Mr Hadley, a leading Perth surgeon.[2] There was no trainee nurse representation as the rules of the federation had not been liberalized to allow this to happen. For the next two years the council functioned with little change in the professional status of its personnel. A major breakthrough came in 1931 when it was decided that 'in future the President be a nurse'. Miss McNevin was elected first 'nurse' president.[3]

Another major achievement was the granting of a request by the commissioner of public health for a nurse to be appointed as secretary to the Nurses' Registration Board. This was only a part-time appointment as the A.T.N.A. still supplied the written papers for the final examinations, which were set in the eastern states. The new appointee was Miss N. U. Lynch, an inspectress with the Department of Health. She was, however, refused a seat on the A.T.N.A. state Council. It would seem that at this stage the association was preoccupied with the politics of nursing, and the promotion of federalism rather than with the affairs and conditions of the average nurse who was fast reaching breaking point. There was mention of reduction of fees both by the Medical Department and the private sector. An interesting side light is the fact that while on one hand the state branch of the A.T.N.A. was urging a federal examination system in the cause of uniformity, it also supported members of the W.A. Secessionist Movement, and encouraged the trainee nurses to participate in this movement.

Dissatisfaction with nursing conditions was not peculiar to Western Australian nurses as shown in a letter from Miss Evans, the federal secretary, to the W.A. Branch secretary in May 1931. Marked personal, it was presented at the June council meeting.

Alas it is too true! some of the misguided members of the pro-

> fession called a meeting of nurses early in April and decided to form a Union— I regret to say that some of the leading lights of the A.T.N.A. were present at the meeting and were in favour of the suggestion some of them even accepting positions on the committee. At present nothing has been done beyond the drawing up of a Constitution and application for registration. I think the stumbling block will be cash as of course the Hospital Employees Union will fight the new Union tooth and nail. I would add that the A.T.N.A.(N.S.W.) was not invited to send a representative and it was only by accident that I heard of it too late to communicate with and warn members...
>
> In spite of the recent troubles and the depression generally things are not quite so bad for nurses as they have been and many of them have been in almost constant work for some time past.
>
> I take it that you are aware that the nurses decided that they would not agree to a reduction in the prescribed fees but it was understood that any nurse might reduce her fees when she thinks its necessary or desirable.[4]

Despite the stand taken by the New South Wales nurses, those in Western Australia were not so fortunate. F. Huelin, the under-treasurer, stated that the staff of Bridgetown Hospital had agreed to participate in an 18 per cent reduction in salary. He contended that if the hospital increased the salaries in these 'days of depression' the government subsidy would be reduced.

On 9 February 1932 Kathleen Yeates was appointed as A.T.N.A. secretary with an honorarium of £10 per annum.[5] A graduate of Perth Hospital and King Edward Memorial Hospital, she was destined to play an important part in shaping the affairs of the association over the next fifteen years. Although she did not hold any post-basic qualifications, Miss Yeates was an educationalist and during the term of her office her aim was higher education for nurses and their involvement in world affairs. In recognition of her work in this field she was awarded a fellowship of the British College of Nurses (F.B.C.N.), the president of the college at this time being Mrs Bedford Fenwick, founder of the International Council of Nurses. (Miss Yeates's diploma is at present held by the author.)

At the twenty-fifth annual meeting held in July 1932 it was noted that this was the first time the council had been comprised of an all-nurse membership, following changes in the constitution which put medical members in an advisory section. It was also decided to abolish life membership, to come into line with other state branches. An important step was that the sections of the council were to be revised and the matrons of all training schools were to become ex officio members of the council. Furthermore the council was to be empowered to elect the office bearers for the ensuing year. The result was that the council as a decision-making body was weighted heavily in favour of the senior members of the profession, many of whom were employers.

There was great concern at unemployment among nurses, and suggestions for its relief included the absorption of trained nurses into training schools and country hospitals. To this end a delegation consisting of Misses Curwood and McNevin, Mrs Walsh and the secretary, Miss Yeates, waited on the minister for health. A report of this states

> that the Minister promised that a circular would be sent to Committee Hospitals asking them to endeavour to employ trained nurses where ever possible. . . . The question of a four years training for General Nurses was discussed and the Government promised to consider the matter with the idea of limiting the number of probationers in order to lessen the unemployment amongst trained nurses.

It should be mentioned that at this stage the hospitals controlled by the Medical Department made it obligatory for their probationer nurses to undertake a four-year period, the last year of which was usually spent as a staff nurse in one of the larger hospitals not designated as a training school. The statutory period, however, was three years. In discussing the proposed four-year training period, the council decided that it could possibly be introduced later, but as a measure to 'raise the standard' and not to relieve the depressed economy. There was also the suggestion that midwifery trainees should be paid.

Another matter of concern was the possibility of allowing paying patients to be treated in public hospitals, particularly obstetric patients, and members from Kalgoorlie strongly protested at the government's decision to build a maternity ward for private patients in Kalgoorlie, because it would come into competition with private enterprise.[6] There was at this stage an all-out effort to promote membership of the professional body and to gain some practical advantages for it. One consideration was the affiliation of the A.T.N.A. with the Civil Service Association, with access to their Board of Appeal, but after inquiry this was ruled out because of the expense involved. The extension of membership to the trainee nurse was more realistic, and it was resolved to admit her as an associate member during the second and third year of training.

The success of the membership drive is reflected in the report of the twenty-sixth annual meeting, held at the Karrakatta Club, with over two hundred present (4 July 1933). Once again the much hoped for affiliation with the International Council of Nurses was threatened by the withdrawal of the Victorian association (R.V.T.N.A.) from the federation. A college of nursing for Australia was to be founded within the University of Melbourne to celebrate the centenary of the founding of the state of Victoria.[7] Although the R.V.T.N.A. approved of this venture, dissatisfaction was expressed when it was found that nurses would not be in control administratively. The upshot of this was that the R.V.T.N.A. withdrew from the Australian Nursing Federation and disbanded. A new body was formed, the Royal Victorian College of Nursing, which combined the professional nursing association with extramural courses for postgraduate study.[8]

In May 1934 the A.T.N.A. Club at 25 Richardson Street, West Perth, was forced to close because it was unable to meet its commitments, that is, loan interest and repayment and the matron's salary. Miss Curwood resigned her position as matron and her services to the association were put on record. The financial position of the club was due to the fact that nurses residing there were unable to get work and had been allowed considerable credit. Even so, some had existed on one meal a day. The club had operated as an 'indoor' and 'outdoor' service to nurses. Most local nurses were on the 'outdoor' list and were able to live home, while those on the 'indoor' list were generally from the country, overseas or the eastern states. The opening up of another 'outdoor' agency without membership limitations contributed to the eventual closure. The club assets were sold but the matron never received her salary.[9]

It was not only the nursing staff who were concerned with conditions of employment in hospitals and in June 1934 a move was made towards the formation of a Hospital Officers' Association covering members of the dispensary staff, X ray department, biochemists, dieticians, clinic sister (diabetic) and trained staff (nursing) of Perth Hospital.[10] The object of the association was to work 'for better salaries and hours of duty'.

This matter was taken very seriously by the A.T.N.A. Council which saw in it a threat to its organization, and as a result a special meeting of the council was held in camera on 12 June 1934. Arising from this meeting it was decided to seek legal advice and obtain all the business records relating to the proposed union of 1921 and 1925. On the advice of Horace Jones, the administrator of the Children's Hospital, Miss Sheila McClemans was asked to undertake the legal proceedings. (Miss McClemans's mother, Mrs McClemans, a trained nurse on the staff of the Public Health Department, was at this time a member of the council and it is noted that there were many spelling errors etc. in the transcript of the minutes of the period, so that it is possible that statements attributed to mother or daughter could be confused.)

Another special meeting was called for 14 June 1934 (with Miss McClemans present as legal advisor) to decide 'whether the A.T.N.A. (W.A. State Branch of A.N.F.) should make application to the industrial court for registration as a Union'.[11] Miss McClemans defined 'industry' as any sort of work, skilled or unskilled, and gave the council directions as to the procedure. The following resolution was carried: 'That this body make application to the register [*sic*] of the Court of Arbitration for the registration as an Industrial Union under the provisions of the Industrial Arbitration Act 1912-1915'. It was decided also that a large general meeting would be held with two speakers, one of whom would be Miss McNevin. It was also decided that the resolution would be put to the meeting by Mrs McClemans and that Mrs Fisher should second it. Miss McClemans explained that if private nurses were included in the award, they would be obliged to accept a definite fixed salary and hours which could not be altered.

The general meeting called by the A.T.N.A. was held at the A.T.N.A. Club on Monday 25 June 1934 but the attendance of 260 was so large that it was adjourned to the Ross Memorial Hall in West Perth.[12] A difference of opinion between Miss McNevin, and Mrs Walsh, matron of K.E.M.H., resulted in Miss McNevin's opening the meeting and then vacating the chair in favour of Miss Bottle. Before the resolution was put, it was explained that the purpose of the meeting was to discuss whether nurses should form a union and whether such a union should be in the hands of nurses themselves or governed by people outside the profession. The resolution was carried. However, the meeting agreed to grant a period of fourteen days grace before putting the resolution into effect so that a conference with the Medical Department and the hospital boards could take place and an opportunity given to the latter to meet the nurses' demands, which were set out in the following schedule:

> That nurses work eight hours a day.
> Lectures to be given in duty time.
> Salaries payable to nurses—all nett.
> First year £26 p.a.
> Second year £36 p.a.
> Third year £52 p.a.
> Pupil nurses in midwifery hospitals to receive the same as first year general trainees.
> Staff nurses £104 p.a.
> Sisters £120-160 p.a.

Extra £10 for double certificate.
Matrons according to the number of beds.
That there be six pupil nurses to every trained nurse.
Overtime not to be allowed.
Maintenance allowance for all nurses while on leave.
Annual holidays for all hospitals 28 days.

Mrs Reid, secretary of the Private Hospitals' Matrons' Association, told the meeting that 'her Association would fall into line with any thing that was reasonable that was granted by the Government'. The meeting then adjourned.

The result of the gesture for a stay in proceedings is contained in the report to a special meeting held on Monday 9 July 1934 at 6.45 p.m. and presented to the general meeting which followed in St George's Hall, at 8 p.m.

> The Council of the A.T.N.A. have to report to you the result of 14 days period of grace granted at the last general meeting of nurses. The Government through Dr Everitt Atkinson was approached and asked to call a round table conference with the various hospital boards and your association, but owing to the Hon. the Minister and the Under Secretary being absent from this State they were unable to arrange anything to commit themselves to any satisfactory finality. The Hospital Boards were then approached with a similar request, therefore we come to you again and ask if it is your wish that the business of applying for registration at the Arbitration Court be proceeded with.[13]

This meeting became the inaugural meeting of the Western Australian Nurses' Association and eventually Industrial Union of Workers was added to its name. (The W.A.N.A. formed in 1909 was long defunct.) Many of the 300 nurses present were trainee nurses. Miss Ethel Brooke Carlin was one of two nominees and was elected the first president. In the matter of appointing a secretary there was some pressure to give preference to a member of the nursing profession, however the eventual appointee was a qualified accountant, Miss Margaret Robertson. Although not a trained nurse she did have connections with nursing through her mother who as Elsie Paltridge had come to Western Australia in the gold-rush days and was attached to the Methodist group of nurses known as Sisters of the People. Though she soon left the group she continued nursing until her marriage.

Ethel Carlin also had medical and nursing affiliations. Her brother was a physician, and she herself was a trainee of Perth Hospital. She became sister in charge of the first Diabetic Clinic at

Perth Hospital and with Dr Bruce Hunt pioneered this field. In addition to supervising the out-patient clinic, Miss Carlin was responsible for the diet and administration of insulin to the diabetic patients in hospital. It often distressed her to see the nurses, who were literally rushed off their feet, having painstakingly to weigh the food, measure the insulin and test the patients' urine several times a day. As president of the new association she became a tireless worker for the betterment of patient care through improved conditions for nurses. When she subsequently appeared in the Arbitration Court she was cited as being the most effective witness to be heard since the court was established.

Following the appointment of its secretary, the Western Australian Nurses' Association was registered as an industrial union by the industrial registrar on 19 September 1923.[14]

The news that nurses had formed a union met with a mixed reception both by the public and some members of the nursing profession. A great deal was said about the detrimental effect unionism would have on future aspirants to nursing due to the belief that it would lower their professional status. This attitude was rather negated by the fact that when the union was first mooted by the A.T.N.A., the Hospital Employees Federation approached that body with a proposition that the H.E.F. would not raise an objection in the court if the A.T.N.A. would agree to allow the H.E.F. control of trainee nurses.[15] This had been given some consideration, but was dropped on the advice of Miss McClemans who said that anybody could object, but there was nothing to say that such objections would be upheld by the court. That the A.T.N.A. was not happy at the turn of events is reflected in the correspondence and interaction between the W.A.N.A. and the A.T.N.A. Council. Clearly the latter expected a much louder voice in the control of union affairs. Although they were two separate organizations, the councils of each had a representative from its opposite number.

The hospitals' administration took a different line of action and there were numerous articles in the press on the hardship which would be inflicted on those institutions if nurses pressed for an award. The secretary of Perth Hospital said that it would necessitate a completely new laundry being built in order to cope with the extra linen involved in employing more nursing staff if hours of duty were reduced. The question of extra accommodation, too, was a key issue.

Failing to obtain by consent an industrial agreement for nurses, the W.A.N.A. took the matter to arbitration following a resolution passed on 4 March 1935. The advocate for the association was Mr A. H. Panton, M.L.A. (speaker of the Legislative Assembly) who had a record of success in appearing for other industrial organizations. The hearing, which extended over many days, commenced early in July 1935 and was given very wide coverage in the press. In the matter of nurses' duties, little was left to the imagination. Over twenty witnesses were called, including nurses, doctors, administrators etc. It is fortunate that this record has been preserved in a scrapbook in possession of the Royal Australian Nursing Federation, W.A. Branch, for it is a saga of nurses' endeavour to overcome exploitation and unbelievable ignorance in relation to their calling. The first awards for trained nurses and trainees were handed down and assented to on 1 November 1935. (See Appendix IV.)

Although far from ideal, it was a start and marked a step in nursing which could only lead onwards and from which there would be no turning back. Of interest is the recognition of the dangers of radium and X ray and the adjustment of hours for persons working in that field. Of significance also is the fact that during the hearing pertaining to the award, Mr Panton made the suggestion that before appointment, probationers to the nursing profession should be sent to a central training school for preliminary schooling in their duties.[16] In replying to this Mr F. J. Huelin, secretary of the Medical Department, said that the suggestion appealed to him personally but he thought objection might be made by matrons who would probably prefer to train the nurses themselves. President Dwyer suggested Mr Panton's objective would be met if the first six weeks of a probationer's service were devoted to personal instruction by a matron or other qualified person, the probationer to be in attendance in the ward but not to do any actual work. Mr Panton said that some such arrangement would be an excellent start.

The initial funding of the Western Australia Nurses' Association to cover its preliminary expenses was met by the A.T.N.A. with a donation of £43 19s 11d, and with the help of numerous cash donations, some of which came from members of the British Medical Association, the union was able to open an office at Room 50, Third Floor, A.M.P. buildings, Perth, on a permanent basis.

The A.T.N.A. was not so fortunate, for when the A.T.N.A. Club in Richardson Street finally closed its doors, it was left without headquarters. For a while the secretary carried on the work from her own home in Rokeby Road, Subiaco, but it was soon evident that to survive and serve any useful purpose a more business-like arrangement would have to be made. In May 1935 a small office was procured in the West Australian Trustee buildings, St Georges Terrace, at a rental of twenty-five shillings per month, light and cleaning extra, for a six months' trial period. The secretary was instructed to buy the furniture. Fund-raising ventures, including bridge evenings at K.E.M.H., were immediately put into action to help cover the cost.

In the interim, council meetings had been accommodated at the Returned Army Nurses' Club rooms in Anzac House, at the corner of Irwin Street and St Georges Terrace, on the former site of the University of Western Australia. The move to the new office emphasized the need for more space if the association were to function effectively. Postgraduate lectures which were organized proved most popular but the cooperation of hospitals had to be relied on to provide a venue. One lecture on 'India' by Mr Gill, held at the Children's Hospital, attracted an attendance of 110.

The secretary, Miss K. Yeates, was employed on a part-time basis, the office being opened during the afternoon. The greatest need was effective communication with members, many of whom were domiciled in the country and rarely if ever came to the city. Dissatisfaction had been expressed with the A.T.N.A. journal, produced in N.S.W., in that it did not have sufficient Western Australian content. Therefore it was decided that the association would produce its own publication, the *Journal of the Western Australian Nurses*, on a monthly basis. The first issue of this appeared on 15 October 1935, edited and produced by Miss Yeates, and was successful.[17] It continued to be published monthly for the next thirty-five years, being replaced by a national journal in 1971. Although small, it gave a wide coverage of local events in the nursing world including reports from the W.A.N.A. supplied by that organization. In addition there was always a fair selection of clinical material. It is fortunate that a full set of volumes has been preserved. This has now been indexed, and is at present in the keeping of the Royal Australian Nursing Federation in this state.

The first issue of the *Journal of the Western Australian Nurses* gave some prominence to the heading 'The Florence Nightingale Club—A Nursing Centre for Perth', followed by the following explanation:

> For a long time there has been a definite need for a Centre for the Nursing Profession in Perth, a social meeting place for trained nurses where members may meet on a common footing.
>
> In order to meet this need, a suggestion was placed before Council of the A.T.N.A. and a committee is being formed to organize a social and educational club in the City.
>
> The Club will be housed in a central position on the second floor of Nestle House, and an invitation is extended to trained nurses through out the State to become members, and by their support make possible the provision of pleasant and com-

> fortable lounge room and library, where nurses may meet their friends and entertain their guests at social and bridge evenings etc. The room is intended to form a centre for the activities of the profession. Arrangements will also be made to hold there the A.T.N.A. postgraduate lectures and the Nurses' Christian Movement meetings etc.
>
> Donations towards furnishing the room have already been received.
>
> *Membership fees*
>
> The nomination fee has been fixed at £1-1-0 and the annual subscription is £1-1-0. The Honorary Organizing Secretary (Mrs Walsh) will be pleased to receive your nomination fee and subscription at the earliest. Be a Foundation Member of this great movement for nurses and you will look back with pride to the day when you helped Nursing a step forward in its progress as a profession.[18]

The cover of the December issue of the journal shows 'a corner of the room and the Office of the A.T.N.A. can be seen at the end'. Elsewhere it is recorded that the A.T.N.A. was paying ten shillings per week as rent to the club, for the use of the office.

In February 1936 a special meeting of A.T.N.A. members was called 'to discuss the Florence Nightingale Club and to obtain permission from the general body of the Association to take over and conduct the Club on behalf of members of the A.T.N.A.'[19] It was stated that the initial steps had been taken and a committee formed which would undertake to establish the club on a working basis for the first year. The vote was in favour of the taking over of the club and allowing the committee to act for the first year. Regarding membership, this was open to any trained nurse but a concession was given to A.T.N.A. members, and the country members fees were to be ten shillings.

The association had now appointed Kath Yeates as full-time secretary because of the extra duties involved in coping with the club and the publication of the journal.[20]

The club was officially opened on Tuesday 28 April 1936 in the presence of some two hundred guests and members.[21] In the absence of Lady Mitchell, the patroness, who was unable to officiate at the opening because of court mourning, Sister Mary Nicolay was asked to declare the club open. Then aged eighty-six she gave an address in which she spoke of her personal association with Miss Nightingale. Details of the Florence Nightingale International Foundation Scholarship Fund, which was being established, and the need to send Western Australian nurses abroad to do the special postgraduate course, were outlined by Miss Yeates. Although the

Florence Nightingale Club had strong links with the A.T.N.A., the club was an autonomous body with its own executive. The first president was Mrs Walsh, with Mrs Weller (née Shapcott) as vice-president, and Miss Alison Davenport as assistant-secretary. The club fulfilled its objective in providing a meeting place for nurses and for the many groups and sub-groups which were formed at this time including the Australian Nurses' Christian Movement, and the ex-trainees associations of the various training schools. A great number of the activities were social combined with fund raising; socially it was a success but financially it was always a struggle for survival.[22] The members were a cross-section of the younger staff members of the hospitals and the more mature women who occupied positions of matrons together with a number who were barred from working for remuneration because their husbands occupied government positions. Nursing was still young and even those who had completed their training in the first Western Australian training schools were still under the age of retirement.

The acoustic properties of the room were not conducive to lectures as the walls were thin, and the vocal efforts of a religious group meeting on the same evenings were not always appreciated by the lecturers, therefore, when opportunity offered, the club and A.T.N.A. office transferred to the top floor of the Mercantile Mutual building further up the Terrace.[23] It was here that over the next ten years the club hosted many overseas visitors and gave hospitality to the groups of nurses passing through en route to the theatres of war.

The Florence Nightingale International Foundation, a living memorial to Florence Nightingale, was inaugurated in July 1934, its stated objectives being 'To establish and maintain a permanent international memorial to Florence Nightingale in the form of an endowed trust for post graduate education'.[24] The idea was first introduced at the meeting of the International Council of Nurses in Cologne, Germany, in 1912—the first meeting held after Miss Nightingale's death in 1910. Mrs Bedford Fenwick proposed and Miss Nutting seconded a motion that an international memorial be established. Following this, in 1914, the *British Journal of Nursing* published a statement signed by the officers of I.C.N. which included the following:

> The international memorial of nurses to Miss Nightingale, which we propose, should take the form of a Chair of Nursing and Health, should be placed in her own country, England in one of its Universities and should open to every woman the door to the rich opportunity of intellectual and technical development along the highest lines of nursing work.

Due to the war the International Council of Nurses went into abeyance from 1914 to 1922. In the meantime, to assist nurses in countries needing public health nursing, the League of Red Cross Societies in 1920 established courses in public health nursing at Kings College, London University, which were transferred to Bedford College a year later. In 1924, in cooperation with the College of Nursing, courses in teaching and administration of schools of nursing were also offered. Students for these courses were usually sent on scholarships provided by the national Red Cross societies or philanthropic foundations.

Following the I.C.N. Congress in Montreal in 1929 a committee was at work on plans for furthering the project when it became known that the League of Red Cross Societies was contemplating closing its courses. It was then agreed that the two interested bodies, the League of Red Cross Societies and the International Council of Nurses, should combine forces in working for the memorial and that the then existing courses should become the nucleus of the new programme when the Florence Nightingale International Foundation should be inaugurated, 5 July 1934. The idea was that nurses from national associations affiliated with the I.C.N. attend the courses and then return to their own countries to disseminate their knowledge and institute programmes. These students eventually became known as 'Old Internationals'. Funds for the foundation were to come from annual fees of the students—usually met by scholarships—and contributions to the endowment fund, the target being £200 000.

In the absence of a national association Australia was unable to affiliate with the I.C.N., but the two associations, the Australian Nursing Federation and its branches and the Royal Victorian College of Nursing, were invited to participate in the scheme, both in fund raising and the provision of scholarships.

In Western Australia, the initial request for the support of the foundation came from the secretary of the Red Cross Society in Western Australia, Miss Abel, in the form of a letter (February 1935).[25] This was discussed and it was decided that an approach would be made to the Commonwealth government to allocate some of the money designed to bring visitors in the health field to Australia, for a fund to enable nurses to go abroad and study.[26] The Red Cross Society was advised that the A.T.N.A. Council would be pleased to meet their representatives and discuss this scheme.

After a further meeting with the representatives of the Red Cross it was decided to take the following steps in launching an appeal: to ask Lady Mitchell or the lady mayoress to call a meeting to explain the cause, and to form a committee to launch the appeal and to in-

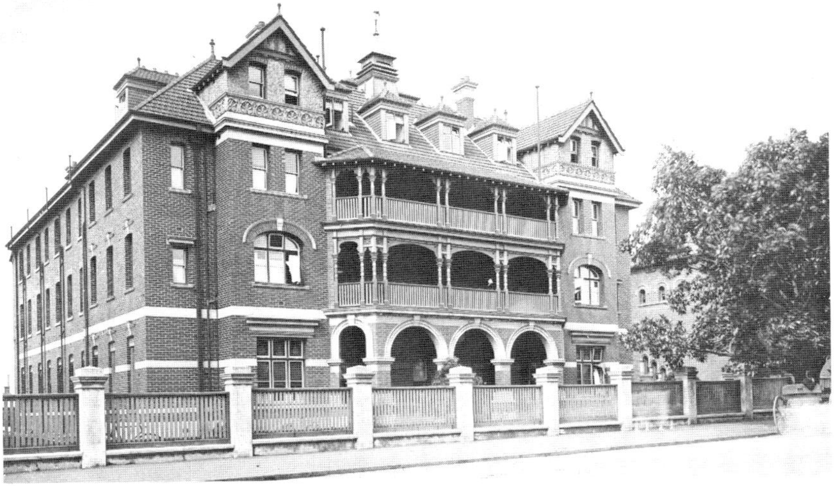

NURSES' QUARTERS, PERTH PUBLIC HOSPITAL, 1909
now Kirkman House.

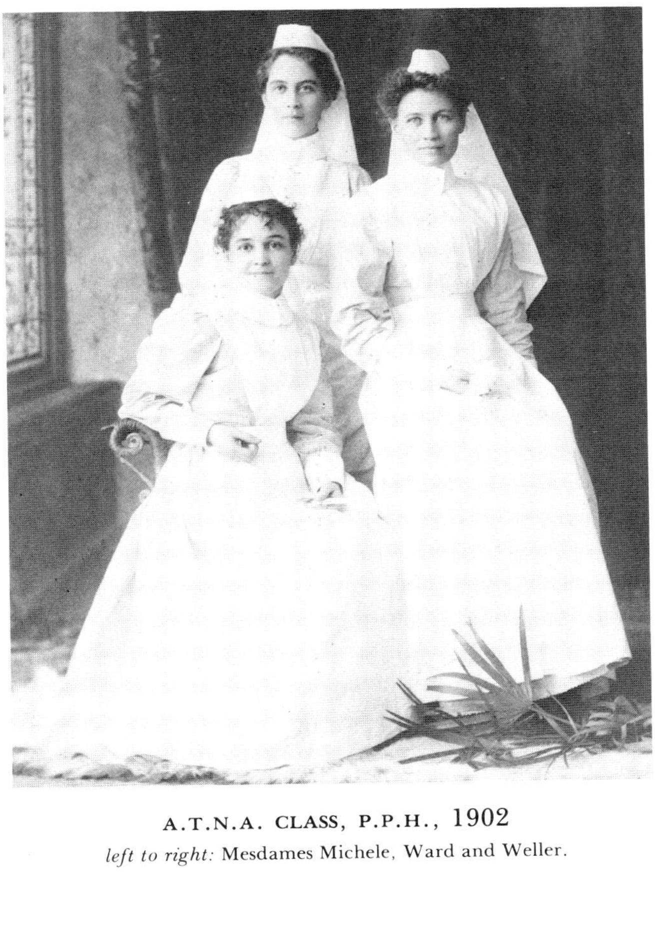

A.T.N.A. CLASS, P.P.H., 1902
left to right: Mesdames Michele, Ward and Weller.

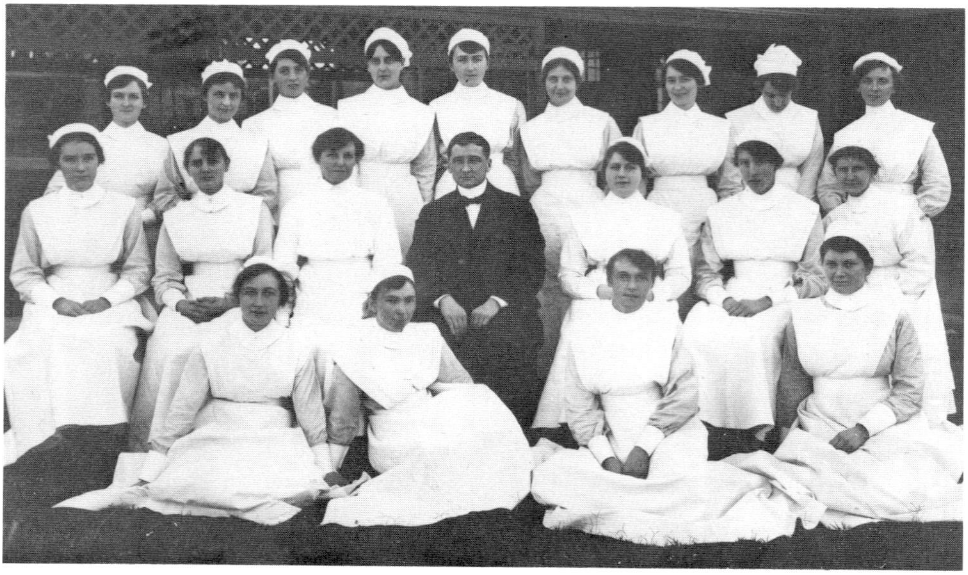

A.T.N.A. CLASS, P.P.H., 1915-18

back row: E. Farrow, M. Buxton, —. Fancy, I. Piesse, M. Burke, G. Ottaway, M. Fowlie, H. Broadhurst, E. Field; *seated:* E. Curwood, A. Strochein, I. Gill (matron), Dr G. Barker, E. Doherty, E. George, K. Muir; *front row:* J. McKenzie Murray, D. Steedman, L. Stokes, A. Pearson.

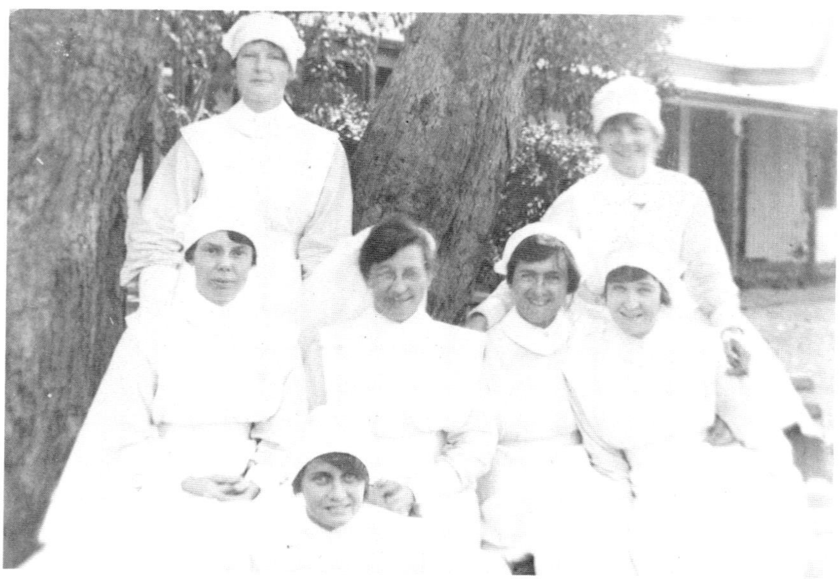

TRAINEES AT INFECTIOUS DISEASES BRANCH, 1921

back row: Cowan, Johnson; *seated:* Daniell, Carnigan (staff nurse), Deakin, Scott; *front:* Hitchings.

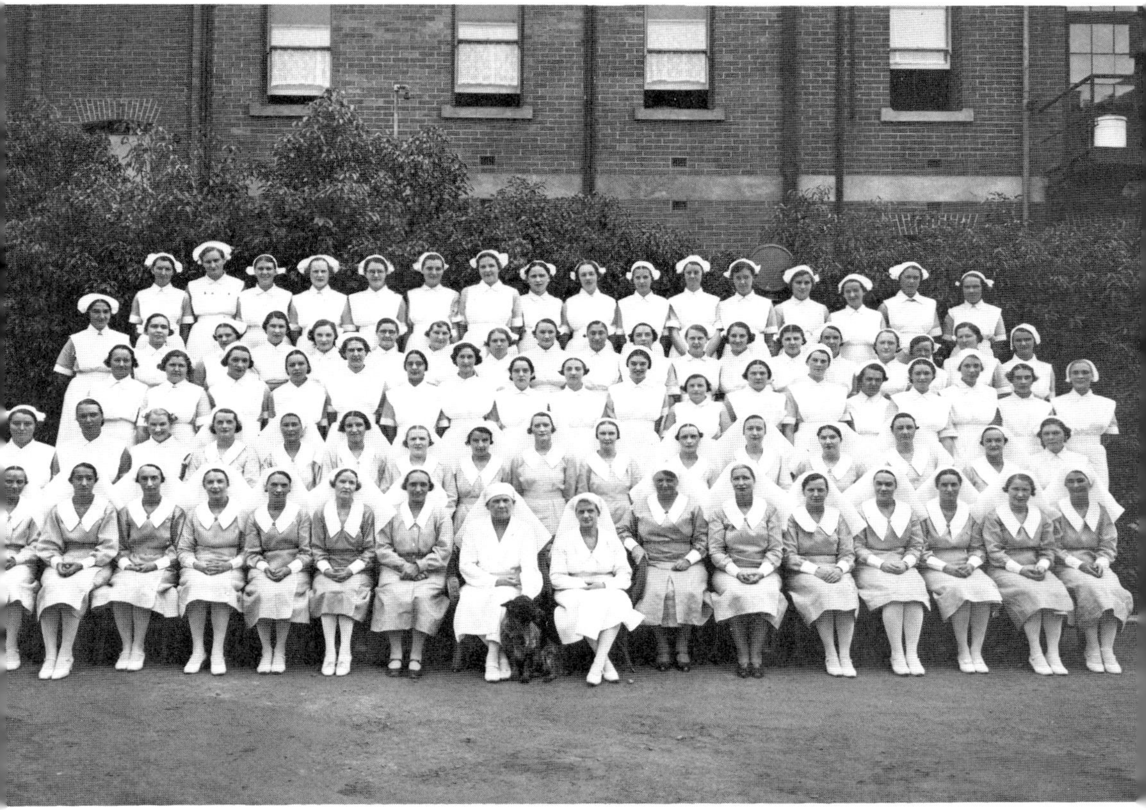

PERTH HOSPITAL STAFF AND TRAINEES, 1937
centre front: the matron, Miss E. McNevin, and her dog, Bunty.

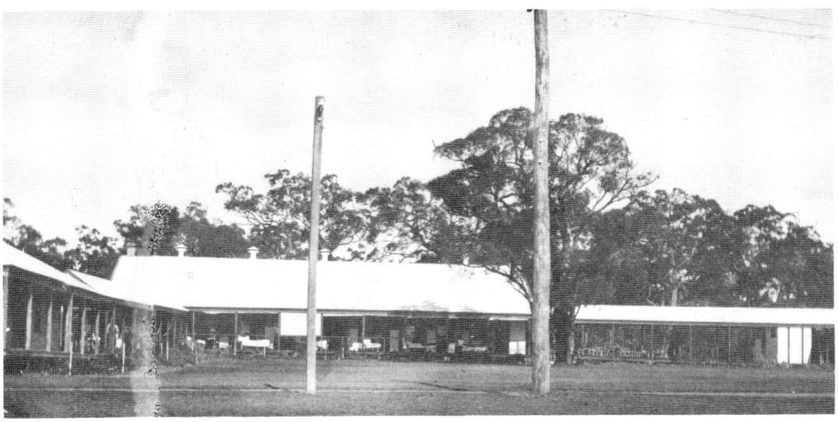

INFECTIOUS DISEASES BRANCH, 1921

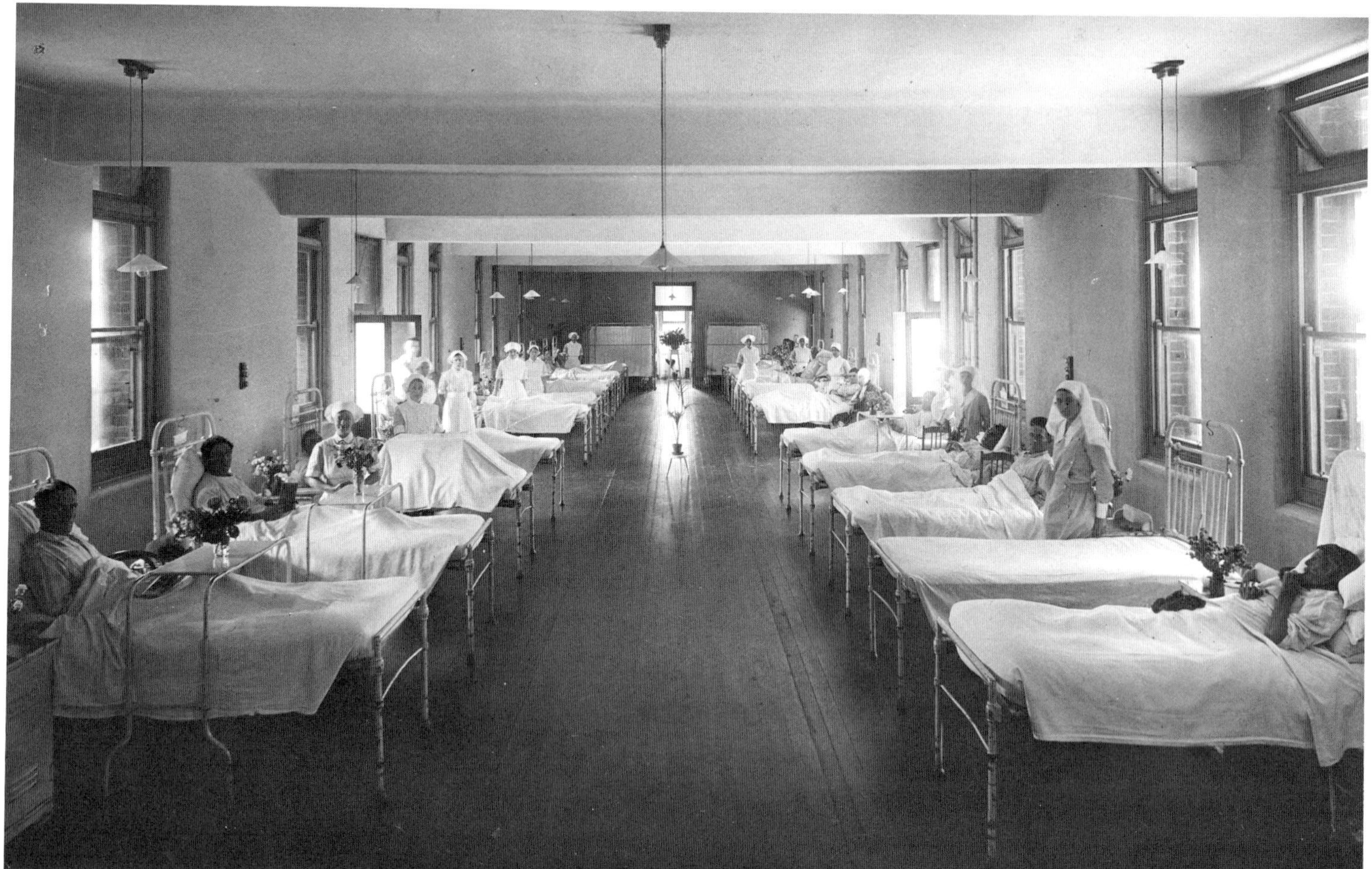

A TYPICAL WARD AT PERTH HOSPITAL, 1930

terest the public in the foundation; and to form a financial committee with the idea of appointing a paid organizer. The secretary reported that already a great deal of publicity had been given in press reports and that Lady Mitchell had consented to be patroness. After several preliminary meetings the matter was left in abeyance as it was pointed out — by Mrs Walsh — that there was already an appeal before the public — the Jubilee Appeal.[27]

However, the *Journal of the Western Australian Nurses* in the April issue of 1936 designated this as a special Florence Nightingale International Foundation Appeal number. The cover, in pale blue, featured the A.T.N.A. badge, on which was superimposed a picture of the statuette of Florence Nightingale holding the traditional lamp. The editorial featured the Florence Nightingale International Foundation and gave details of the proposed fund, although it is not clear at this stage whether the money raised was to go directly to the Nightingale Fund or form the nucleus of a fund sponsored by the W.A. Branch of the A.T.N.A. for a scholarship for a Western Australian nurse. To quote:

> It is the desire of a number of women in W.A. that we should also have the advantages of advancement in nursing education that a Scholarship gives to a country. Nurses are asked to make their donations to this on Florence Nightingale Thanksgiving Day (May 12). If every nurse who has been trained sent one shilling towards this fund, it would be a great beginning to a worthy cause. All donations will be acknowledged through this Journal . . .
>
> Stamps for sealing the back of letters are available from the office of the A.T.N.A. . . . These may be procured at 1/- per dozen. We ask all nurses to buy them and use them so that the fund may be built up. A statement of the finances of this fund will be published next month.

July, 1936. F.N.I.M.N. Fund opened.	£ s d
Sale of stamps at the A.T.N.A. office	3-15-0
Proceeds of Bridge Party	17-1
Total	4-12-1

There was at this time a certain amount of confusion among nurses as to the roles of their nursing organizations and to some extent resentment towards the A.T.N.A. This was certainly not helped by the attitude taken by the dean in his sermon on the occasion of the Florence Nightingale Thanksgiving Service held at St George's Cathedral on Sunday, 10 May 1936. To the congregation of some two hundred nurses, most of whom were students, the concluding remarks were to say the least untactful:

> At one time it had been necessary for prospective nurses to pay

> a premium before they could enter the training for the profession. To-day the tendency was to make the profession more attractive. The Nurses Union was formed to obtain justice for women who had previously been overworked. While he would not pass judgment on this action he hoped there was no likelihood of nursing becoming a matter of so much work for so much pay. If that happened the profession would fast deteriorate.[28]

Resulting from this, an embarrassed Nurses' Christian Movement decided that perhaps in future it would be better to alternate the venues for the annual event, a practice that has continued ever since.

The first approach to the public for support of the fund came in September 1936 when a meeting was held at Government House at the invitation of Lady Mitchell, wife of the lieutenant governor, to form a Florence Nightingale Memorial Committee, of which she kindly consented to be patroness.[29] The aims and objects of this committee were to provide scholarships for nurses to undertake studies towards gaining postgraduate degrees. The committee was representative of organizations other than nursing but with similar objects and included the Red Cross Society. Through this committee a scholarship fund was formed, the first fund-raising effort being the organization of a White Angel Ball for 2 October 1936. Held in Government House Ballroom, the idea was promoted by the screening of a motion picture, *The White Angel*, starring Kay Francis and based on the story of Florence Nightingale. The amount raised from this effort was £83. S. J. Perry, the fund organizer, and for many years an active member of what was eventually to become the Florence Nightingale Committee, made it possible for all nurses to preview the film at the Regent Theatre through his connections with the film industry. It was over two years before sufficient money was raised (£300) to provide a scholarship from Western Australia, the first recipient being Miss Maud Campbell.[30] On her arrival in England, the outbreak of World War II disrupted the programme and she was unable to continue with the project. During the war Miss Campbell served with Princess Mary's Royal Air Force Nursing Service.

The duties of secretary for the Florence Nightingale Memorial Committee were undertaken by Miss K. Yeates, who continued with this for many years. She was also a member of the select committee formed to assess applicants for scholarships.

It is perhaps unfortunate that so many nursing organizations came into being at the same time for this has led to confusion both then and now. The following is aimed at some clarification. In 1930 the two organizations dealing with the affairs of nursing were the Nurses' Registration Board (a statutory body for the registration of general nurses) and the A.T.N.A. (state branch of the Australian Nursing Federation), the professional organization. The registration of midwives was still carried out by the Midwives Board under the provisions of the Health Act of 1911. The A.T.N.A. Club functioned as an employment agency and also provided a residence for its members. Although an independent body, it was supported by the A.T.N.A. and provided a venue for council meetings. The Military Nurses' Club was also residential, mainly for the purpose of leave and recreation, and was exclusive to nurses who had served with the military forces. The function of this club was largely social and it was the forerunner of the Returned Sisters Sub-branch of the Returned Services League of today.

The viability of both the A.T.N.A. and the W.A.N.A. depended on membership which, after the granting of the first award in the Arbitration Court,[31] tended to favour the W.A.N.A. It was a bid to counteract this that prompted supporters of the A.T.N.A. led by Mrs Walsh to found the Florence Nightingale Club.

The Nurses' Christian Movement with headquarters in the eastern states formed a Western Australian branch about 1934. Undenominational, it strongly supported nurses serving in hospitals in the mission field at home and abroad.

And to add to all of the above was the formation of ex-trainee associations, for nursing had always been sectarian as far as training schools were concerned. At one stage this had almost amounted to rivalry as each 'school' strove for the accolade of 'topping the state' in the final Registration Board examinations. When this tended to get out of hand, the board ceased to publish the marks gained by the individual candidates, an action which was sharply criticized by the medical men responsible for the lecture programmes in the hospitals.

All associations had a membership fee and in the day of an economic depression the view of some nurses was that nursing had become too expensive.[32]

Perth Children's Hospital nurses were the first to form an ex-nurses association, the inaugural meeting of which was held at the hospital on 21 June 1930.[33] Its aim was to bring together ex-nurses and to further the work of the Children's Hospital. One of its projects was to raise £1000 for a life endowment of a cot. Mrs King, née Waterhouse, had the distinction of being the 'earliest trainee' present, having gained one of the first four certificates given by the hospital in 1912.

The origin and motto of the badge adopted by the Children's

Hospital is not known but it is obviously based on that appearing on the nurses' certificates of training—a red cross with cherubs' wings surmounted by a ribbon bearing the words 'Healing in its Wings', presumably a misquote from a passage in the Old Testament. In the 1920s it was stated that some of the trainee nurses became frustrated at the delay in providing them with a distinctive badge, and so had one made to their own design, depicting a knight on a charger in red enamel, a copy of the 'buttons' sold in an Appeal Day for the hospital. These rebel badges became something of a status symbol for their wearers, and were eagerly sought after. At that time the nurses responsible for the inauguration of an ex-trainee association produced a journal, published annually, firstly in 1930 as *The Magazine* and in 1931 as *The Optimist*, but unfortunately it did not survive. Copies are held in the nursing archives of the Princess Margaret Hospital, which has now given its name to the ex-trainees association.

Perth Hospital Ex-Trainees Association was inaugurated at a meeting held at the Florence Nightingale Club on 23 September 1936, with Mrs K. Weller, M.B.E., as president.[34] Mrs Weller, who had a long and distinguished career in nursing, was an ex-trainee of the hospital and had been in the second A.T.N.A. class of 1902. Apart from providing an opportunity for social get-togethers, the objective of the association was to raise money for amenities for sick nurses in the hospital. In 1936 Perth Hospital was still very much a hospital for the sick poor, the equipment was 'utility' and there were few refinements. There were no food trays and meals were served in thick china mugs and plates placed on the lockers or overbed tables. Some preferential treatment was given to sick staff members, who were nursed in the 'Specials' of Wards 3 and 8, and it was traditional to extend this courtesy to any ex-trainee who was admitted as a patient. Special china, trays and tray cloths, and floral screen covers were provided for, to a great extent with money derived from fining nurses for carelessness in breaking equipment, chiefly thermometers. The one shilling fine for each thermometer was equal to one-fifth of a week's salary. To break a large syringe was financial disaster. An indication of the economic climate of those days was the increase in the number of nurses admitted and there was need for some alternative method of obtaining finance. The legality of fining nurses was also in question as members of the domestic staff were not required to be penalized for breakages.

Perth Hospital, too, had acquired a badge, the design of which linked it with its origins of the colonial days, but more in keeping with an affluent society. Executed in gold, it depicted the red cross of St George on a white shield within a gold and blue enamel circle, and a small black swan surmounted by a crown, the motto, *Servio*. The cost was £1 10s and it was available at the discretion of the matron to trained staff only. During the war years the badge was changed to an oblong in white metal, and each trainee received one from the hospital on graduation. In the 1950s it was returned to its former design. The prefix 'Royal' was added when this was conferred on the hospital in 1946.

With the passing of the years, the venue of the R.P.H. Ex-Trainees Association, now known as the R.P.H. Ex-trainees and Associates, was found to be unsuitable and the association was invited to meet at the hospital.

The term 'government nurses' referred to those who trained within the framework of the hospitals controlled by the Medical Department. Because all had to spend eighteen months of their term of training at Kalgoorlie Hospital, their loyalties were to that hospital. On graduation comparatively few remained in the Kalgoorlie area and so reunions were not a practical solution to commencing an ex-trainees association. Nevertheless a group was formed in Kalgoorlie, and known as the Kalgoorlie Past Nurses' Association. Its badge was an enamelled square of gold and its members supported the hospital in providing amenities for the patients and the nurses' quarters. Membership was not restricted to graduate nurses and nurses who had completed only part-time training at the hospital were accepted for membership. Just when this association was formed officially is not known, possibly the early thirties.[35]

The *Journal of the Western Australian Nurses* in its September issue of 1936 carried the following announcement:

> Government Nurses interested in the formation of a Past Nurses Association are invited to meet at the Florence Nightingale Club Rooms on Tuesday September 22 at 8 p.m. to discuss the formation of the Association and to elect officers.

In the November issue, under the heading 'Kalgoorlie Past Nurses' Association', there is a notice that a reunion would be held at Anzac House on 7 December and that all government nurses would be welcomed. Under the same heading there is an account of the annual meeting in December 1937, but office bearers are not mentioned. There is a notification in January 1938 that the association would meet quarterly at the Florence Nightingale Club and from subsequent notices it seems as if the association in Perth was to be named Kalgoorlie Past Nurses' Association. It is of interest to note that in 1938 Miss Fyfe was re-elected president and Mrs Breydon, vice-president. From a sum of money left to the association by the latter, a prize has been awarded yearly to a government nurse who has been nominated as outstanding in the practical field of nursing. The Kalgoorlie nurses did not have a hospital badge at this time.

The following is an extract from the *Journal of Western Australian Nurses*, 20 April 1937.

> At a representative meeting, held at the Florence Nightingale Club Rooms on April 2, it was decided to form a Fremantle Hospital Ex Trainees' Association. The following ladies who were present formed themselves into a committee to establish the Association—Miss Bottle (Chairman), Miss Perryman (Secretary), Misses Carroll, Carson, Cocks, Egan, Gill, Kiernan, Lefroy and Mrs Henderson.[36]

At the following meeting, held at the hospital, it was stated that 'the Association intends to interest itself in social activities and to assist sick nurses'. The badge of Fremantle Hospital is blue and silver depicting a shield with the letters F.H. surmounted by a Maltese Cross. The motto, *Vive Valeque*.

The oldest nurses to qualify for membership of these associations by virtue of training in the respective hospitals would have been at the most in their early sixties and the bulk would have been in the forty age group and younger. As new training schools were formed within the framework of the newer hospitals, so did further ex-trainee associations arise. With the development of schools of nursing affiliated with a group of hospitals the tendency has been to belong to the hospital rather than the school although this is changing with the evolution of the independent school. In the 1930s this closeness to the hospital was deeply rooted to the extent of creating a clan. The matrons were invariably made special honorary members of the organizations and acted as hostesses when the hospital precincts were used as venues. At this time only one matron qualified for membership of two associations, Miss Balding of Fremantle, who had trained at Perth Hospital.

Two other nursing societies also operating were the Catholic Nurses' Guild and the Guild of St Barnabas, the latter for communicants of the Anglican persuasion.

Although the membership fees for the nursing organizations were small they did have a limiting effect on membership and those who had to travel any distance to the city found that they could not keep up with the cost.

Of interest is a large tablecloth, now in the possession of the Nurses' Memorial Centre. The cloth, which was donated to the Florence Nightingale Club by Janet Chalmers of K.E.M.H., has embroidered on it the names of members and visitors to the club and provides a fascinating record.

In 1934 the state of Western Australian hospitals and their inability to provide facilities for the adequate training of nurses came under fire from members of the medical profession and the A.T.N.A. The matter was given wide publicity in the press.[37] Much of this criticism was directed at Perth Hospital and the Infectious Diseases Branch. The matron stated that the nurses were receiving insufficient training and it had become very obvious that there was a 'definite falling off in the qualities of the nurse'. In August 1934 a special meeting was convened between members of the A.T.N.A. Council and representatives of the B.M.A. Many suggestions were put forward to alleviate conditions prevailing at the hospital, including the employment of more domestic staff, or meeting the problem of accommodation by allowing trained staff to 'live out'.

Miss E. Carlin suggested that a tutor be appointed to relieve the tutorial duties of the ward sister. Miss McNevin (the matron) wholeheartedly supported this. She had been on a fact-finding tour of the eastern states and was impressed by the establishment of preliminary training schools. Resulting from this and possibly spurred on by mounting criticism over the next months, the Preliminary Training School was commenced at Perth Hospital in June 1935.[38] It was to be of four weeks duration for groups of 'probationer' nurses who would receive their theoretical and practical instruction before being sent to the wards. The tutor sister appointed was Miss E. J. Bowe who had been an assistant tutor at Royal Melbourne Hospital. (Following World War II 'Jessie' Bowe became matron in chief of the Royal Australian Army Nursing Corps.) The first student nurses to enter the school were Mary E. (Mollie) Brady, who subsequently became the first matron of Perth Dental Hospital, Ruth Huggett, Eileen Forrest and Grace Walker.[39]

The establishment of the school was given a lot of publicity and featured in the *West Australian* with photographs and a lengthy article by 'Ixia' together with other announcements. The commencement was also marked by a social function in the Murray Street nurses' quarters when a grandfather clock was dedicated to the late Miss Gill, Miss Mary Ann Nicolay performing the ceremony. Those present were introduced to Miss Bowe and invited to inspect the school, which was located in the lecture hall adjoining the quarters. Among those present are listed Sister Mary Nicolay; Mesdames J. Thompson, Head, Downe, Brooking, Weller, Robinson, Watkins, McClemans, Bennett, Walsh, Gillett, Larkin, Dargin, Cook, Bremner, McLeod, A. Hill, Freeman, McKay and H. Thompson; and Misses C. Phillips, Wignall, Perkins, O. Hall, Balding, Jones, Nicholson, Ashton, Simson, Yeates, Piesse, Monger (2), Homan, Stokes, Curwood, Hawke, Mulgrave, Bonham, Tate,

Fyfe, Gordon, Ure, Urwin, Caporn, Hedges, Mead, Cowan and Darch (unfortunately initials have been omitted).

The following is an undated extract from the *West Australian* (June 1935):

A Schoolroom for Nurses

By 'Ixia'

Members of the nursing division of the St. John Ambulance Brigade last week inspected at the invitation of the matron of the Perth Hospital (Miss E. McNevin), the preliminary school for nurses and its equipment. For four weeks before beginning their actual ward training, probationers there receive instruction enabling them to start their nursing careers with considerable valuable knowledge in various branches of curative treatment.

For demonstrations a section of the nurses' lecture Hall has been partitioned off. In addition to samples of regulation ward furnishings, there are lifelike composition models of perfectly jointed limbs, and the upper part of a body, firmly mounted at a suitable height for bandaging practice and lessons on the proper application of poultices or dressings. Before being allowed to experiment on sufferers in the wards, new nurses become skilful in the school at making the poultices they learn to apply aright.

Life Size Model

Better than diagrams for acquainting probationers with the working interior of the human body is a life-size anatomical model, naturally coloured. Outer parts of the torso and throat, when removed reveal the various vital organs, and each of these may be lifted out for examination. The top of the brain can be opened and the brain taken out, also the eyeball with its controlling muscles. Each of the many sections is numbered and the names and particulars of all are detailed in the printed lists. Half of . . . this marvellous model is moulded to represent the normal flesh development; the other shows the muscles and sinews.

This carefully cased treasure is jealously guarded by the matron, fearful that parts of it may 'walk off' as the skull of the school skeleton has done. The keys of its double-locked cabinet are always held either by Miss McNevin herself or the instructing sister. A Sydney hospital is the only other institution to possess a similar model for nursing instruction.

In the two beds of the miniature ward repose lifelike dolls. One of these, recently acquired, is naturally jointed to the finger-tips and as useful for nursing practice as a real man or woman. Several orifices in the softly flexible body with rubber tubes leading to waterproof bags in the interior permit the

> internal liquid treatment drill. The rubber bags can be withdrawn through a door opening in the back of the figure and emptied. Practice in feeding a patient artificially is also possible. The same arrangements in the head enable the eyes to be bathed and nasal douches, throat or ear treatment to be given.
>
> *A Dummy Baby*
>
> A dummy baby, charmingly and chubbily realistic occupies the adjacent white cot. It has a washable body and limbs as soft and pliable as those of a living child. Everything necessary for the care of an infant also is at hand.
>
> The school training for probationers starts at 8 every morning and finishes at 6 p.m. unless three hours off are given through the day to get the girls accustomed to working time variations. Then the lesson time ceases at 8 p.m. Usually six probationers work under a sister in the school. Each sits at a small table in the middle of the room in front of the sister's table when class instruction is given on preliminaries essential for nursing success. Matron McNevin is enthusiastic about the Nursing School and would prefer that three months instead of one be spent in the demonstration room by probationers.

Not all trained nurses were as enthusiastic about the venture as Miss McNevin. Even the ward sisters had reservations about it and were sceptical of its beneficial effect on nurse training. In some areas it was considered that it was a possible threat to authority and that it would cause a division of loyalties between staff of the school and staff of the hospital. The emphasis in nursing was on expertise in the performance of practical procedures and the promise that P.T.S. nurses would be well versed in these and be able to perform without supervision, was not valid. The opportunities for perfection in the wards were not those available in the schoolroom; no model, no matter how perfect, can equate with a living person. Even the cleaning techniques which were practised by the P.T.S. nurses on the bathrooms and toilets of the nurses' quarters were vastly different from those encountered in the pan-lavatories and lotions rooms of the wards.

Third-year nurses who had been given earlier lectures by the matron admitted to being confused when it came to tutorials by the tutor, and a feeling of insecurity when it came to taking the finals. There was one thing for certain, and that was that schools of nursing had come to stay. Basically the pattern of experience did not alter and the pattern was laid down before the commencement of training. The word training is used here advisably for procedures were carried out with a 'drill-like' precision, and the emphasis was on 'how' rather than 'why'.

Not all training schools were alike, for structure had to be adapted to function. A constant criticism of Perth Children's Hospital was that the trainees were lacking in adult experience and there was a demand for a special Children's Register. Country hospitals, too, differed in that they lacked 'specialization' and the honorary system of practitioners, with junior resident doctors. Ancillary services such as social welfare, physiotherapy, pathology, etc. were generally confined to hospitals such as Perth and Fremantle.

However, taking the above into consideration, the pattern of training given below, which was that of Perth Hospital, was broadly speaking that used in the other training schools.

Built at the turn of the century, Perth Hospital was designed in the conventional manner, with blocks of long wards opening on to verandahs. The ablution and toilet areas were situated at one end and the ward pantry and 'lotion' rooms the other. Even when the Military Block was built in the 1920s the building was designed as a replica of the older buildings. The verandahs, originally for convalescent patients, had for many years been in permanent use and generally accommodated the longer-term patient and those with conditions such as gangrene, colostomy, etc. and suppurating wounds, which were considered better in the 'open air'. There was also a tendency to use the verandah beds for patients in traction and such appliances which tended to make the ward look 'untidy' but with the increase of orthopaedic surgery wards were coming to be specialized for patients requiring this type of treatment.

Originally the wards, which were strictly 'male' and 'female', were built to accommodate twenty patients, ten on either side with some ten extra patients being accommodated in the smaller wards or 'specials'. There was a further subdivision according to the type of treatment being carried out, e.g. medical, surgical, genito-urinary, gynaecological, etc. The old colonial building of 1855 was used as the out-patient department and casualty. What had been the basement was used for out-patient treatment of patients with venereal disease, and was commonly known as the 'caves'. Other departments, such as operating theatres, X ray, dispensary, pathology, administration, etc. were a fair distance from the wards and to be sent on an errand to these meant time lost from ward duties. Furthermore no patient was allowed to go to any of the departments without being accompanied by a nurse.

The pattern of nurse training was embodied in the staffing of wards which entailed a sister and staff nurse in charge of each ward supported by a team of 'probationer nurses'. The tasks allotted were graded in relation to experience. The two most senior nurses had assigned to them the two most junior to join the team, and were held responsible for their instruction. For the first year nurses wore a green uniform and for the first three months wore a 'bobtail' cap after which they 'signed on' and acquired a cap with a frill. At the end of the first year they wore a pink uniform and were rated as senior nurses. Eight nurses were allocated to each ward for day duty and two for night duty—a junior and a senior nurse. On night duty there were only two trained nurses for the whole hospital. Lectures and examinations were taken in 'off duty' time, and for those who happened to be on duty it was mandatory to excuse them from the ward if this was feasible. Every nurse was required to do at least three months training at the Infectious Diseases Branch, and as the majority of patients there were children, it gave 'children's' nursing experience. On paper the training programme looked reasonable, affording a wide experience in all types of patient care, but it was the over-occupancy of the wards and the extra-curricula duties which, together with the advances in medical technology, made the position almost impossible. As there was only one wards-maid allocated to each ward, the bulk of the domestic work fell on the shoulders of the nurse, especially in her first year of training, and the list of duties expected of her left no time for emergencies and little time for nursing care. If a nurse could not keep up the pace, or decided to discontinue training, there was always another waiting to be called up immediately and put in her place. However with the introduction of the Preliminary Training School, the single replacement idea was rendered obsolete and the waiting period for a number to emerge from the school did place the staffing of the hospital at a disadvantage. The advent of the union and the award for shorter hours seriously disrupted the training pattern, and although nurses were actively discouraged from signing for overtime, the relief from pressure resulted in a slowing down by the workforce. Although the specific tasks allotted to each member of the ward team were posted on the wall of the duty room, the time allowed for these was totally unrealistic. Those expected of the first junior probationer are listed as an example.

5.45 a.m.	Report for duty, and sign on. (As all staff signed on at this time, and the book was then removed to the matron's office it was necessary to start much earlier to get into the queue.) Read the reports and have a cup of tea.
6.00	Each nurse was allotted five patients or rather 'beds' and these had to be bathed and toileted in bed. It was rare to have any who were able to go to the only two bathrooms and toilets on the wards.
7.00	Give out 'tooth mugs' and/or attend to mouth toilets

	of patients on one side of the ward—usually 10 to 12. Sort and count the soiled linen.
7.10	Go to breakfast.
7.20	Return to ward and help give out the breakfasts, i.e. porridge, or bread and milk, bread and butter, and tea, which had milk added and was dispensed in large jugs, and which was made by the junior nurse. Sugar was rationed and in the male wards always at a premium. Helpless patients needed to be fed.
8.00	Return the used dishes to the ward pantry and scrape and stack for washing up. Scrub the patients' lockers on one side of the ward. Fold the towels precisely, and straighten the window blinds and align the beds, fill the water jugs.
8.45	Each junior nurse had to sweep one half of the ward, and all patients were offered toilet facilities. Dust and polish the ward sister's desk, wash the pen nibs and fill the ink wells.
9.00	The ward was required to be ready for inspection by the matron or sister, and the honorary doctors began their official rounds. Cleaning duties. All enamel ware scrubbed and boiled, copper sterilizers polished, benches and sinks, etc. thoroughly cleaned. Rubber mackintoshes were 'carbolized' and blood-stained linen rinsed before being sent to the laundry.
9.45	Prepare morning tea for the ward staff. Give out soup and beef tea.
10.00	Off duty for three hours until 1 p.m. which included the midday meal time. If working a 'through' shift, take over the duties of the second junior nurse which were alternative and included getting patients up on the lounges, attending to pressure areas, toileting and sweeping the whole of the ward by midday.
12 md.	Give out the dinners as directed by the sister or staff nurse, who personally served them. The light diet of jelly and junket was prepared on the ward beforehand. All dishes had to be returned to the ward pantry and scraped and stacked for washing up by the wardsmaid.
1.30 p.m.	Dinner in the nurses' dining-room. This was a formal meal presided over by the senior trained staff. Between 1 and 2 p.m. the patients and the ward were prepared to receive visitors.
2.00	Take and record all temperatures. Refold and put away all clean linen.
3.00	Attend to the patients' basic needs. Those on lounges

	returned to bed. Quilts removed and folded over the end of the beds.
	Prepare staff afternoon tea.
4.00	Evening meal given out by the wards-maid. Bread and butter and an egg. Cup of tea.
4.45	Collect and deliver dishes to pantry. (As the wards-maid's duties ended at 5 p.m. any dishes collected after that time had to be dealt with by the duty nurse.)
5.00	Each nurse swept half of the ward.
5.30	Off duty for evening meal.
6.00	Basic care of patients—toileting etc.
6.30	Evening visiting hour twice a week.
7.00	Give medications in form of aperients.
	Empty and refill sterilizers.
	Check and record 'foul' linen ready for laundry.
8.00	Off duty.

In addition to the general duties as laid down, the junior nurse was required to assist when needed with preparation for operations, dressings and procedures, last offices, admission of patients, listing and recording their belongings. In the surgical wards she had to accompany the patient to the operating theatre, help during anaesthetization, position the patient, and check the 'packs' with the ward sister who was required to assist with all patients from her particular ward. As the nurse progressed in seniority, her duties were just as demanding but orientated more to nursing techniques and nursing care although still responsible for some domestic chores. The amazing thing was that all trained nurses, having experienced the situation, took so long to do anything about the matter, and strangest of all, that many condoned it as a necessary adjunct to the training and discipline of the nurse.

In contrast with the wide coverage given in the press to the establishment of the first Preliminary Training School the announcement in the *Australasian Nurses' Journal* of 15 October 1935 in the Western Australian section is in low key:

> Preliminary School—Perth Hospital is to be congratulated on being the first hospital in Western Australia to open this important school for the preliminary training for the benefit of the trainees. The idea of Sister Tutors and Preliminary Schools has been advocated by the A.T.N.A. for some years.

(It is noted that in the *Journal of the West Australian Nurses*, Jubilee issue of 1951, and the *Perth Hospital Journal* of September 1940 the commencement of the P.T.S. is stated in 1936, which is incorrect.) The other hospital training schools were in no hurry to introduce the P.T.S. idea. A Preliminary School was established at Wooroloo Sanitorium in 1938 where trainees attended for a six to eight week period. The first tutor was Miss M. Attwood. It was not until 1944 that Perth Children's Hospital (Princess Margaret Hospital) commenced a P.T.S., and arrangements were made for trainee nurses from Fremantle Hospital to attend for six weeks prior to commencing at the hospital. The tutor appointed was Kathleen Reidy. Fremantle Hospital inaugurated its own School of Nursing in 1946 with a modified Block System, the tutor appointed being Helen Bailey.

Between the years 1935 and 1940 so much happened which affected the theory and practice of nursing that it is difficult to list the events in sequence. The three main career areas for women were clerical, teaching and nursing. With the retrenchment in teacher training by the Education Department there had been a swing towards nursing, but with the slight easing of the economic situation there was a tendency for the girl with the higher academic qualification to lean towards teaching. The nursing authorities interested in recruiting staff with higher qualifications feared that the evidence given on nurses' conditions in the Arbitration Court was calculated to have a detrimental effect on the recruitment of nurses as did the demand for a revised method of selection.

After a tour of the country and 'Board' hospitals, the A.T.N.A. secretary suggested to the Medical Department that an inspecting matron be appointed to advise matrons of the hospitals how best to improve conditions for their staff. Arising out of this the commissioner for public health, Dr Everitt Atkinson, gave notice of a conference to be held and invited the A.T.N.A. to send representation.[40]

The conference was held on Monday 9 December 1935 and reported on in the *West Australian* as follows:

> *Training Nurses*
> *Suggested Central School*
> *Conference discusses Methods*
>
> A report concerning a recent conference at which representatives of eight bodies discussed the better training of nurses was submitted to the Perth Hospital Board yesterday, by Mr. J. W. Tyson, who was one of the Board's delegates at the conference. The Commissioner of Public Health (Dr. Everitt Atkinson) presided at the conference, which was attended by representatives of Perth, Fremantle and Children's Hospitals, the West Australian Branches of the British Medical Association and the Royal College of Surgeons, the Nurses' Union, the Nurses' Registration Board and the Australian Trained Nurses Association.

Mr. Tyson's report stated that after a lengthy discussion the conference recommended: — (a) that the age of commencing training be 19 years in all hospitals; (b) that a certificate from the headmaster that a girl had passed the eighth standard (sub-junior standard in secondary schools) be accepted for admission and that any girl not having this certificate should be required to pass an equivalent examination before being accepted by the Nurses' Registration Board.

The Perth Hospital Board concurred with this section of the report although Mr. A. H. Panton expressed the opinion that examinations were often tommy rot. It was more a question of type, he said.

Mr. Tyson's report further stated that it had been suggested at the conference that a central training school should be established to prepare trainees for all hospitals and that a post-graduate course should be instituted to assist sisters to become better teachers to probationers in country hospitals who had completed their first year. The matter had been referred to the advisory committee of the Australian Trained Nurses' Association. A suggestion by the representatives of the Perth Hospital that the hospital would doubtless agree to train a proportion of the country trainees was not well received, as the provision of a Central Training School was considered to be more important.

At yesterday's Board meeting, Mr. Panton said that a Board of three matrons should select girls to enter the proposed central school.

The secretary of the Perth Hospital (Mr. V. C. H. Eagleton) expressed a fear that unless each matron was allowed to select trainees to suit her requirements, the personal touch would be lost. The Perth Hospital, he said wanted to maintain its nursing traditions. Consideration was being given to the possibility of issuing distinctive badges to girls who had completed training at the hospital and the giving of prizes as an incentive to proficiency.

The report further stated that the conference was of the opinion that it was undesirable to send untrained girls to the Wooroloo Sanitorium. A suggestion by the Trained Nurses' Association that a supervising matron should be appointed to country hospitals to maintain a more efficient service had been referred to the committee dealing with training schools.

The Australian Trained Nurses Association referred to in the above was in fact the Australasian Trained Nurses Association (W.A. Branch of the Australian Nursing Federation). Many of the suggestions in the report were based on those submitted by the A.T.N.A. whose representatives were Miss E. A. Harvey (president), Mrs A. M. Walsh and Miss K. Yeates (secretary). The Western Australian Nurses' Association was represented by the president, Miss E. B. Carlin, who was also a council member of the A.T.N.A., and the Nurses' Registration Board by Miss F. Bruce. The names of the other nurse representatives are not known.

The report was very favourably received by the A.T.N.A. Council, but it is not quite clear whether the subsequent advisory committee requested to go further into the matter was that of the A.T.N.A. or appointed by the commissioner. It is stated in the minutes of the A.T.N.A. Council of 10 December 1935 that a committee comprised of the matrons of the training schools, the president and secretary (?), Misses Bruce and Carlin, should go into the matter of the suggested preliminary training school and report back to the council. In the minutes of the meeting of 11 February 1936, under the heading 'Preliminary training for nurses', it is stated that a report from the committee appointed to deal with this matter was received and it was decided that it be forwarded to Dr Atkinson, the chairman of the conference.

Much of the work involved in this report was done by Miss K. Yeates who through her connection with the British College of Nursing, of which she was made a foundation fellow, formulated the scheme of university training for nurses and initiated correspondence with the University of Western Australia. This scheme was presented to the university by Dr D. D. Paton, an eye specialist. Professor H. Whitfeld's reply makes it clear that although he favoured higher education for nurses, the limiting factor was lack of finance:

> So far as I can judge, the number of lectures which it is suggested should be given at the University is roughly as follows:- Preliminary School, four series per annum of 18 lectures, equals 72; Second Year, two series of 42 lectures each, equals 84; Third Year, two series of 42 lectures each, equals 84. The cost of such lectures would probably not be less than about two guineas each, and it would be advisable to have something extra to cover books, preparation of synopses, clerical work, etc. From the University point of view, therefore, it looks as though the cost would be about £500-£600 for the provision of the lectures and examinations as set out in the draft.
>
> I have not consulted any of the University Boards or Officials about the proposal, as I understand it is still only a draft. I do not know, therefore, whether the University would at this stage undertake the responsibility of joining in the scheme, provided that the University grant could be increased to cover the cost. It would, of course, be out of the question for us to undertake it with out present grant, which is insufficient for our present teaching faculties.

Speaking personally, I may say that I hope that you will succeed in your effort to provide a better training for nurses, and I am sure that the University also would wish you success.

The lectures enumerated in the plan did not differ greatly from those already given in hospitals as part of the general training programme.

It is difficult to assess which of the advances in medicine had the greatest influence on medical and nursing care. The year 1936 saw the use of a drug, 'red' prontosil, the first of the sulphonamides, which had a dramatic effect in the treatment of patients with infections caused by some groups of pathogenic micro-organisms. The prontosil was administered by intramuscular injection, its colour being apparent in the excretions of the patients treated, and the subsequent staining of the bed linen. The sulphonamides which followed were administered orally and marked the beginning of treatment of people with such conditions as acute lobar pneumonia at home without the services of a nurse over a long period. It marked an era where the classic pattern of a disease no longer determined its diagnosis or its rule of thumb management. The introduction of the Soluvac flask and the replacement of body fluid both rectally and intravenously by the drip method meant expertise in the management of new equipment as did the wider acceptance of the routine of blood transfusion. The tablet was taking over from the standard mixture for sedation and analgesia, and measurements were translated from 'tablespoon', or 'half an ounce', to grains.

The responsibility placed on the nurse for the preparation for the administration of drugs alone warranted a higher educational standard for acceptance for nurse training. In the field of anaesthesia, induction rectally of substances such as paraldehyde and avertin was usually commenced in the ward and left to the nurse for administration. It was inevitable that mistakes did occur through ignorance, but the miracle is that there were so very few. Nevertheless when this did happen, the whole of the nurse's training background was brought into question and explanations demanded as to what a nurse was 'taught', without consideration being given as to what was 'understood'.

The position of the graduate nurse was giving both the W.A.N.A. and the A.T.N.A. cause for concern as the avenues for employment in the private sector were closing. One of the main reasons for this was the acceptance of compensation cases by the public hospitals and the building of community wards which accepted patients without a means test and under the care of their own medical practitioner. This was particularly so in Fremantle and to a lesser degree in Kalgoorlie. The staffing of these sections was largely by probationer nurses. The largest privately run hospitals both in the country and in the city were those administered and staffed by the Sisters of the Order of St John of God, without secular staff. Mount Hospital, administered by a group within the Anglican Church, employed trained staff until it became a general training school. Devonleigh Hospital in Cottesloe, privately owned by Miss Florence Grono and supported by a group of doctors, employed trained staff only, as did St Helen's Hospital in East Fremantle. However both the latter catered for midwifery as well as general patients, so staff required double certificates.

Arising out of this situation, there was a tendency for nurses to travel either to the eastern states or overseas on what could be termed a working holiday, many electing to further their experience and obtain post-basic certificates. Singapore and Malaya were within easy reach, the shipping lines made a feature of very reasonable fares, and chances of employment were good. The coronation of King George VI in 1937 was an incentive for nurses to visit the United Kingdom, as was also the Quadrennial Congress of the International Council of Nurses being held there that year, and to which Australia was being admitted as a member-nation. Mrs Agnes Walsh and Misses Irene Dunne, Norma Monger and Olive Jones were among those who attended, from Western Australia. The Australian Army Nursing Service was represented at the coronation by a group comprising the principal army matrons of all states. Western Australia was represented by Miss J. McDonald, matron of Lemnos Hospital, West Subiaco, and principal matron for Western Australia. Miss McDonald was not from Western Australia and there was some feeling because a Western Australian ex-army nurse had not been chosen. World events were stimulating interest in building up the Army Reserve, and many nurses were 'putting their names down' for active service, as war seemed to be inevitable. The acceptable group was between the ages of twenty-five and thirty-five years for overseas service, which virtually ruled out nurses from World War I, although they were acceptable for home service.

In 1937 the most important event in professional nursing was the acceptance of the Australian Nursing Federation as the national body to represent Australian nurses in the International Council of Nurses.[41] In Australia this was an achievement and ended the stalemate which had developed between the Royal Victorian College of Nursing and the A.N.F. on the matter of amalgamation. This matter, which had dragged on since 1935, was finally solved by a conference held in Melbourne and attended by delegates from all states.[42] Western Australia was represented by Eleanor Harvey and Kathleen Yeates, both of whom travelled at their own expense. When unity was established, a document indicating this was signed by a delegate from each state. (Kathleen Yeates signed for the A.T.N.A. branch in Western Australia.)

Prior to this conference Miss Harvey had suggested at the Western Australian council meeting that I.C.N. membership be used as a lever to bring about affiliation—a united association in Australia. The amalgamation was achieved on 1 June 1937, barely in time for the delegates to get to England to attend the congress opening in London in July. The leader of the Australian delegation was Miss Jane Bell of Victoria, accompanied by Miss Hall of New South Wales. Miss Bell acted as proxy for Miss Kellett, president of the newly formed Australian Nursing Federation. The world president of I.C.N. was Miss Effie Taylor of Canada, and details of the congress are given in the *Australasian Nurses' Journal*, September 1937. The programme is of interest not only because of its content of nursing affairs, but because many of the member nations were to disappear within a very short time.

To the rank and file of nurses, however, there was still some confusion as to the role of I.C.N. and the benefits conferred on member nations through the professional association. They believed it gave world-wide acceptance of the certificates of its members for general practice without taking into account the laws of registration of nurses in each country. Many nurses were disillusioned when, trying to register with the General Nursing Council of England and Wales, they found that their training background was lacking in some areas.

It must be admitted that differences did exist between the W.A.N.A. and the A.T.N.A. regarding their respective roles in professional nursing, but they were equally concerned at the seeming apathy of nursing legislation. In 1937 the first major amendment to the Nurses Act was introduced and assented to in January 1938.[43] The areas affected were:

(a) The Infant Health Certificate of training was accepted.
(b) The introduction of a Children's Register for those who wished to continue paediatric nursing, and the provision of a six months period to be undertaken in a general hospital to qualify for inclusion on the General Register.
(c) The registration of the traditional veil as head covering, restricting its use to registered nurses only, in the sphere in which they were working.

(d) Annual registration of general trained nurses and payment of a fee of one shilling. Provision was made for the removal of names from the register if not renewed after a two year period. However names could be restored to the register on application. Nurses' Registration Board certificates were signed and stamped on the back for each year registered, and registers were published in the *Government Gazette*. By this measure it was hoped to keep a 'live' register, and although registration was not compulsory it was a means of recognition for salary and status.

The composition of the board still remained at five, members being Dr E. Atkinson (chairman); Dr Hector Stewart, medical member; Miss J. Fyfe, succeeded by Miss I. Dunne, representing the Medical Department; Miss E. Simons, who succeeded Miss E. McNevin as matron of Perth Hospital; Miss E. I. Curwood, member elected by nurses. Miss Dunne and Miss Simons were new members. Before her appointment to the Perth Hospital, Miss Simons had been matron of the Queen Victoria Hospital for Women in Melbourne. She was a member of the Royal Victorian College of Nursing and a past president of that organization, and an examiner for the Registration Board of Victoria. Miss Simons had served for two years with the Australian Army Nursing Service during the Great War and was a member of the Returned Army Nurses' Club. Miss E. McNevin had resigned as matron of Perth Hospital to take up a position as matron of the Coast Hospital (now Prince Henry, New South Wales, her own training school).

Factors which increased the pressure on hospital administration were many but can be summed up as follows.

The old Victoria Hospital (I.D.B.) could not cope with an increase in infectious diseases, including an epidemic of diphtheria. The conditions under which patients were being nursed caused a public outcry and a demand for a new hospital. The local authorities who were responsible for the financing of the institution under the Health Act felt that they were unable to do this and it became a question as to whose 'baby' it was, the Department of Public Health or Perth Hospital. At one stage it was suggested that the hospital be removed to Blackboy Hill, which had been the site of the army camps during the World War. Questions were asked in the house at government level and after much debate it was decided to build a new hospital on the present site in Shenton Park. In June 1937 tenders were called and that accepted was for £38 992 with the proviso that the building be completed in six months.[44]

The sister in charge of I.D.B. for many years was Miss Elizabeth

Spring whose name had become synonymous with the institution by the many trainee nurses who had been under her care. In 1938 ill health forced her to retire and her place was taken by Miss Mollie John.

The high incidence of diphtheria in the community could have been partly attributable to the lack of an immunization programme. Some years earlier a happening in Queensland known as the 'Bundaberg Disaster' had made people wary of presenting their children for immunization and seriously retarded the implementation of a programme in Western Australia. However in 1937 some of the local authorities decided that it was safe enough to reintroduce it with the result that the disease lessened dramatically over the next decade. Plans for rebuilding and additions to other hospitals, including Fremantle, Perth Children's Hospital, Northam, K.E.M.H. and a new maternity ward for Kalgoorlie, were put into action. Kalgoorlie also acquired a new Women's Ward, but this was by accident rather than design as the old wood and iron building was gutted by fire. A relic from the gold-rush era, it stood little chance when the kerosene stove used for boiling the ward sterilizer exploded. Fortunately all the patients were safely evacuated as it happened during 'visiting hour'. The staff nurse in charge, Dora Culmsee, showed great initiative in moving the oxygen cylinders away from the blaze.[45]

Funding for these projects was helped considerably by legislation which enabled the setting up of the State Lotteries Commission for the purpose of supporting charitable institutions. Known as 'Charities', a 2s 6d ticket offered to people the chance of a lifetime to attain a 'fortune'. One of the first grants made by the commission was to Perth Hospital, enabling the board to send their pioneer social worker, Sister Aimee Eakins, to Melbourne to undertake a degree course, and to upgrade the Social Service Department of the hospital. Another source of revenue was the distribution of the Jubilee Appeal for youth and motherhood. Two institutions which benefited were King Edward Memorial Hospital and Kalgoorlie Hospital, which received a new maternity ward.

The building of a new Perth Hospital on the old site was deferred, but when pressure was brought to bear on the government by the hospital's refusal to admit patients, building was commenced in 1939. However, because of the intervention of war, the first half (East Wing) was not completed until 1948. (It is recorded that the Hospital Fund Act, introduced in 1930, provided for a hospital tax of 1½d in the £ on all income in excess of £1 per week. The proceeds which had amounted to £275 000 were paid into a trust fund and were used for both construction and maintenance of hospitals.

Because of uniform Commonwealth taxation arrangements introduced in 1942 the state hospital tax was abandoned.)[46]

In 1939 there was a change in administration at Perth Hospital which was to have a far-reaching effect on the nursing profession and remove the dominance of the position of the matron for ever. The appointment of a hospital manager meant his taking over of the domestic running of the wards, issuing of equipment, supervision of linen and laundry services which had hitherto been the province of the matron as recognized 'head' of the institution. The manager has now become hospital administrator and the position is now an integral part of all large health institutions.

The matron, however, did retain her prerogative in the selection of nursing staff and probationer nurses. Service needs demanded an increase in intake of the latter and there was concern that many had to be deferred because they were unable to cope with the educational standards required. A conference with headmistresses of secondary schools resulted in a suggestion that those who failed the entrance examination conducted by the Nurses' Registration Board be given an intelligence test—this to apply to selected students only. The university was approached regarding this matter but replied that the department dealing with this was overcommitted and could not help.[47]

The increase in the student intake resulted in an alteration in the final examination pattern and a system of three state examinations a year was introduced. The N.R.B., which was responsible for setting and marking the examination papers, had relied on the A.T.N.A. for submission of material, as the examination fulfilled a dual purpose, that of N.R.B. registration and of acceptance for membership of the association. This was now discontinued. The A.T.N.A. welcomed the change because it clarified the situation regarding membership. Many nurses who passed their final examinations were under the impression that they automatically became members of the association, and failed to make application and pay the necessary fees.[48]

An attempt to help the nurse teachers by the introduction of a postgraduate course in psychology and methods of teaching through Adult Education was not successful,[49] nor a further effort to establish a central training school using the combined resources of Perth Hospital, Children's Hospital and King Edward Memorial Hospital.

There is mention in the minutes of the A.T.N.A. at this stage of a national health insurance scheme on both a state and federal level, but details are not clear, and it seems to have fallen through.[50]

Two important projects suggested to the hospitals by the N.R.B. and the nursing associations in 1939 were the compilation of a national register of nurses and a roll of assistant nurses, and a re-training of nurses to care for the chronically ill. However both these schemes were thwarted by the fact that war was imminent.

October 1939 saw the death of Sister Mary Ann Nicolay whose presence had dominated the nursing scene for fifty years.[51] She was in her eighty-ninth year. When matron of the Colonial Hospital in 1890, the 'new' Perth Hospital was still on the drawing-board, when she died there, demolition had already begun to replace the 'new' with yet another 'new'. For nursing and for the hospital, it was the end of an era.

CHAPTER FIVE

THE WAR YEARS
1939-1945

The organization of the Australian Army Nursing Service followed the same pattern as that adopted in World War I. It functioned within the framework of the Royal Australian Army Medical Corps, and the head of the nursing service was the matron in chief, responsible directly to the director-general of medical services. Nurses were not given military rank, but were designated as matrons, sisters and staff nurses. The courtesy title of 'sister' was given to both of the latter groups. For purposes of administration a principal matron was appointed to the command in each state and matrons were appointed in charge of the nursing staff of hospitals for both home and overseas service. In Western Australia the principal matron appointed was Miss Margaret Dorothy Edis, and the matron of the Base Hospital, 110 Australian Military Hospital, Miss E. M. (Mollie) Nickoll.[1] Both of the above had served in World War I, and had seen overseas service.

Australian general hospital units for overseas were raised in the eastern states, with some medical and nursing staff from Western Command to supplement the largely state of origin team. Because of the small number of Western Australian nurses chosen, it followed that all A.G.H. matrons were appointed from the eastern states and the only Western Australian trained nurses to be appointed as matrons for overseas service during the war were Miss Eileen Kenny and Miss Ann Jewell.[2] Miss Jewell was matron of the ill-fated hospital ship *Centaur* which was sunk by enemy action on 14 May 1943 off the Queensland coast, and in which ten other nurses lost their lives. A trainee of Perth Hospital, Miss Jewell had been domiciled in Victoria for a number of years and was appointed from the Army Reserve in that state. The nurses' home of Royal Perth Hospital was subsequently named in her honour.

During the first year of World War II only thirty-five Western Australian members of the A.A.N.S. proceeded to the Middle East and the United Kingdom for war service. Later this number increased as the theatre of war changed to include Ceylon, Malaya,

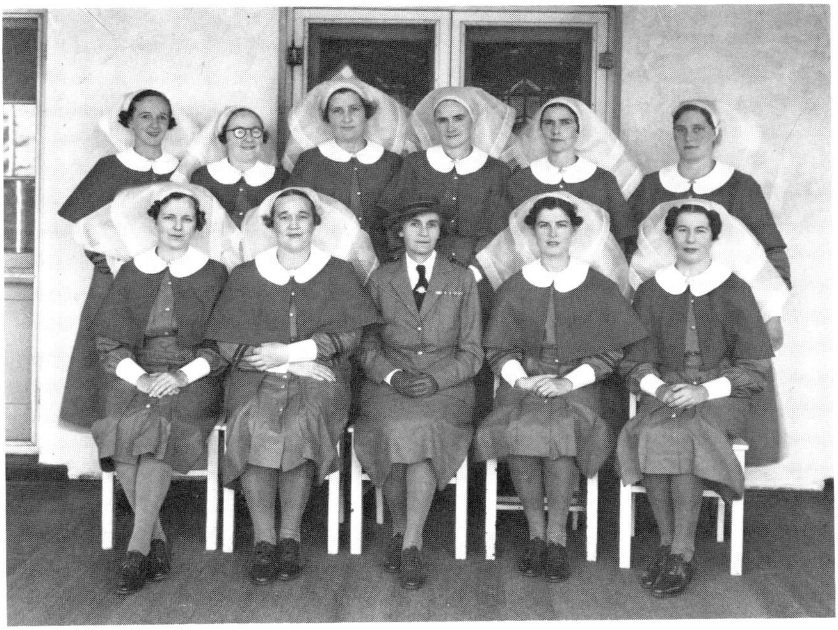

WORLD WAR II ARMY NURSES

The first group of A.A.N.S. to go overseas: *standing:* Staff Nurses E. Ong, R. Warner, M. Dunman, E. Youd, K. Barnes, E. Goff; *seated:* S/N E. Roberts, Sr D. Clinch, M. Edis (principal matron), Sr D. Burgess, S/N I. Membery.

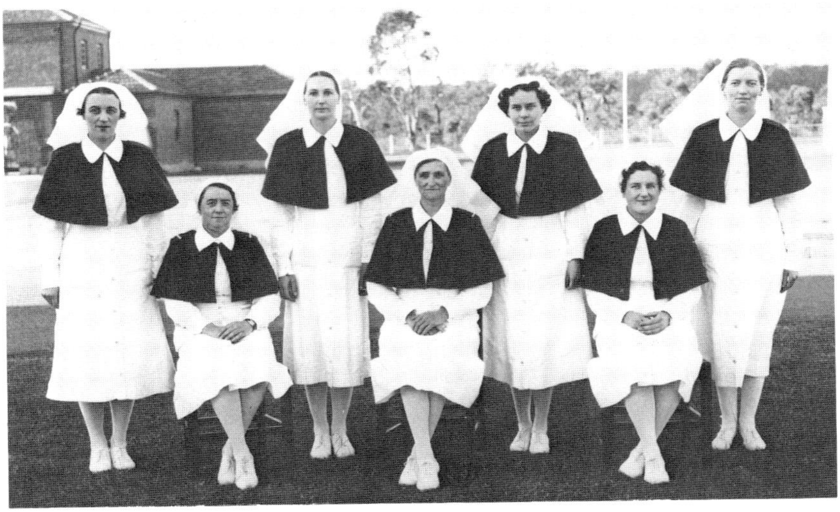

WORLD WAR II AIR FORCE NURSES

The first group of R.A.A.F.N.S. to be called up: *standing:* Staff Nurses P. Bryant, J. Heaney, A. Bennett, M. Vance; *seated:* Sr A. Fiedler, N. Monger (matron), S/N F. Shaw.

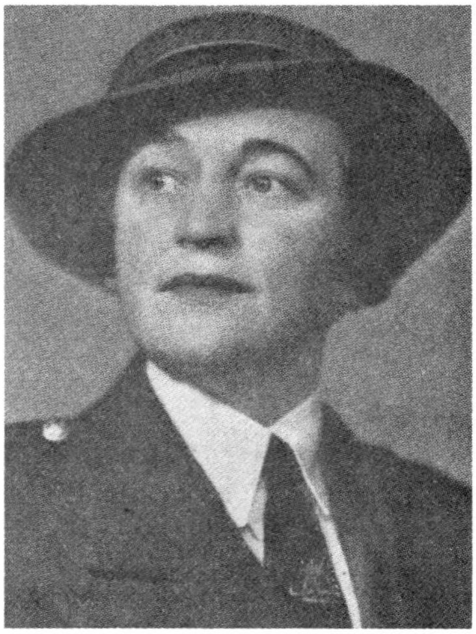

ANNE JEWELL

DIED IN ACTION

Nurses who lost their lives in World War II as a result of enemy action. Anne Jewell was matron of 2/3 Australian Hospital Ship *Centaur*, the others died in Malaya. 'We will remember them.'

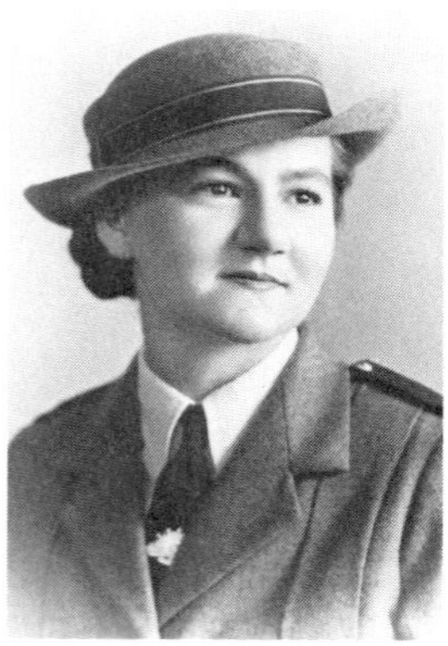

BESSIE WILMOTT

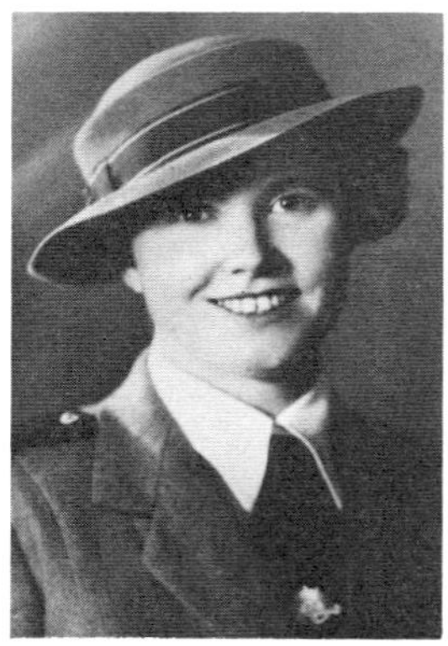

LOUVIMA BATES

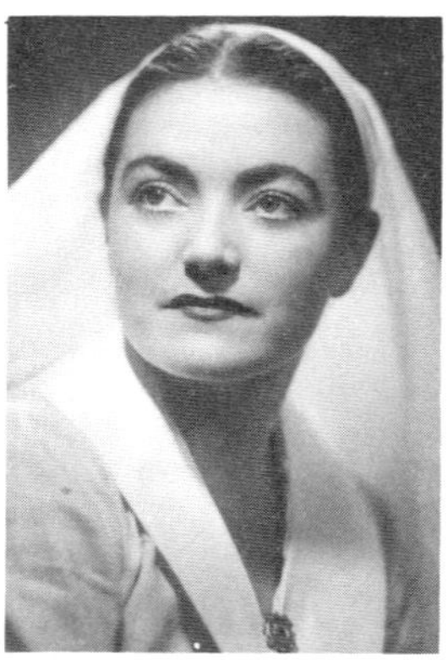

ALMA BEARD

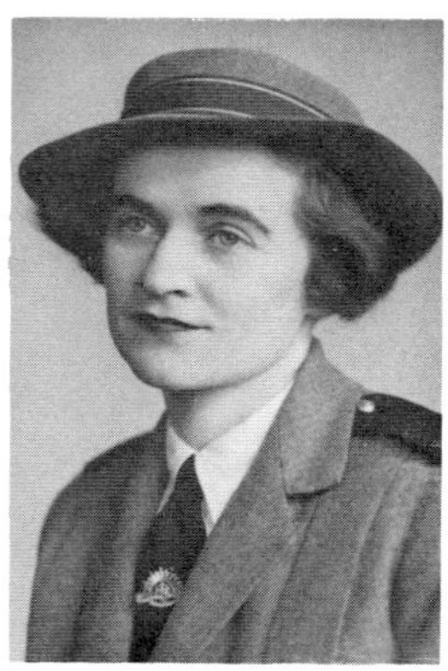

MINNIE HODGSON

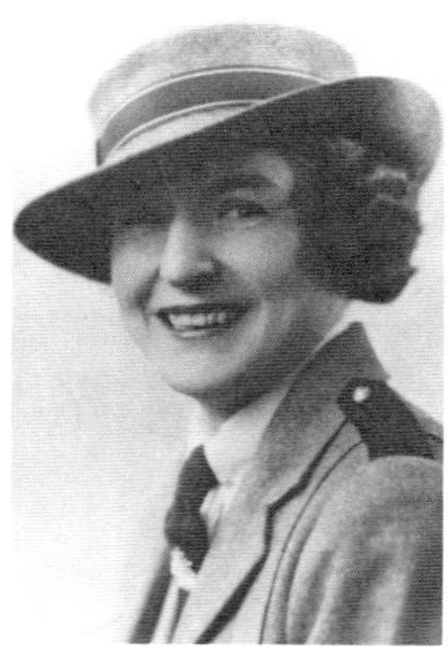

PEG FARMANER

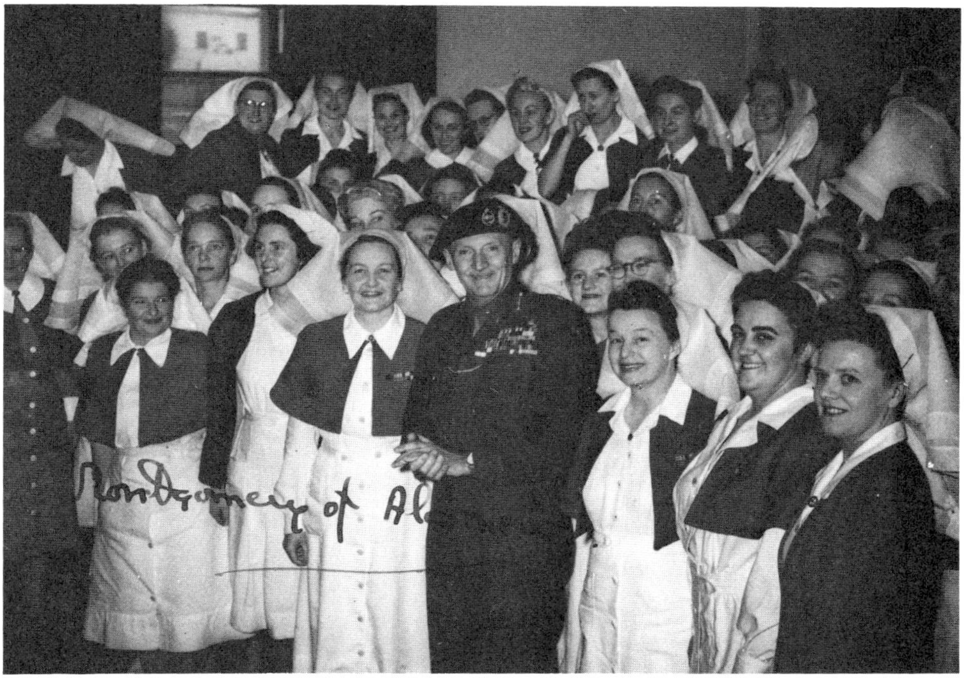

REPATRIATION HOSPITAL, HOLLYWOOD
General Montgomery and nursing staff, 1947.

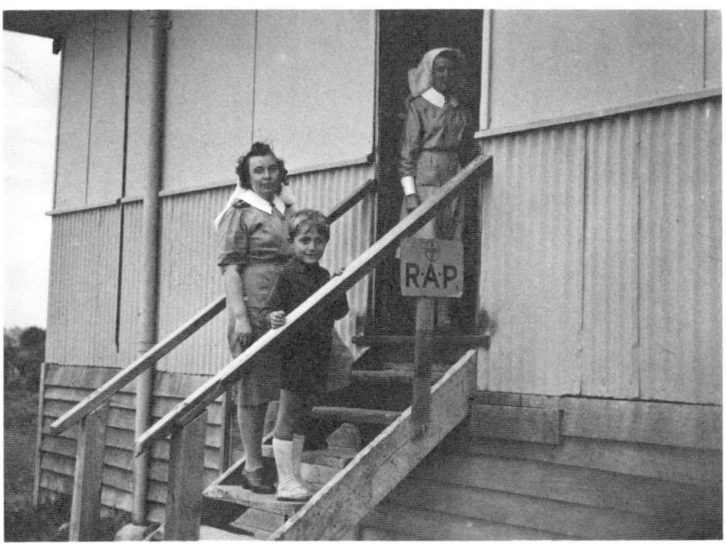

R.A.P., GRAYLANDS MIGRANT CENTRE, 1948
Lieutenant E. Membrey, Captain V. Hobbs and young patient.

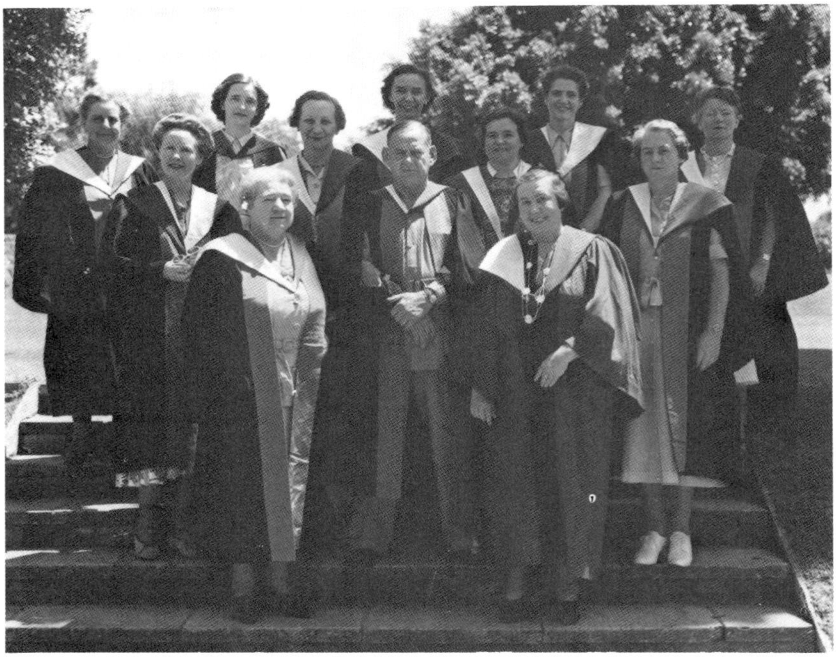

COLLEGE OF NURSING, AUSTRALIA

First annual meeting, Perth 1951. *Back row:* C. Rout, P. Church, V. Steel, G. Williams, V. Gibbs; *centre:* H. Barton, A. Sage, K. Scrymgour, E. Hughes-Jones; *front row:* A. Walsh, General Kingsley Norris, J. Townsend.

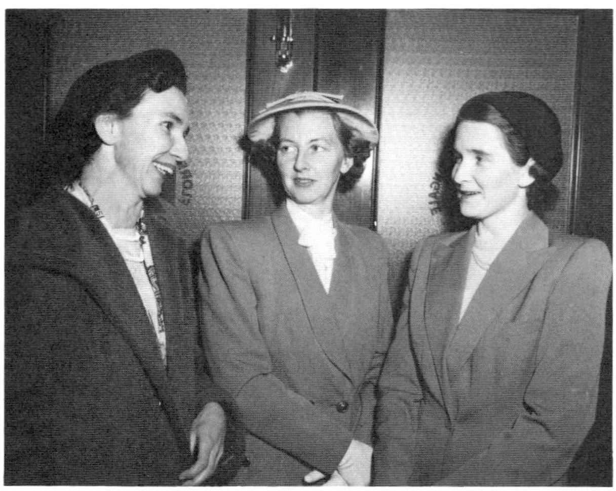

FIRST W.A. FLORENCE NIGHTINGALE SCHOLARS, c. 1950

left to right: V. Steel, B. Gordon, P. Church.

New Guinea and islands of the south-west Pacific. In the Malayan campaign four Western Australians, Peg Farmaner, Bessie Wilmott, Minnie Hodgson and Alma Beard, were among the twenty-one nurses who were shot on the beach of Banka Island, 15 February 1942, the only survivor being Vivienne Bullwinkel, who was later taken prisoner. Another nurse, Louvima 'Vim' Bates, was drowned when the ship she was on received a direct hit and was sunk. She was one of ten to lose their lives. Iole Harper was one of the thirty-two nurses who spent three years in a Japanese prisoner of war camp in Sumatra until liberated in 1945. Nine of them died during that time.[3] Of the six nurses taken prisoner by the Japanese in Rabaul and transported to Japan, there were no Western Australians. These nurses were released on the cessation of hostilities. A composite memorial to all nurses lost due to enemy action was erected in Augusta, Western Australia, in April 1978.

In 1939 the problem arose of finding a suitable hospital or building for conversion to a military hospital. The old Base Hospital at Fremantle had ceased to exist, and the Military Block at Perth Hospital was needed for the civilian population because while the old wards had been demolished, the new building had not been completed. After inspection of many suggested sites, 'Lucknow', a private hopital in Stirling Highway, Claremont, was selected to become the 10th A.G.H. Later another hospital of the same name in Queenslea Drive, Claremont, was converted to a hospital for the women's services and known as 'Knutsford'. The staffing of the military hospitals was maintained by those members of the A.A.N.S. awaiting movement overseas, but as time went on a stable staff of those ineligible for overseas service was maintained.

Changes in the pattern of warfare and the build up of troop concentrations in camps such as Northam and Melville brought the problem of sickness associated with crowded conditions. Influenza, infectious diseases such as measles, with complications, meant the opening of camp dressing stations, afterwards upgraded to field hospitals. In 1940 there was an outbreak of cerebro-spinal meningitis. A newly completed hospital block at Claremont Mental Hospital in Davies Road was taken over by the army. Fortunately most of the patients responded to treatment with the drug M & B 693, although there were some deaths.

Quarters for the army nurses were a secondary consideration, and those who occupied them can now look back in retrospect and laugh for after all there was a war on. From the beginning staff of the hospitals was augmented by members of the Voluntary Aid Detachment which subsequently became the Australian Army Medical Women's Service (A.A.M.W.S.).

The military hospital at Hollywood was built in 1941 and occupied in the middle of that year. It was a pavilion type hospital spread out over a large area, and designated the 110th Military Hospital. The grounds were prepared and the trees planted by the Italian prisoners of war brought from the Middle East following the campaign in the Western Desert.

In 1941 the Royal Australian Air Force Nursing Service was formed, the first nurses from Western Australia being Norma Monger, principal matron, Jean Wheatley, senior sister, and Audrey Bennett, Mary Vance, Florence Shaw, Phyllis Bryant and Jean Heaney. After being equipped at Laverton in Victoria, they returned to Western Australia and were posted to Pearce Air Base, and were later joined by others. A ward at Hollywood was allotted to them for members of the air force service.[4]

Nurses entering the armed services had to cope with generally unfamiliar disease conditions en masse. Wards of anything up to a hundred beds were designated for the treatment of patients with a specific infection, i.e. malaria, gastro-intestinal conditions such as dysentery, 'scrub' typhus, infectious hepatitis, glandular fever, etc. Following the New Guinea campaign, the wounded were usually suffering from the above as well as their surgical conditions. Infestation with parasites such as hookworm was common.

It was chemotherapy on a large scale, with hitherto unknown drugs such as atebrin, insoluble and soluble sulphonamides. Atebrin, which was used extensively as a prophylactic against malaria, coloured the skin a bright yellow, which masked signs of other conditions, so the onus for diagnosis was placed on pathological findings. The collection of specimens became the responsibility of the nursing staff, as were the initial patient records of the results. It was pointed out that these could have an important bearing on the patient's entitlements for repatriation benefits due to war service. In 1943 penicillin became available for general use by the Australian army, but it was not used in a Western Australian civilian hospital until 1944. The effect can be described as nothing less than magic, changing as it did the approaches to medical and surgical treatment.

Blood transfusion as supportive treatment meant the setting up of blood banks on an unprecedented scale and the discovery of blood components such as the Rh factor was the forerunner of the exchange transfusion which was to play such an important part in the lives of mothers and babies.

For civilian nursing the dominance was more on the everyday surgical and medical conditions of the older age group in the community, with surgery of election rather than that of emergency.

People evacuated from Malaya and Ceylon did introduce some tropical conditions, and the build up of both the civilian and service population resulted in an increase of venereal disease. Generally it highlighted the fact that nurses needed more nursing education to equip them to cope with the rapidly changing structure of their profession.

The work of the plastic surgeon and his team of specially trained staff came into prominence during the war years. Their experience was to be of untold benefit to people during the post-war period and has progressed ever since. In Britain, the Middle East and other theatres of war, injury from burning led to a revolution in the treatment of burns and their repair by skin grafting, and with the advent of penicillin the lessening of infection scarring and contractures, which had been a foregone conclusion for those who had been severely burnt, were reduced to a minimum in many instances. Prosthesis, pioneered by the facio-maxillary units, has led to the reconstruction of limbs and joints, and the continued research for materials acceptable to the body plays a major part in the rehabilitation of people in today's world.

Despite the fact that war was dangerously near, there was an acute shortage of nursing staff which persisted long past the 'duration'. The most badly hit areas were the country hospitals so that in the end government direction of manpower in nursing was inevitable. Among the suggestions put forward to cope with the situation was one to place the control of nurses under the Medical Department and this was effected by the appointment of two senior members of the nursing profession, Misses Mary Reid and Ivy Curwood, as 'manpower' officers.[5] On completion of training nurses were directed to areas most urgently requiring their services. Unfortunately the salary structure was not commensurate with the positions, and this created problems for the W.A.N.A.

Married nurses were asked to return to nursing. It was suggested that the number of babies 'delivered' to obtain the Midwifery Certificate be reduced from twenty to ten, a move that was strenuously opposed. The closing of Hillcrest Hospital at Fremantle as a midwifery training school meant that K.E.M.H. was the only obstetric nurse training school in the state. To cope with the acute nursing situation, Mount Hospital was accepted by the N.R.B. and the A.T.N.A. as a three year general training school in 1941.

A scheme was put forward for the utilization of military hospitals as training schools by interchanging the civilian student nurses with the V.A.D.s so that the latter could get experience in the women's wards. However it was decided that the venture would not be acceptable to the students who would be disadvantaged by the greater uniform allowance and pay packet of the V.A.D. (A.A.M.W.S.). It was also envisaged that if such a scheme became a reality, prospective trainees nurses would take advantage of the army training with the inevitable decline of entrants through hospital channels. This would have had serious repercussions in the government hospitals, which were not included in the scheme. It was also suggested that an outdoor uniform be approved for the civilian nurse but the problem of the decision as to the entitlement of the wearer in addition to obtaining extra ration tickets became the deciding factor against it.

One group of nurses not dissatisfied with food rationing were the trainees at King Edward Memorial Hospital who remarked that with the introduction of rationing their tea and butter allowance had greatly improved on what it had been previously.

In 1942 accommodation had become a major problem, especially for nurses. People from Malaya, returning servicemen from the Middle East, and service personnel from the United States made the acquisition of even a room impossible. The War Nurses' Hostel fund was opened and a building purchased in Ord Street, West Perth, in 1943 and converted into a hostel for service nurses on leave and requiring accommodation.[6] There was at this time a further A.G.H., the 118th at Northam of almost a thousand beds, and the 1st A.G.H. returned from the Middle East and was set up in Merredin. Guildford Grammar School, too, was taken over and converted into a hospital for United States servicemen.

The hostel was governed by a committee which subsequently became the War Nurses' Memorial Association, and Miss I. T. Borwick, A.R.R.C., a First World War sister, voluntarily undertook the management as part of her war effort. In the post-war period the property was sold and the hostel was moved to Mount Lawley. When it ceased to be a viable proposition this property too was sold and the money obtained converted into a trust fund, administered by the War Nurses' Memorial Association.[7]

On the civilian side, the problem of accommodation for the aged nurse was causing concern to both the W.A.N.A. and the A.T.N.A. According to Miss Bottle, then A.T.N.A. president, some of the women were desperate, as they could no longer afford the high rental being asked for the poorest of rooms. One contribution to the situation was the fact that many servicemen married while on leave but could not provide homes for their wives, so that in many cases the young wife and often a child boarded with the parents and grandparents, some of whom in other times might have let rooms, a situation which continued well into the post-war period.

The fund inaugurated by the A.T.N.A. in 1924 in line with the

Constitution for the relief of aged and incapacitated nurses was handed over to a specially formed committee which in 1941 became the nucleus of the organization known as the Society for the Care of Aged or Incapacitated Nurses (Western Australia) Incorporated, the objective being to raise additional funds towards the establishment of 'a home which will serve the needs of all nurses who through age or infirmity require such consideration'.[8] The original sum was £456 4s 9d and thirteen War Savings Certificates. Membership was set at ten shillings per annum and anything not less than ten guineas paid in a single sum entitled the subscriber to 'life membership'. The first six 'life members' were Mr F. Hadley, Mrs A. M. Walsh, and Misses R. Bottle, M. D. Edis, K. Yeates and Mr. E. Gillett.[9]

It was not until August 1943 that a house was purchased at 25 Davies Road, Claremont, and a home established. It was named Eleanor Harvey House as a memorial to Eleanor Harvey, who had died on 17 January of that year. All the nursing associations combined to provide for the furnishings and upkeep of the home and have done so ever since. The first guests were not charged any fees but over the years and with the improvement of social services a modest rental has been charged to cover the overhead expenses.

Although the question of a new home for aged women in the community had from time to time received much comment in the press and other agencies, the Women's Home, or Old Women's Home as it was usually referred to, was still housed in the original Lunatic Asylum in Fremantle. For many years the matron of the institution had been Miss E. Jenkins, assisted by Miss Helena Hutton, who became matron on Miss Jenkins's retirement.[10] Although the function of the home as a maternity hospital had ceased, the grim old building was still thought of as having been a poorhouse.

During the war the inmates were evacuated to Woodbridge, near Guildford, and the Fremantle building occupied by American servicemen. It was not until 1951 that the concept of a modern home for aged women took shape in the Mount Henry Home at Como overlooking the Canning River. Today it is looked upon as one of the most modern extended care centres in the community but, even so, in the minds of some people there is still the stigma of its origin, the poorhouse. Miss Hutton has explained that nurses who had to become inmates of the Women's Home through force of circumstance, and there were quite a few, were given some preferential treatment involving responsibility for such tasks as taking charge of the bread and butter, etc. Earlier attempts to provide a home for retired nurses was always hampered by lack of funds. It is recorded that one retired nurse offered her home to the association on the condition that she be allowed to live there and be cared for. The offer was refused because it was felt that in the event of her death the association might not have been able to meet the expense of her funeral.[11]

At this time, the A.T.N.A. and W.A.N.A. each had delegates on the council of the other body. A problem which did not make for the happiest of relationships between them was the fact that the trainee nurse members of the W.A.N.A. had full voting rights and were entitled to be elected to the council of that body, while in the case of the A.T.N.A. the trainee nurse was an associate member and not entitled to a place on the council. This was, as stated in a letter from Miss Norma Monger, an A.T.N.A. Council member, 'a trained nurses' association' and therefore the acceptance of the W.A.N.A. president was out of order as there was the possibility of her ineligibility for full membership of both organizations.[12] A request from A.T.N.A. members that they form their own council seems to have been dismissed out of hand. A strong supporter of both organizations was Miss Olive Anstey of Perth Hospital. Realizing the personality and potential of this dynamic young woman, who was to become the world leader of nurses, Miss Carlin lost no time in getting her interested in nursing affairs. Almost from the minute she completed her basic training in 1944, Olive Anstey was elected to the Council of the A.T.N.A. as a full member of the Australian Nursing Federation.[13] Like Norma Monger, Olive Anstey had a strong political background which was to prove invaluable in her future service to nursing. In 1943 Miss Simons resigned her position to be married, and Miss G. Siegele was appointed matron of Perth Hospital. That same year Miss Olive Jones was appointed matron of Fremantle Hospital on the resignation of Miss S. Jones, who had followed Miss M. Balding as matron.

August 1944 was a time of crisis for nursing when the staff of the Claremont Hospital for the Insane walked out in protest at being unable to get sufficient staff for the female wards. Although nurses at Claremont Hospital were given on the job instruction and issued with a certificate of competence, the hospital was not an accredited training school for mental nurses and did not come under the control of the Nurses' Registration Board. The mental nurses had their own industrial union, which was affiliated with the Australian Labor Party. There was no shortage of nurses in the male wards, possibly because most of the attendants had been there for a number of years and were outside the age of recruitment for the services. However, with the women it was a different situation as the institution had relied heavily on the assistant nurse and those waiting to be called up for general training. Most of the nursing was custodial care, and attendants had to have attained the age of eighteen years. With the large number of young women being recruited into the women's services or manpowered into essential employment, there were very few indeed who wanted to work in mental institutions, where the conditions of work left a great deal to be desired. For the immediate period student nurses from Perth, Fremantle and the Children's Hospitals were seconded to Claremont, but this was ruled out by the Nurses' Registration Board because of the disruption of their training, as Claremont was not a training school. The use of army personnel was also ruled out by the prime minister, John Curtin, because it was illegal.[14]

As the situation became more desperate, Minister for Health Panton stated that he would over-rule the Nurses' Registration Board by bringing down legislation which would result in nurses within the state being directed to nurse where ever needed. This did not eventuate but he did introduce an amendment to the Nurses Act to provide for the acceptance of a training programme in mental nursing resulting in state registration and final examination by the board.[15] Those nurses who already held the in-service certificate of the Claremont institution were given recognition of their status and registration. Training in mental nursing was offered to any who wished to undertake the course irrespective of their educational qualifications. The representative of mental health on the N.R.B. had stated that if all entrants needed to have the same standard as for general training, they would chose to undertake the latter course and the mental institutions would be without staff.

In the same amendment the Midwives Board was abolished and the registration of midwives and control of their training was transferred from the Health Act to the Nurses Registration Act. The membership of the board was increased to nine members, appointed by the governor: the commissioner of public health, ex officio, and chairman of the board; the inspector-general of the insane, ex officio; two medical practitioners, one of whom was practising as an obstetrician, both nominated by the British Medical Association; two senior registered nurses on the staff of a nurse training school or hospital, in active practice as such, one of whom was trained and experienced in midwifery nursing and infant welfare nursing; a general trained nurse, a mental nurse and a midwifery nurse who were registered in accordance with the requirements of the act and who were nominated respectively by the general trained nurses, by the mental nurses, and by the midwifery nurses who were also registered under the act.

With the promise of improved working conditions, pay increase, etc., members of the Mental Nurses' Association returned to work.

As was pointed out, the hospital was outdated and the new block which had been occupied by the military was unoccupied, due presumably to lack of staff. A programme of renovation and upgrading of facilities was put into operation. Just how desperate the situation had become is shown in the headline news of the *Daily News* of 5 August 1944:

> *City Staffs*
> *Comb-Out Goes On*
>
> Comb out of City business houses by the Manpower Directorate to secure staff for the Claremont Mental Institution will continue until that institution is fully staffed. Those interviewed will be women employed in work that is considered less essential than the work of caring for inmates of the hospital. Despite the fact that these measures have been taken over the past three weeks without respite the Manpower Directorate has not yet been able to supply sufficient numbers for the work . . .

The placing of unskilled people in charge of those mentally ill and the inevitable effect on both is indicative of the level of care of the mentally ill at that time.

Some of the infant health sisters were also not happy with changes in departmental policy which meant that one nurse could no longer be permanently attached to one particular clinic in the metropolitan area.

A question which arose indirectly from the industrial action taken by the Mental Nurses' Association, was whether the W.A.N.A. would affiliate with the Australian Labor Party as a means of obtaining security.[16] A meeting was held to debate the proposal and the majority of members voted against joining a political organization. Rather, it was suggested that it would be more beneficial if the A.T.N.A. and W.A.N.A. in this state were to amalgamate.[17] However, nothing further was done at this time.

With the end of the war in sight, it was envisaged that there would be large numbers of nurses in Commonwealth employment in the Department of Repatriation, and these would need to be covered by an industrial award. In Western Australia there was already an association with access to the Arbitration Court at state level, the W.A.N.A., and it was suggested that the organization investigate the possibility of gaining federal recognition. However the Federal Council of the Australian Nursing Federation did not favour this move and felt it better that federal recognition be achieved by the federal body. In 1921 the Victorian Trained Nurses' Guild had gained recognition by the federal court and there was a movement to make this the Federal Employees Section of the

A.N.F. This was opposed by the Hospital Employees Federation, which had a nurses' section and federal recognition in the eastern states. What followed is complicated and long drawn out. Over the ensuing years, the guild became the Australian United Nurses' Association, and eventually the Australian Nursing Federation Employees Section of the A.N.F.[18] and some twenty years were to elapse before agreement of a type was obtained from the various nursing bodies in all states.

In 1946 nurses who returned from serving in the Australian and British services found a hostile environment in the community brought about by the acute shortage of nurses in civilian hospitals,[19] especially in the country, and the unfulfilled expectations that this would be alleviated by the discharged service personnel. Until such time as the army establishments were taken over by the Repatriation Department, nurses were retained and discharge from the services was slow. The first to be released were the married women who, now reunited with their husbands, were anxious to settle down and have a family. Secondly, those who wished to join the Repatriation Nursing Service were given an accelerated discharge. The department's policy was the employment of qualified nurses, and terms of employment were most attractive, including transfer with seniority and the privileges of service time to count towards long service leave. The hospitals were modern and there were exciting advances in medicine and surgery. Furthermore there was an empathy and a nurse-patient relationship based on shared experience and a pattern of nursing care integrated with the discipline of the army hospital which they both understood. There was also that indefinable something which is born out of war, and forms a bond between those who serve which can never be broken.

Other factors which affected the shortage in Western Australia were the rehabilitation programmes financed by service authorities whereby nurses could undertake further training to obtain post-basic certificates, in approved hospitals offering midwifery and infant health training. As King Edward Memorial Hospital was the only training school for obstetric nursing in the state, and its intake was limited, there was a drift of nurses out of the state. Because of the structure of the course, infant welfare training at K.E.M.H. had not been acceptable to this scheme and was therefore discontinued.

Deferred pay was paid in a lump sum, and this gave opportunities for travel and furthering of experience. A large number of nurses went to South Africa and the United Kingdom, and there were some who used this opportunity to undertake postgraduate courses in teaching and nursing administration overseas. The army and air force too both retained nursing personnel for service in the establishments associated with the post-war service and the occupation force in Japan, and later during the war in Korea. There were also those who returned to their former positions with the Medical Department, but there was not enough of them and conditions generally were unsatisfactory. There was a shortage of equipment and the buildings themselves needed upgrading. There was also the inevitable shortage of domestic and ancillary staff resulting from the lifting of manpower restrictions.[20]

The reaction of the general public through the press, the Medical Department, and even some members of the medical profession is unbelievable. Headlines in large black print appeared daily giving stories of closure and inability to maintain a sufficient number of beds. In 1946 the successful application to the Arbitration Court and the granting of an award with substantial increases in pay and a forty-four hour week gave rise to statements by hospital administrators that hospital finances were near breaking point and there would be an added burden on the taxpayer. A long-term solution was the encouragement given to members of the A.A.M.W.S. to undertake general training under the rehabilitation scheme, but here again numbers were limited by the standard of educational entrance.

A more immediate solution was the employment of the male nurse. There were men who had been nursing throughout the duration in the A.A.M.C. and the naval and air force medical services. These were credited by the Nurses' Registration Board with part of the time served, the remaining period to be served in an accredited training school. Here again the educational aspect presented problems, and at Hollywood Hospital a school was inaugurated to help. A number of male nurses were employed at Wooroloo Sanitorium, but the general attitude towards the male nurse was that his employment must be confined to the nursing of male patients, which limited his use in the country hospitals which had a comparatively small bed average. In 1946 the male nurses formed their own association,which embraced the trained as well as the assistant nurse and which was accepted in the Court of Arbitration.[21] It ceased to exist in the fifties when the male trained nurses joined the state branch of the Australian Nursing Federation.

The following extract from a letter to the *West Australian*, 31 January 1946, sums up the attitude to the situation. Under the heading, 'A Doctor's Suggestion', and signed Dr G. Hall, Cunderdin, it reads:

> The widespread shortage of hospital nurses and domestics has

> revealed that there is a shortage of female labour throughout Australia . . . . Why should such a shortage have suddenly arisen after a war in which thousands of young males from Australia were killed and in which very few females lost their lives? There can only be one conclusion—that there are at present many women holding down jobs which they should turn over to men who have returned from the war and are unemployed. During the National Emergency these women did a patriotic service by doing a man's job but now they are doing their country and their boys in particular a dis-service by remaining on . . .

The inference is clearly that nursing and domestic work are solely female occupations.

Tuberculosis, or T.B. as it is commonly referred to, had always been a contributory cause to the numbers of people who were chronically ill and in need of hospitalization. However, unless the patients had nowhere to go, such hospitalization did not usually become effective until they exhibited some positive signs and symptoms of the disease or their condition was such that their families were unable to cope. Wooroloo Sanitorium, built in 1916, in the hills some thirty-two kilometres outside Perth, was constructed on the pattern of open verandah type wards, and the treatment was based on that practised in other parts of the world, i.e. rest, open air and a nourishing diet, and above all, good basic nursing care. Very few of the nurses at Wooroloo contracted the disease in contrast to those at Perth Hospital who nursed the patients during their referral stage.

With recruitment for the services it was found that one in every 300 healthy young men showed signs of T.B. on the chest X ray which was part of the medical examination, thereby pointing to the fact that the incidence of the disease was much higher than previously thought. Among those accepted for service, there was again on discharge the tell-tale radiological evidence of possible lesions, either missed in the very early stages or acquired during war service. To cope with the situation, in 1946 the army reopened the Military Hospital at Northam for the purpose of confirming diagnosis by pathological tests, and for the treatment of those found to have the disease.[22] The move met objections both from the people of Northam, who did not want a T.B. hospital in their area, and from the men who were forced to go there and be separated from their wives and families. Everything was done to help in the matter, and the people from the town and surrounding areas rose magnificently to the occasion once the situation was explained and they were assured they would not be exposed to infection.

For the patients it was a calamity which most of them could not believe had happened as they did not feel ill and had no outward signs, not even a cough. The treatment was soul destroying—complete bed rest for weeks or months on end and in some instances, surgery. Minor procedures were carried out at Northam, but for major surgery the patient was transferred to R.G.H. Hollywood. For the nursing staff, who were all Army Nursing Service, assisted by nursing orderlies from the R.A.A.F. and the R.A.N.S., it was an experience in health care which involved the patient, his family and the community and the patient ceased to be thought of as a disease statistic and became very much a person.

Every Sunday a free train was provided for families and visitors (cars were still at a premium) and all members of the medical and nursing staff were made available to help with hospitality and counselling, and to care for the children under fourteen who were not allowed contact with their fathers. On the civilian side, the Wooroloo community began a special care programme which involved a sheltered workshop and a small farming community where families could live together and the children have medical supervision.[23] This of course did not happen immediately, the immediate problem being the detection of T.B., which could only be achieved by an organized programme of mass X ray, and which the Anti-tuberculosis Association, formed in January 1946, had as its first priority. Political pressure and advances in chest surgery resulted in the closure of Northam Military Hospital and the transfer of the patients to a block in R.G.H. Hollywood. It was envisaged that the Commonwealth would build a specialized chest hospital for the treatment of all T.B. patients, both civilian and service, and Dr L. Le Soeuf advised that the land adjoining the Repatriation Hospital would be the most suitable location. Ironically when this became a reality in 1958, the 'fight against T.B.' was almost over.

The seemingly higher incidence of tuberculoses among miners could have been due to the fact that all those in the industry were required to have annual chest X rays, which led to early detection. The classical question, 'What are the signs and symptoms of early T.B.?', and the answer, 'There aren't any', could have applied.

During the war years the headquarters of the International Council of Nurses had been transferred to the United States, but with the cessation of hostilities it was decided to return to London, and the Florence Nightingale International Foundation was reformed within the structure of the I.C.N.[24] Changes in nursing theory and practice brought about by the rapid advances in medicine and surgery and their complexities more than ever emphasized the need for an extended curriculum and qualified nurse teachers and administrators to put it effectively into practice. At the end of the war, there were no nurses in the above category, with recognized qualifications on an international level, in Western Australia. In an attempt to solve the problem, the Royal Victorian College of Nursing had earlier introduced an extra-mural course for sister tutors which was undertaken by Miss Constance Livesey but this course did not entirely fulfil the requirement.

The Australian Red Cross Society had made money available for six scholarships to enable a nurse from each state to undertake the Sister Tutor Diploma course at the Royal College of Nursing in London, covering a two-year period. The scholars were chosen by the Florence Nightingale Memorial Associations in each state, which conferred on them the honour of being 'Florence Nightingale Scholars'. The recipient in Western Australia was Miss Patricia Church, a tutor at Perth Hospital where she had completed her basic training, and also a graduate of the University of Western Australia, where she had gained a Bachelor of Arts degree. In 1947 the nursing associations in the state, supported by the staffs of all hospitals, held a large exhibition which created widespread interest and was also successful as a fund-raising venture. This was coordinated by the state Florence Nightingale Committee and enabled another student, Miss Verna Steel, to be sent overseas, to undertake the sister tutor course at the Royal College. The following year Miss Kathleen Johnson was awarded a Florence Nightingale scholarship which took her to London, to study for the course in hospital (nursing) administration. Miss Johnson was also a graduate of the University of Western Australia, and was eventually to become Royal Perth Hospital's first and only Western Australian trained nurse to hold the position of director of nursing (formerly matron) of her training school.

Two other students were also awarded scholarships for post-basic study in New Zealand. They were Barbara Gordon, who returned to become senior tutor at R.P.H., and Alice (Jenny) Mattinson, who succeeded Mrs Walsh as matron of K.E.M.H. A condition of acceptance of a scholarship was that the recipient was bonded to give two years service in a specific area associated with her field of study.[25]

It was realized that postgraduate nursing education was of great importance to Australia and to further this objective the formation of a Florence Nightingale National Committee was essential. Discussion with the council of the Australian Nursing Federation was held, the outcome of which was that the A.N.F. agreed to act as a national council until the states each had time to form or re-form a Florence Nightingale Memorial Committee at state level for the specific function of raising funds for post-basic education and in co-operation with organizations with a similar interest to found an Australian college of nursing for the purpose. There were however two schools of thought on such a venture, based mainly on its possible situation and overall administration. Some of the state nursing bodies favoured a separate college in each state with a federal co-ordinator. There was also the suggestion that if one college was formed it should eventually be located in Canberra. In Western Australia, Miss Connie Livesey's suggestion that the college should be along the same lines as that of the Royal Victorian College of Nursing, extra mural, that is, as an extension of the University of Western Australia, was favoured, but an approach to the university ruled this out as the university had no provision for such a course. The idea of separate state colleges was favoured by the nursing organizations of New South Wales to the extent of their forming a committee to bring this to reality. The secretary of this committee was Olive Anstey, who had transferred to New South Wales to undertake midwifery training and to obtain wider experience in nursing practice. She was also organizer of the New South Wales Nurses' Association for a year, and it was because of her office experience that she was asked to act as secretary for the proposed college.

On 26 February 1949 the *Sydney Morning Herald* featured an article headed 'Special Training for Nurses' in which it was stated that it was proposed to set up a college in New South Wales and that it had been formed by the four professional nursing bodies, the A.T.N.A., N.S.W. Nurses' Association, the Institute of Hospital Matrons (N.S.W. and A.C.T.) and the Trained Nurses' Guild, N.S.W. Branch. In view of the fact that a national college was about to be launched, with headquarters in Melbourne, reaction to the New South Wales college was not favourable and resulted in the withdrawal of the A.T.N.A. (N.S.W.) from the venture, to support the national organization, and the creation of some animosity in Western Australia which was reflected in the refusal of Miss Anstey's request for publicity in the *Journal of the West Australian Nurses* on the grounds that it might jeopardize support for the national venture.[26]

On Saturday 2 April 1949 a conference was held in Melbourne at the Women's Hospital, convened by the special subcommittee of the National Florence Nightingale Memorial Committee of Australia and plans were finalized for the founding of an Australian college of nursing. The Western Australian delegates and observers to the conference were Mrs Agnes Walsh (National Florence Nightingale Memorial Committee of Australia), Miss M. D. Edis (Australian

Nursing Federation, W.A. Branch A.T.N.A.), and Miss Jean Freeman (Trained Nurses' Guild). The only state not represented at the conference was Queensland, an apology being received from Miss J. Abbott. Delegates to this conference were made foundation members of the college and also members of the Interim Council. The Western Australian delegate to the Interim Council was Miss M. D. Edis who was accompanied by Mrs Garnsworthy. The simultaneous press release to all states read as follows:

> Last Saturday week 25 nurses, leaders in their profession from all over Australia and representative of all nursing organizations were present at a conference in Melbourne when plans were finalized for a new educational body—College of Nursing, Australia. This college is to provide post graduate education; ward sisters, sister tutors and administrators will be specially trained for their positions—and will fill a very great need in Australia.[27]

Regarding the founding of an Australian college of nursing, the following extract from A.T.N.A. minutes is of interest as it would appear that in any event the state of Victoria was to have a college, either state or national, preferably the latter:

> Miss Crawford asked if any reply had been received regarding information of the War Nurses Memorial Centre in Victoria.
> A letter from Miss Lindsay, regarding this matter reports:
> Re War Nurses Memorial Centre
> (a) Would the scheme benefit nurses throughout Australia? Yes, it is visualised that the proposed centre will be of benefit to nurses throughout the Commonwealth.
> (b) Is it only for the State of Victoria? No, it is Victoria's effort as a memorial, but the Constitution provides that the Centre's facilities shall be open to all nurses in Australia.
> (c) Is it intended to become the Royal Australian College of Nursing in the future? While it might well become the Royal Australian College of Nursing, this is not the present intention.[28]

Yet on a souvenir programme of a huge function held on the St Kilda Cricket Ground, on Sunday 14 March 1948, sponsored by the media, the following statement was made.

> The objective of the War Nurses' Memorial Appeal is to establish in Melbourne a centre at which nurses may undergo post graduate training for higher administrative and executive positions without having to go overseas, and where amenities

including accommodation, library and recreation facilities will be offered to all nurses. There will be special facilities for disabled war nurses and nurses awaiting or recovering from hospitalisation.

The centre will fittingly commemorate the 75 Australian nurses who died for their country in the Second World War and its utilitarian purpose will benefit not only the nursing profession as a whole, but also the community in general.

(signed) Miss E. Hughes-Jones
Honorary Secretary[29]

It is small wonder that the nurses themselves were confused on the issue.

The first president of the newly formed college was Miss A. M. Sage, R.R.C., and matron in chief of the Royal Australian Army Nursing Service, from Victoria. She was followed by Mrs A. M. Walsh, O.B.E., who was elected at the inaugural meeting of the College of Nursing, Australia, on Saturday 18 February 1950 at the Royal Australian College of Surgeons, Spring Street, Melbourne. The official guest was Dame Katherine Watt, D.B.E., R.R.C., nursing advisor to the Ministry of Health, U.K., and the guest speaker, Dame Enid Lyons, D.B.E., M.H.R., vice-president of the Executive Council.[30] The founding of the college coincided with a highly successful public appeal for funds for a memorial to honour those nurses who had lost their lives during the war. It resulted in the purchase of a large house set in extensive grounds in St Kilda Road which was designated the Nurses' Memorial Centre, created for the use of nurses and nursing organizations. A substantial part of this building was offered to the College of Nursing, Australia, and adapted to its use.

The year 1946 heralded a change in the pattern of nursing education in the training hospitals, when a modified block system of teaching was introduced into Fremantle Hospital by Miss Helen Bailey, who had been appointed as sister tutor. This system operated along the same lines as that proposed in the 1930s and allowed for nursing students to be withdrawn from the wards for the purpose of a study block at intervals throughout their training. In this way it was possible to have lectures and tutorials in an organized manner without the pressure of having to be released from ward duties. The result was reflected in their high performance at state registration examinations.

Dora Helen Bailey had been in England just prior to the outbreak of war, her 'profession' being that of wool classer, for which she was attending a convention. Her interest stemmed from the family farming property near Beverley in Western Australia. She also had teaching experience. Her stay in England during the war years induced her to undertake nursing training at Queen Elizabeth Hospital in Birmingham and her midwifery with Queen Mary's Maternity Hospital, Hampstead Heath. Her basic and post-basic experience before returning to Western Australia in 1946 made her well equipped for the organization and introduction of modern trends.

After sixteen months at Fremantle, Miss Bailey resigned and joined the Medical Department where, with the then commissioner of public health, she organized a scheme of nurse training to meet the needs of the smaller country hospitals. The plan was to set up a central training school for nurses undertaking training in hospitals controlled by the Medical Department. It was to be a complete block system — the first of its kind in Australia — and was designed to give the essential theoretical and clinical instruction in a series of study blocks associated with a particular hospital chosen for the purpose. In order to implement the plan, a special appointment was made within the Medical Department, and designated 'organizer of nurse training', the appointee being answerable only to the commissioner of public health. Miss Bailey was the first to hold the position, which not only involved planning and taking charge of the nurse training programme, but required her to visit schools in the capacity of a recruiting officer, for potential nursing students.[31]

An unsuccessful quest for premises in the metropolitan area resulted in the Central Training School being accommodated at Northam Hospital, the unused children's ward being converted into classrooms and the old isolation ward being used as quarters. In its initial stages three hospitals, Northam, Narrogin and Collie, were the first to be associated with the Central School and for the purpose were upgraded by the Nurses' Registration Board to full-time training schools, the period of training being dependent on the clinical material available and the average number of occupied beds exclusive of those occupied by maternity patients. It was planned that more government hospitals would participate, the limiting factor in the beginning being lack of accommodation.[32]

The school opened on 15 September 1947, and during the remainder of the year nineteen nurses — one male and eighteen female — completed the preliminary course. As part of the plan, the clinical instructors (junior tutors) from the school accompanied the students to the various hospitals to become resident tutors. In 1948 it is recorded that additional nurse training schools were established in connection with hospitals at Geraldton (29 March 1948) and Merredin (12 November 1948). The hospitals at Katanning and Busselton were also approved by the N.R.B. as training schools.

Kalgoorlie was visited by the organizer of nurse training on three occasions to give the senior nursing lectures. Ninety-three students passed through the preliminary training school at Northam. Of this number three female and ten male students were appointed to Wooroloo Sanitorium and two male nurses to Royal Perth Hospital. Seven discontinued training during the year. Some of the students were ex-service personnel who had been nursing orderlies and who were training under the rehabilitation scheme. In all hospitals, lack of stability of trained staff and inability to obtain modern essential equipment adversely affected the training programme.

The decision of the Nurses' Registration Board to introduce a first year examination as from July 1948, known as the First Professional, necessitated premises being found in Perth to accommodate students returning to the First Year Study Block which coincided with the N.R.B. examination. As a temporary measure use was made of the Country Women's Hostel at Cottesloe and, later, an unused building at King Edward Memorial Hospital was used to house the nine students for the first 'block' school, following which the vacated army officers quarters opposite the university at Crawley were converted into temporary classrooms.

During 1948 the search for a site for the Central Training School was continued without success. Finally arrangements were made for the purchase of Devonleigh Private Hospital at Cottesloe. The midwifery section was retained as a maternity hsopital, but the general wing became the Central Training School and was used for both preliminary students and those coming into First, Second and Third Year Blocks. Pending the erection of a large prefabricated classroom, a marquee was used. The school at Northam was closed and the Kalgoorlie students joined the blocks. Miss N. Tant, well known to the nurses over many years, was appointed home sister and part-time tutor.

As the teaching load increased and the work of organization opened up it was realized that there was need for a suitably qualified person to take charge of the training school and leave the organizer free to do the work intended. Ministerial approval was granted for the appointment of such a tutor, but it did not materialize as no other tutor was available. This meant that the teaching responsibility fell on to one person, leaving little time for school visiting and advance recruitment of nurses. However wireless broadcasts to interest girls in nursing were given and lectures in psychology, physics and chemistry arranged for the junior tutors.

An earlier amendment to the regulations by the Nurses' Registration Board had ruled that under certain circumstances the period of training in a smaller training hospital could be shortened provided that six months of the student's time was spent in a larger A-class hospital. Metropolitan hospitals were approached regarding cooperation, but the plan for using them did not materialize and students from Collie and Narrogin Hospitals were transferred to Kalgoorlie Hospital after their First Year Block for the final two years of their training thereby making the training period of all students three years. Geraldton and Northam Hospitals remained the full three years training schools. The other smaller hospitals were phased out. Two badges were also designed, one for the Central Training School and one for Kalgoorlie Hospital. The badges were almost identical and it seems to indicate that the two establishments were originally intended to be two separate institutions.

In 1950 Helen Bailey reported that the close proximity of a school to a midwifery hospital, e.g. the Central Training School at Devonleigh, was undesirable and another site for either of the above should be obtained as lack of space hampered the teaching programme. No alternative was made available at this point.

In 1951 Helen Bailey resigned to go overseas to further her post-graduate education in Edinburgh, and Edith Harler was appointed organizer of nurse training in her place. Another appointment was Verna Steel, to the position of principal tutor. The school continued to function as the Central Training School until its transfer to 18 Colin Street, West Perth, in 1955 when the name was changed to Government School of Nursing. When Verna Steel resigned to take up an appointment in Melbourne in 1954 Vicki Hobbs was appointed in her place and occupied the position for the next sixteen years until her retirement from nursing in 1970.

Although nurses through their nursing organizations had been pressing for years for a better system of nurse education, they were far from happy with the introduction of the Central Training School and its method of implementation, which they considered a retrograde step. They felt also that the Nurses' Registration Board had yielded to outside pressure. The concern arose following the 1944 amendment to the Nurses Act when the Nurses' Registration Board was enlarged and assumed control of the midwives and mental nurses. New members appointed to the board, because of their positions, were considered to have a bias towards the Medical Department. The first regulations framed to administer the act were presented and withdrawn. The reason for this is not known as copies do not seem to have survived, but the board functioned for the next three years without new regulations. When the setting up of the Central Training School was imminent the regulations were prepared and gazetted 10 February 1947, having been assented to 22 November 1946. Changes contained were clearly in favour of the establishment of a method aimed at providing staff for the smaller country hospitals. The first regulations under the provision of the Nurses Registration Act 1921 contained the following:

> Three years is prescribed as a course of training provided that the Board may require the period of training to be longer . . .
> In respect of the Government hospitals approved by the Board, the wards of Wooroloo Sanitorium shall be regarded as medical wards, and the period of training in the said wards shall not exceed one year . . .

There is no mention of a definite number of daily occupied beds needed but hospitals were required if they desired approval as training hospitals to make application through the medical officer in charge or the matron giving specific details. Following the first major amendment to the Nurses Registration Act 1921-1937, gazetted on 2 August 1940, the rules were drastically revised and in the 'general section' hospitals were classified as 'A' and 'B'. For the purpose of such classification

> (a) Class A general training hospitals, shall be those which have an occupied bed average of not less than 40 adults of both sexes, excluding midwifery cases; and
> (b) Class B general training hospitals, shall be those which have an occupied average of not less than 30 adults of both sexes, excluding midwifery cases.

Under the 1947 regulations the revisions are as follows:

> (a) Class A general nurses' training hospitals shall be those which have a daily average of not less than forty occupied beds, excluding midwifery cases . . . when the whole of the course of training is undertaken in such a hospital . . . a minimum period of three years . . .
> (b) Class B general nurses' training hospitals shall be those which have a daily average of not less than twenty occupied beds excluding midwifery cases. . . . when the whole of the training is undertaken in such a hospital a course of training is provided for a minimum period of four years.

There was little change in the curriculum, the anatomy and physiology section still had no mention of the reproductory system, male or female, and the number of lectures required to be attended by the student remained the same—two-thirds of the lectures and demonstrations given, the minimum number given in the major subjects to be twelve.[33] On the other hand the average daily number of occupied beds required by a midwifery training hospital had to be sixty, which ruled out any but King Edward Memorial Hospital.

Regarding mental nurse training, the applicants were not required to pass the educational examination of the N.R.B. before commencing training but were allowed to take the examination any time before sitting for the registration examination. The advantage in passing the examination was that on completion of training, a state registered mental nurse could be granted a remission of one year's training should she wish to undertake general training.

Since the retirement of Nellie Ursula Lynch from the Medical Department, the position of secretary to the Nurses' Registration Board had reverted to being a Public Service appointment according to seniority, which meant that the appointee was not necessarily a nurse. In spite of requests from both nursing organizations, the A.T.N.A. and the W.A.N.A., the position remained unchanged. However the main cause of discontent was the title given to Miss Bailey's position, that of organizer of nurse training.[34] Members of the Matrons' Association, an independent autonomous body, made a formal protest to the minister and enlisted the support of the matrons' associations in other states, as well as the A.T.N.A. The main cause of their concern was fear that while Miss Bailey was carrying out her recruitment programme, people might be misled into thinking that she controlled the training of nurses for the whole state including the metropolitan training schools, which did not come under her jurisdiction. However the protests were of no avail and the title continued to be used. The matrons of the country hospitals were also resentful. Although they welcomed the relief from staff shortage, they felt that they had not been completely put in the picture and that the position of organizer of nurse training was a threat to their status, and also that the whole thing was a fait accompli.

Another matter of concern was the power given to the minister to lower the age limit for commencing nursing training. This was dropped to 17½ years and in special circumstances, seventeen years. As nurses were unable to register until they were twenty-one years of age, this meant a nurse might have completed her training period and passed the registration examination but would be employed as a fourth year nurse until reaching the required age. It was also a matter which would affect her salary and status.

A further amendment to the act to allow short-term training was not considered a wise move. A two-year programme for tuberculosis nurses in 1946 and mothercraft nurses in 1948 were looked upon as short-term solutions to the immediate problem of staffing the hospitals, but not in the best interests of the trainees in those fields because there was a slim chance of future employment once the vacuum had been filled.[35] The W.A.N.A. accepted the short-term trainees, reluctantly, for membership but the A.T.N.A. had difficulty in equating it with membership of the I.C.N.

In the late forties and early fifties changes in the pattern of treatment of illness required the professional nurses to master new skills. Acute anterior poliomyelitis struck savagely and produced an illness of long-term management. Immunization programmes and penicillin had drastically reduced the numbers of patients with scarlet fever and diphtheria, but in their place were those with polio to whom the tank respirator had necessarily become a way of life. The management of these patients and the complex mechanisms of the machines used in their care was a long and difficult process. It marked the beginning of long-term resuscitation and changes in the management of people with spinal injuries and other neurological conditions. Nurses had to be taught to cope with the situation.

The migration programme planned for the early post-war period promised some relief from the shortage of staff in government-controlled hospitals. People entering the country under this scheme had to be directed for two years in essential work and this temporarily solved the shortage of domestic and auxiliary nursing staff in hospitals.

The first migrants arrived in Western Australia in October 1947 and for a very short time occupied temporary quarters at Graylands. However they were mostly men and boys and were moved on quickly to the eastern states by train, the ship turning around to return for more passengers. In the first intake there was one English family, the rest being from Malta and other Mediterranean countries. Most had been living under crowded conditions in concentration camps and the immediate health problem was 'scabies' for which they were treated en masse by the staff of the Regimental Aid Post, set up by the army and staffed by two members of the Australian Army Nursing Service, Captain V. Hobbs, and Lieutenant E. Membrey. Before the arrival of the migrants the nursing post acted as a first aid establishment for the exhibitors, especially in the animal section, of the Royal Agricultural Society's annual show. Many of these attendants were girls who had worked on the land, and with the lifting of rationing, had made their first purchases of fashionable shoes, the result being that there was a constant stream for medical attention for 'blistered heels'.

Subsequent ships did not disembark their passengers at Fremantle but went straight on to the eastern states. The Graylands establishment closed and the nursing staff along with other members of the A.A.N.S. were transferred to New South Wales and Victoria to become the nucleus of the nursing service attached to the Interim Army, and served in the camp hospitals and the military establishments with the Occupation Forces in Japan and the Long Range Weapons Establishment at Woomera, South Australia. When migrants finally arrived for settlement in Western Australia they were accommodated at Holden Camp at Northam, where a maternity section was set up and administered by Miss H. G. Doyle, a First World War sister. Most of these migrants were from Baltic countries and were 'displaced persons'. They were eager to work and accepted positions on the domestic staffs of hospitals or as assistant nurses. The main difficulty was that they spoke little or no English and the language problem together with the fact that they could not produce papers to prove their nursing experience precluded their acceptance by the Nurses' Registration Board as state registered nurses. However under a system of assessment in hospitals, many were subsequently able to register.

All hospitals had to adjust to a large migrant intake, and especially the maternity hospitals, such as K.E.M.H., and it was in this field that Miss J. Mattinson, with the cooperation of migrant staff, was able to inaugurate an interpreting service which was of immense value to these people. Migration was not a one-way exercise, for in addition to those coming into the country, there were the wives of the United States and Canadian servicemen leaving to join their husbands. Quite a number of these were nurses.

CHAPTER SIX

THE FIFTIES

The years from 1949 to 1959 marked the attainment of unity within nursing and adjustment to changes in the pattern of nursing care and nursing education in a rapidly changing world. Following the combined conference of the Australian nursing organizations which marked the inauguration of the College of Nursing, Australia, in 1950, it was felt that in Western Australia there was the opportunity for the unification of the Western Australian Nurses' Association and the Australian Trained Nurses Association (W.A.) to form one nursing body. After long discussions and legal interpretations the amalgamation of the two associations was assented to by the members of the combined councils of the two organizations on 12 January 1954 in the Florence Nightingale Club Rooms.[1] 'Miss Siegele opened the Meeting, giving a resume of what had been done to achieve the amalgamation of the two bodies. The first meeting to discuss this project was held in 1949 and it had reached finality in December 1953 when the Constitution had been accepted by the Court of Arbitration.'

Those present were as follows: Members representing A.T.N.A.: Miss Siegele (president), Mesdames Walsh, Ferguson and Green, Misses Edis, Crawford, Stokes, Leslie, Johnson, Mattinson, Harris, Harler, Richardson, Lee, Spencer, Youd. Members representing the W.A.N.A.: Miss Broadway (president), Misses Wells, Guilfoyle, Campbell, S. Martin (proxy for Miss Wallace) and Reidy. (Unfortunately no initials are given.) An interim committee was formed and a special general meeting was called for 4 February 1954, to be held in the Royal Perth Hospital main lecture hall. It was pointed out that all financial members of the A.T.N.A. who were not members of the W.A.N.A. needed to be enrolled in the new association before they were eligible to vote or be elected to council. The name of the association was to be the Royal Australian Nursing Federation (W.A. Branch) Industrial Union of Workers. The question of an office was debated, and the merits of the A.T.N.A. office in the Florence Nightingale Club were compared with the room occupied by the W.A.N.A. in the AMP building at the corner of William

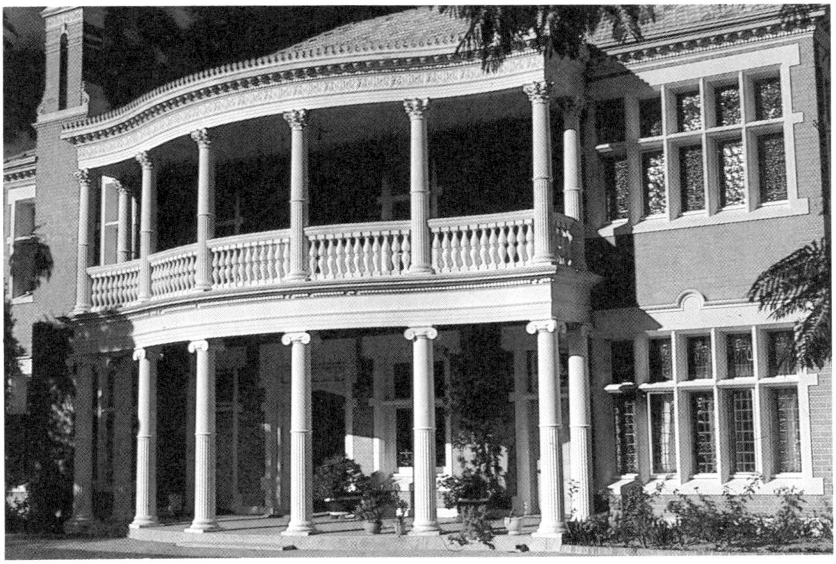

GOVERNMENT SCHOOL OF NURSING, 1955
Collins Street, West Perth

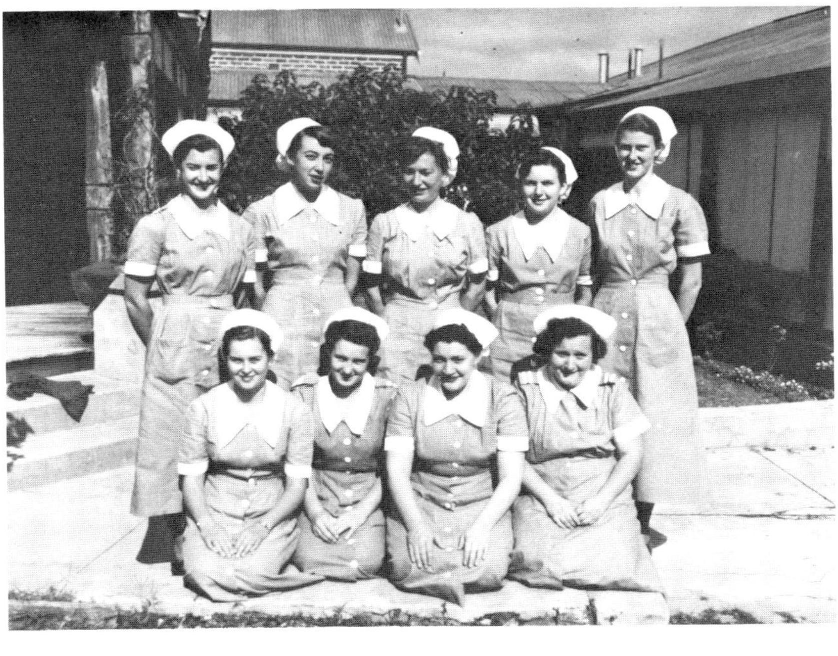

CENTRAL TRAINING SCHOOL
First Year Block at Devonleigh Hospital, 1950. *Back row:* —, J. Betts, J. Prendergast, P. Collings, J. Jones; *front row:* B. Longworth, —, D. Giblett, F. Wiley.

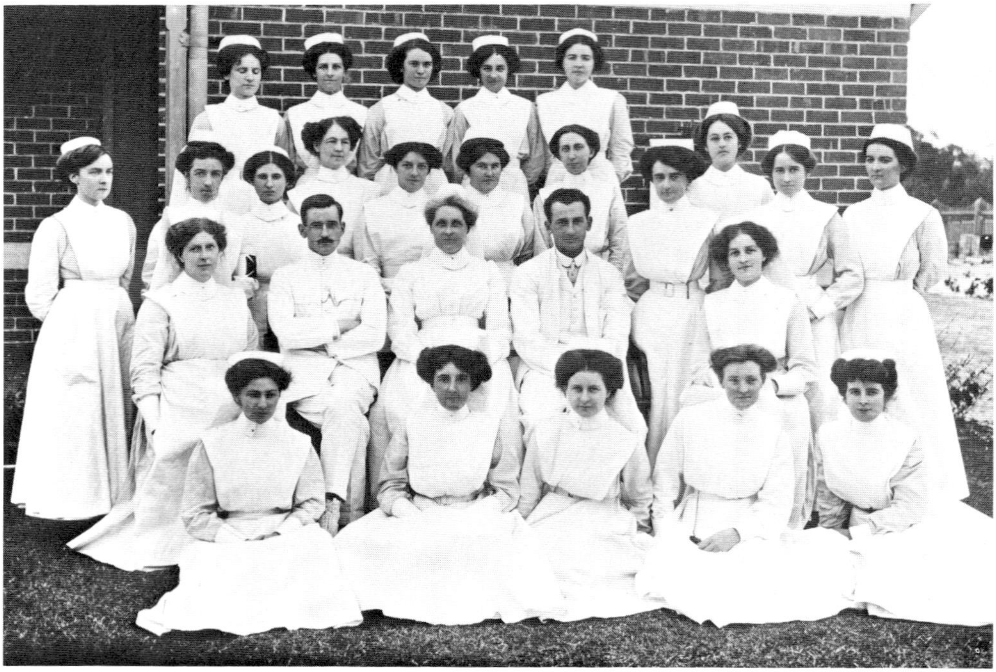

PERTH CHILDREN'S HOSPITAL, 1911

back row: D. Paterson, G. Cook, C. Smith, M. Bailey, E. Hamersley; *second row:* S. Fitzpatrick, —. Green, M. Miller, P. Pustkuchen, M. Hunt, A. Williams, M. King, H. Homan, H. Williams, M. White, D. Bell; *third row:* J. Cassell, Dr H. Gray, A. Anderson (matron), Dr M. Cave, E. White; *front row:* I. Proudfoot, A. Brown, I. Jefferson, M. Peake, A. Burton.

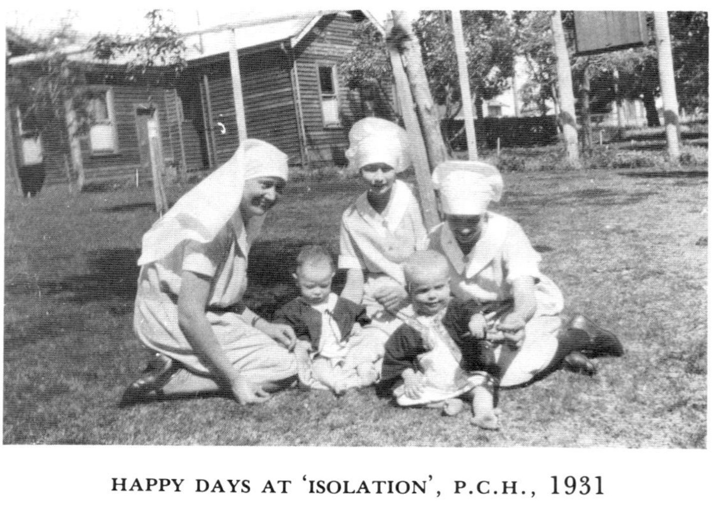

HAPPY DAYS AT 'ISOLATION', P.C.H., 1931

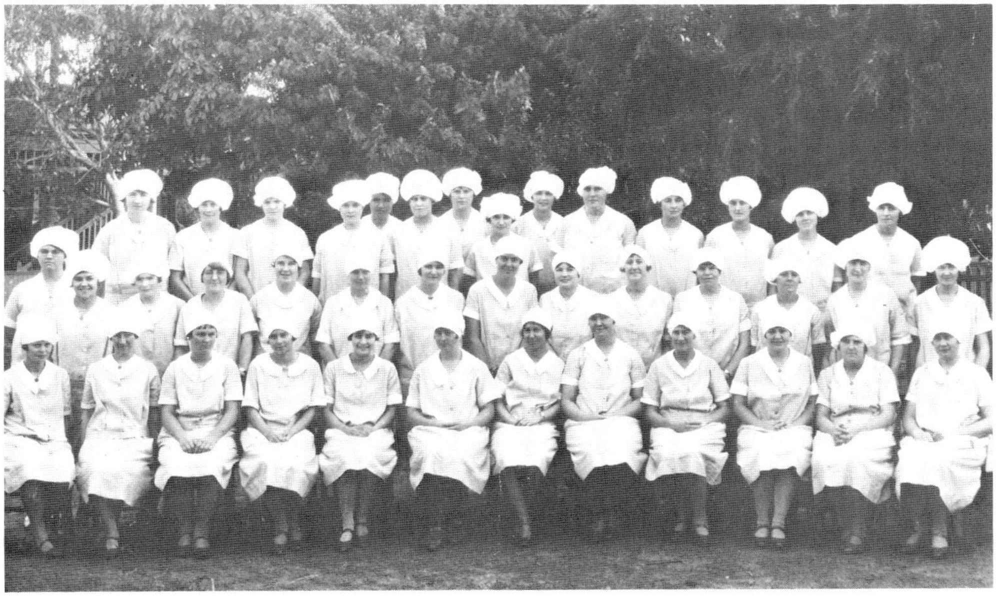

P.C.H. TRAINEES, 1928

back row: P. Fowler, U. Wright, —. Delaney, D. McGrath, O. Edeson, J. Solomon, B. May, F. Inkpen, K. Newman, E. Corteen, M. Copley, K. Moore, G. Boundy, R. Williams; *centre:* J. Pullen, M. Inkpen, P. Beecher, R. Warner, L. Clinch, N. Liveright, J. McGrath, G. Kidd, M. Cranfield, D. Wallace, W. Hawkesley, J. Thomas, R. Stebbs, A. Schurman; *front row:* E. Robertson, A. Blackett, M. Wickham, J. McDonald, —. Blair, E. Gibbs, M. Young, M. Bergin, L. Keeper, M. Leishman, J. Wren, G. Morrell.

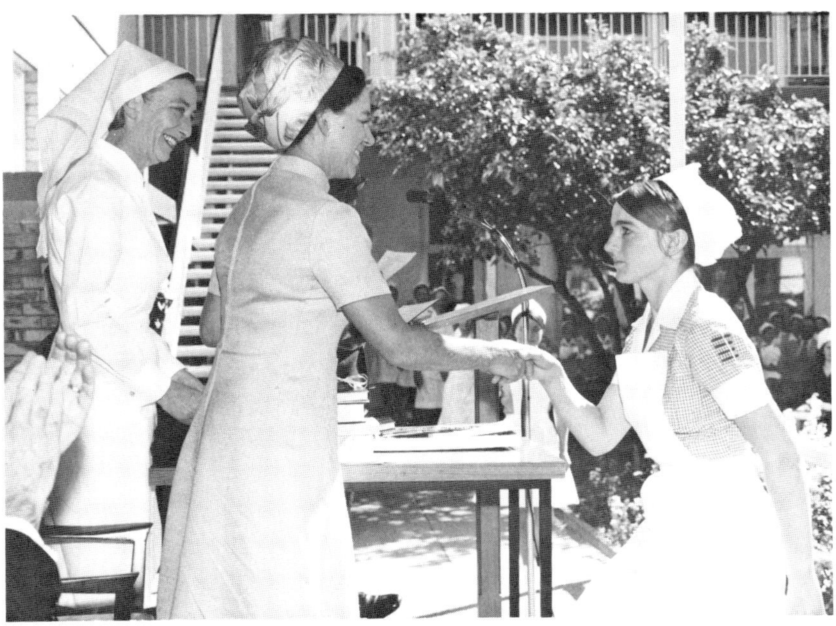

PRINCESS MARGARET HOSPITAL, OCTOBER 1972

formerly P.C.H. Here H.R.H. Princess Margaret presents S. Armstrong with her certificate, with J. Butt (matron), left.

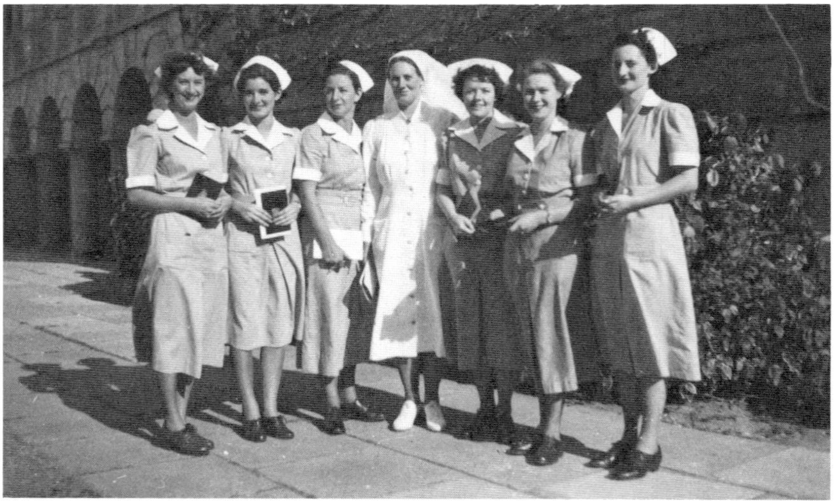

MOUNT HOSPITAL GRADUATES, 1950

left to right: M. Underwood, N. Nix, —. Marsden, A. Harris (tutor), B. Stewart, —. Drummond, B. Howells.

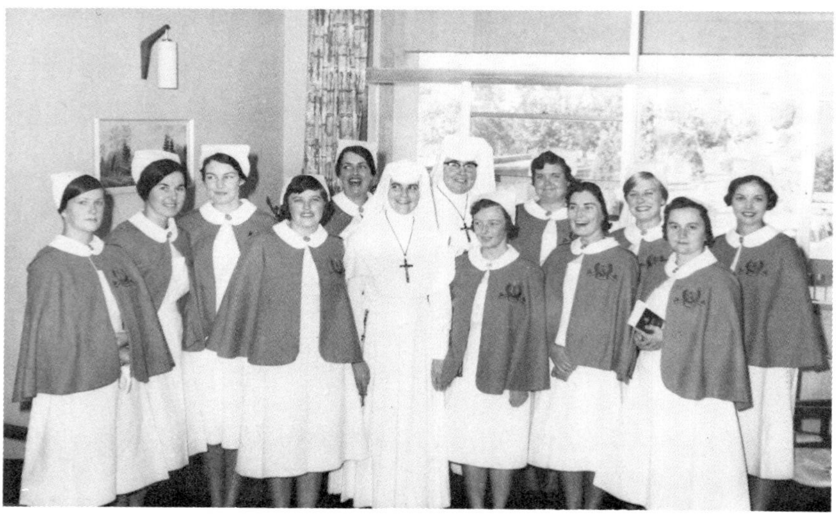

ST JOHN OF GOD HOSPITAL, 1965

Sisters Evaristus and Cecily with the first group of secular graduates.

Street and St Georges Terrace. The latter was the eventual choice. Miss K. Reidy, secretary of the W.A.N.A., was appointed secretary of the new association.

The positions of nurses who qualified for the federal award was less satisfactory because of the lack of unanimity between the Australian United Nurses' Association and the federal body of the Australian Nursing Federation, which was in the process of reconstruction with the appointment of a full-time organizing secretary following the transfer from Sydney to Melbourne in 1951. To facilitate matters the A.U.N.A. applied for a change of name and became the Australian Nursing Federation Employees Section (A.N.F.E.S.) and was registered in the federal Court of Arbitration and Conciliation under that name. Branches of the A.N.F.E.S. were set up in most states and operated within the framework of the state branches of the Australian Nursing Federation. In Western Australia members of the committee of the A.N.F.E.S. automatically became members of the council. What it meant was that the A.N.F. was supporting two organizations and a common membership fee was charged. In 1956 the A.N.F. was granted the prefix 'Royal' and became the R.A.N.F. A visit from the secretary-general of the federal body, Miss Avery, resulted in the setting up of sub branches of the A.N.F. in some of the larger country centres to stimulate interest among nurses living and working in these areas. A peculiar situation developed in Kalgoorlie where a very vigorous ex-trainees association had been functioning for a number of years, when it was found that many of its members, although ex-trainees in the true sense of the word, had never completed their training and were therefore ineligible to join the sub branch. However the two functioned well.

The move to the A.M.P. buildings was completed in 1956 after the closure of the Florence Nightingale Club rooms in the Mercantile Mutual building which was under a process of reconstruction. For some time the club had not been a viable proposition and its existence relied on the A.T.N.A. office attached. With the expansion of hospitals and their teaching departments and new nurses' homes there was a move for the ex-trainees associations to be accommodated in their respective training centres, where visual aids and hospitality of the boards of management together with parking facilities made a convenient location for lectures and social gatherings. For R.A.N.F. Council meetings, the A.M.P. rooms proved adequate, but for the larger meetings there was a problem, and although the hospitals were generous in providing venues, it was felt that the time had arrived to procure permanent offices and a centre for nursing activities. At the annual meeting of the state branch held 26 July 1956 the budget was presented by Miss A. J. Mattinson, who in conclusion stated as the 'Aim of the Federation in the future':

> A nursing centre where all meetings large and small could be held. A place of dignity with room for expanding office staff, a reception room for rental and bringing in a certain income. Flats or rooms to let.
>
> We must aim at prestige in the community.[2]

At the annual meeting of 1957 there is no mention of progress towards a centre either in business arising out of minutes or the president's address. But there was an appeal by Mrs J. E. Ferguson to support the War Nurses' Memorial Hostel in Queens Crescent, Mount Lawley, which was providing accommodation for convalescent and visiting nurses. A possible reason for this was that the annual meetings of both the College of Nursing, Australia, and the federal meeting of the R.A.N.F. were being held in Perth that year and council members were preoccupied with these events. There was also an industrial award before the Arbitration Court.

In 1958 the matter of a nursing centre again came up for decision when it was stated 'that because of the expansion of the R.A.N.F. it is necessary to think of owning our own building; therefore a committee has been formed to investigate the possibility of this' (the names of those on the committee were not given).

Following on this a special general meeting was called, and held in the lounge of the Perth Chest Hospital on 18 November 1958. The meeting was presided over by Miss P. Lee, president of the R.A.N.F. (W.A. Branch). It was stated that following the setting up of the special committee to investigate the possibility of providing a centre, it was brought to their notice that a building was on the market which might be suitable for purchase for their purpose, but that the council had no power to place an option on any building and it was desired at this meeting to confer upon the council the powers necessary to purchase a property. Ways and means of raising finance were discussed and it was decided that there should be an appeal organizer and that the existing investigating committee should form the nucleus of an appeal committee. Members of the committee have been identified as Maude Anderson, theatre sister P.M.H.; Olive Anstey, matron Perth Chest Hospital; Stella Boxsell, senior staff member R.G.H. Hollywood; G.(Biddy) Dodd, assistant matron R.G.H. Hollywood; Beryl Grant, subsequently matron Ngal-A; Rose Broadway, sister in charge of casualty R.P.H.; Mavis Leworthy, matron Northam District Hospital, subsequently matron Fremantle Hospital; John Mullaley, senior staff member R.G.H.

Hollywood, rep. A.N.F.E.S. Those elected were Doris Richardson, organizer Friends of R.P.H.; Joyce Gilbert, assistant matron Perth Chest Hospital; John Brett, principal tutor Perth Chest Hospital; Margaret Beard, deputy to principal matron Medical Department; Hilda Jury, supervisor Maternal and Child Health. It had been decided that the centre be known as the Nurses' Memorial Centre and that the committee be empowered to carry out the work of setting up the centre and to make decisions without having to call a further meeting.[3]

In 1959 Miss Anstey, in an address at the Conference of Student Nurses, outlined the aim and function of the Memorial Centre: to erect a memorial centre dedicated to all nurses who had served Western Australia in war and peace. The centre would house the administrative office of the R.A.N.F. and any other nursing bodies such as the Western Australian Committee of the College of Nursing, Australia, the Florence Nightingale Committee, the Student Nurses' Association, and any other body that might be formed in the future. The educational, cultural and social activities of the various bodies could take place at this centre; and it would accommodate visiting nurses whether actually engaged in nursing or not. A property large enough for future expansion was needed, with a building on it that could be adapted into offices with very little cost. The property should be close to the city and easily accessible and be situated so that parking facilities would be available:

> this sounds like a tall order, a hard task, in fact just the type of task that the Nursing Profession is used to . . . . tall orders and impossible tasks are more or less every day occurrences in the life of a nurse.[4]

In January 1960 a suitable property, situated at 34 Kings Park Road, West Perth, came on the market at a cash price of £18 000, and thanks to a generous grant of £5000 from the Lotteries Commission, a loan of £5000 from the R.A.N.F. and the balance of £7500 from the Commonwealth Bank on mortgage, the property was purchased. Building went ahead and the centre was opened by the Hon. Lady Gairdner on 18 June 1960, when a plaque dedicating the centre was unveiled. In the ensuing years the money borrowed from the R.A.N.F. and the mortgage to the bank was paid off by the efforts of nurses from all parts of the state of Western Australia. Owing to the fact that a War Nurses' Hostel was already operating, administered by the War Nurses' Memorial Association, the centre was designated the R.A.N.F. Nurses' Memorial Centre, to avoid confusion between the two. The upward trend in salaries lessened the need for accommodation to be supplied by the centre—

the War Nurses' Hostel was already proving that it was not a viable proposition — therefore the original idea of making such additions to 34 Kings Park Road was shelved.

The College of Nursing, Australia, had a far-reaching effect on the progress of nursing in Western Australia for not only did it provide for a greater number of students to undertake post-basic education, by virtue of financial assistance which would have otherwise because of the distance and cost of overseas venues have been limited to a few, but also its structure as a national venture allowed for more involvement on a policy-making level.[5]

Under its constitution the college was administered by a council composed of three fellows from each state elected by their fellow members. In order to get off the ground, foundation fellowships were conferred on people in each state who had contributed to its founding materially and professionally. These included most of the matrons of training schools and sister tutors who had gained their diplomas overseas. In each state a college committee was set up and designated in this state W.A. State Committee (College of Nursing, Australia). In addition to providing representatives on the college council, one of the functions of the state committees was to provide a 'refresher week' each year with the aim of enabling nurses to keep abreast of the many new developments in nursing.

The annual meetings of the college are required to be held in a different state each year on a rotating basis, in the state of origin of the retiring president. The 1951 annual meeting was held in Perth, as Mrs A. M. Walsh had followed Miss A. M. Sage as president. The venue was Winthrop Hall, University of Western Australia. In organizing this, a small subcommittee of the state branch of the Florence Nightingale Memorial Committee was formed, which subsequently became the nucleus of the W.A. State Committee of the College of Nursing.

The first courses conducted by the college began in March 1950 and were as follows: Ward Sister Diploma course, six months; Sister Tutor Diploma course, nine months; Nursing Administration Diploma course, nine months. The first students from Western Australia to attend were Miss Alice Harris and Sister Mary Kearnan, Sister Tutor Diploma course, and Misses M. Fraser and Ozanne, Ward Sister Diploma course. Those first attending the Nursing Administration Diploma course the following year were Misses Phyllis Lee and Nina Simpson.

Under the terms of their Florence Nightingale scholarship agreement students were 'bonded' to undertake service where directed for two years after the completion of the course. Miss Harris returned to her training school at Fremantle Hospital to become principal tutor of the school of nursing. Misses Lee and Simpson returned to their former positions on the staff of Royal Perth Hospital. Subsequently Miss Simpson was posted as matron of Kalgoorlie District Hospital, while Miss Lee was appointed to the newly created position of principal matron with the Medical Department. It was largely due to her influence that the department agreed to award scholarships through the Florence Nightingale Committee for students to undertake further courses, and also assist with finance those who did not meet the criteria of that organization. The metropolitan training schools also adopted this policy with regard to senior members of their staff.

By 1954 all of the nurse training schools had at least one teacher with a Sister Tutor Diploma and these were the people who carried the teaching load and were held responsible for the theoretical and practical instruction of the students, aided by the clinical instructors. Unfortunately there were very few who wished to undertake the Sister Tutor Diploma course which entailed an increased study programme and higher academic qualifications.

Ways and means of attracting nurses to this field included the granting of three weeks special leave taken in periods of one week at a time during the year. This was assented to by the employing authorities under the terms of a gentlemen's agreement outside the arbitration award, but unfortunately created dissension on the part of those employed in other categories who felt that they were being unfairly treated. It is doubtful if the measure attracted more nurses to the teaching field, but it did give those already practising some respite.

Changes in the field of medicine were demanding the knowledge of new techniques, but there was a reluctance to discard the time-honoured procedures practised over the years which had become synonymous with what many people understood as 'nursing'. To mention a few, hot foments, mustard pastes, turpentine stupes and a variety of enemata remained in the curriculum to be taught and learnt. Enamel ware had been replaced by stainless steel and trolleys with equipment for carrying out seemingly simple procedures were set up in a elaborate detail. The student was required to memorize every piece of equipment needed for each procedure. The challenge came when she faced the examiner in the course of the practical examination at first year and again at final level.

The shortage of nurses to staff the metropolitan and country hospitals persisted. Married nurses were given the opportunity of employment but there was some resistance to this as it was felt that the unmarried nurse who lived in was rostered for the evening and night tours of duty, and the married nurse who lived at home was given preference for day duty. Student nurses who married before completing their training time invariably left and their loss was classified as 'wastage'. Examinations also took their toll and the First Professional examination conducted by the N.R.B. at the end of the student's first year was primarily designed to assess those who might have too much difficulty in completing the three year course. Two attempts only were allowed at this examination, which consisted of three written papers, on anatomy and physiology, hygiene, and general nursing. The first papers were set and marked by medical men appointed as examiners by the N.R.B. and the paper on general nursing was a combined effort on the part of the tutor sisters, all of whom were appointed as examiners. At one stage these papers were set in the eastern states but marked locally. Resulting from this, the Sister Tutors' Section of the R.A.N.F. became a virtual forum where each examination was debated, often hotly, and recommendations were forwarded to the registering authority. A prerequisite for entrance to the examination was that the student had to have a certificate in the practice and theory of invalid cookery. For practical purposes, examination rooms were set up in each training centre with all the equipment used in basic nursing care within the hospital. For student and examiner it was an exhausting business but it did tend to form an overall pattern of nurse teaching, in addition to bringing to light many of the fallacies still persisting in the hospitals regarding the practice of nursing care.[6]

An attempt to examine finalists using the ward situation was also introduced, but discontinued later when it was found that the number of the more sophisticated nursing procedures did not exist in relation to the number of students being assessed. The appointment of an educationalist to the Nurses' Registration Board was of great assistance, the first appointed being Dr Neal, who was responsible for introducing the 'objective' or 'short answer' type of assessment which covered a wider selection of subjects and gave more scope. Dr Neal also pointed out that the criterion for entry had been misconstrued as a pass in two subjects only, arithmetic and English at second year high school level, which had replaced the former Nurses' Entrance examination conducted by the board. The actual criterion was a minimum of a pass at second year high school level which included the subjects of English and arithmetic. The training schools had the power to set their own standards, which depended very much on the number offering for studentship. Representatives from all nurse training schools visited the schools and colleges. The Central Training School, which fared badly as girls were not particularly attracted to the country, moved to new premises in 1955 in a lovely gracious old home in 18 Colin Street,

West Perth, and was renamed the Government School of Nursing.[7] A film was made based on the activities of the school and the advantages of training in a rural setting. Students in the Study Block at the time provided the cast with one of their number as 'leading lady'. They all agreed that the experience killed any aspirations they might have had for a change of career as a film star.

In 1952 the Nurses' Registration Board decided to sponsor the training programme of another grade of nurse, whose function would be the care of the less acutely ill patient and those in homes or hospitals for the chronically sick. This was the nursing aide, who was accepted with a lower standard of basic education and was to receive a less intensive training. She was in charge of a clinical supervisor and received the greater part of her instruction at the patient's bedside under the supervision of trained staff.[8] The first school of this type was set up at Merredin Hospital, and in 1953 at Royal Perth Hospital. The original period of training was twelve months, but this has been extended.

Although accepted by the N.R.B. the nursing aide did not by training qualify for membership of the R.A.N.F. The reason for this was the possibility of conflict with the membership of the International Council of Nurses, which stipulated that the nurses of member national associations must have had a recognized general nurse training. It was envisaged that, when qualified, nursing aides would be able to staff the hospitals, to give basic nursing care under supervision of trained staff, and thereby allow the student nurses in time to acquire full student status. It was also hoped that the nursing assistant who was untrained would be phased out. However, mostly for economic reasons, this has not materialized.

Sponsored by the Commonwealth government, the Colombo Plan allowed students from Asian countries to undertake a variety of training courses at approved institutions and universities. They were given limited visas and it was planned that they would return to their countries of origin on completion of their education, to work in the education and health fields. Such students had to be carefully selected and had to have a high level of general education. Students undertaking the nursing course had to be female, and for the basic course they were accepted by Royal Perth Hospital. The first group graduated in 1957. There were also some who undertook post-basic training in specialized areas such as midwifery.[9] Under the same plan, a group of seven graduate nurses from Perth Chest Clinic were seconded to Ceylon in 1956 as clinical instructors in the field of tuberculosis control.

The establishment of Perth Chest Clinic and its community involvement in conducting the compulsory chest X ray and immunization programmes was playing an outstanding part in the early detection of the disease. Nurses from the clinic visited the patients and their relatives, and supervised the taking of medications, which meant that fewer had to be admitted to hospital. Treatment was free and the payment of a TB allowance was a factor in lessening the stress. To cope with the advances in chest surgery and diagnostic procedures, a new hospital, funded by the Commonwealth but controlled by the state, was built. Designated Perth Chest Hospital, it was built on land adjacent to the Repatriation General Hospital at Hollywood, and opened in 1958.[10] Olive Anstey was appointed matron and John Brett principal nurse educator.[11] The Nurses' Registration Board's registration of the two-year course in tuberculosis nursing was transferred from Wooroloo, and patients and staff were transferred to the new hospital. Wooroloo was phased out to become a general hospital for the district and then a geriatric unit. Today most of the hospital has been taken over by the Department of Corrections as a minimum security prison and part of their rehabilitation process.

The new two-year programme introduced at Perth Chest Hospital was upgraded to include a lengthened Preliminary Training School and a system of study days. Registration was also granted for a six months' post-basic course in tuberculosis nursing. Students undertaking the two year course were able to sit for the First Professional examination and continue at another training school to complete their General Nursing Certificate in two years. Realizing the value of student membership of the professional organization, Miss Anstey was successful in having them accepted for membership of the R.A.N.F., a move that was opposed by some who felt that such nurses should conform with other nurses at the Chest Clinic who came under a Public Service award.

Other categories of nurses accepted by the R.A.N.F. for student membership were those undertaking a three year course of study at Perth Dental Hospital. The school, which was established in 1949, was registered by the Nurses' Registration Board in 1953. The matron was Mollie Brady, a graduate of Royal Perth Hospital and one of the students in the first Preliminary Training School.[12]

In 1959 the Alexandra Home, which had succeeded the House of Mercy, was transferred to new premises in Jarrah Road, South Perth, and became Ngal-A Mothercraft Home and Training Centre.[13] It was registered with the N.R.B. for the training of nurses in mothercraft—short-term training—and also training for the post-basic certificate in infant health. Beryl Grant was appointed matron.[14] Although subsidized by the government, the home is still administered by an independent authority.

An event which was to have a far-reaching effect on nursing was the founding of a medical school within the University of Western Australia. The first students were accepted in 1957, and degrees were conferred for the first time in 1959.

The dramatic effect of the use of penicillin and other chemotherapeutic substances cannot be measured. Infections and 'laudable pus' seemed to disappear overnight, only to reappear again in a more sinister form, as pathogenic micro-organisms began to become drug resistant. One of these, *Staphylococcus aureus*, 'golden staph', became a killer, invading hospital wards and nurseries. The emphasis was on cross-infection and how to control it, and in the investigations many nursing procedures became suspect, particularly the methods employed in the disposal and handling of infected material, bed linen and blankets. Facilities for hand washing were also suspect, as was the indiscriminate use of antiseptics and detergents, which were gradually replacing soap and water. The need to understand more about the nature of micro-organisms and to devise methods for their destruction led to the reconstruction of the nursing syllabus to include a section on microbiology in what was formerly known as 'hygiene', and which was renamed 'communal health'.

Extensions to hospitals and the newer ones being built were incorporating laboratories and technicians, which was necessary not only from the point of pathology, but for the biochemistry involved in the administration of the newer drugs and their side effects. The benefit derived from the use of these drugs was being reflected in the disappearance of much that was unpleasant in the wards, and it contributed to the extension of the life of the patients. This, however, has created a problem of long-term hospitalization for greater numbers, and for many more frail and aged patients.

CHAPTER SEVEN

THE SIXTIES

Overseas recruitment had resulted in the appointment of additional qualified tutors to the major metropolitan hospitals. As some of the appointees were male and accepted for full membership of the R.A.N.F. it meant adjustments to the award. It also meant that the Male Nurses' Association went out of existence.[1] Dissatisfaction with the curriculum content resulted in the forming of a special committee from the R.A.N.F. Council and the Sister Tutors' Section of the association, to review the matter and make recommendations to the Nurses' Registration Board. The result was that new regulations were drawn up and promulgated in the *Government Gazette* (No. 87) of 25 October 1960. This is quite an extensive document and deals with all categories of nurses, the curriculum in all cases being restructured and upgraded.[2]

The occupied bed average of hospitals deemed acceptable as training schools rose to fifty in the general A-class hospitals, but the B-class hospitals were unspecified, except that should they be under fifty and the time spent in them during training limited to twelve months followed immediately by two years in an A-class hospital. In the field of mental health the average daily occupancy of beds was set at 1000 with a minimum of 500 admissions annually. For the general certificated nurse undertaking post-basic experience in a mental institution additional experience was needed in 'acute', 'long stay' and 'day hospitals with bed averages of 100 persons'. (The Claremont Hospital for the Insane, as it was designated, had the highest number of occupied beds of any hospital in the state and reflects the slow progress being made in caring for the mentally disabled, a situation which was to change drastically in the following decade.)

In the field of midwifery, training time for the midwife had been extended to two years for the post-basic course and the acceptance of those only for midwifery gradually ceased. Previously legislation had been passed to require those practising midwifery to be proficient in the administration of analgesia and to have qualified by examination. This had become necessary because of the installation of more sophisticated equipment in hospitals which replaced the 'rag and bottle' method.[3]

To help students cope with the revisions, the educational requirement for professional entry were once again reviewed and although the standard remained at a Second Year High School Certificate of the Education Department of Western Australia with a pass in English and arithmetic, other subjects were added. The basic requirement became a pass in five subjects, with either history, geography or social science, and two others from the following list: a science subject (general science, physics, chemistry, biology, physiology and hygiene), art, home science, music (fourth grade practical and theory AMEB), a language (other than English), algebra, geometry, or such other qualification as the board deemed equivalent or higher qualifications. The above were the minimum requirements of the N.R.B. but training schools were able to, and did, set their own standards of acceptance which fluctuated according to the number of applicants.

The age of entry had been lowered to 17½ years, but the school leaving age was fourteen, and for some, to continue for the next 3½ years constituted economic hardship. For those who visualized nursing as a practical experience, and who were not orientated to classroom study, the temptation to take a job was an overruling consideration. To counteract this the state government, through the Medical Department and other agencies, introduced a scheme of awarding bursaries for tertiary education, to offset the financial loss of remaining at school. Acceptance was by assessment and the recipient had to enter into a bond of two years service on completion of the training course. Statistics regarding this are not available but it is known that many took advantage of the opportunity, and there were a number who 'bought themselves out'.

In July 1960 a new appointment was made to the Nurses' Registration Board, that of education officer, and Miss D. H. Bailey became the first to hold this office.[4] The position of secretary continued to be a Public Service appointment based on seniority. Miss Bailey's role was to take over matters dealing with education in relation to nurse training. Her former position of principal tutor at R.P.H. was taken by Dorothy Clarke.

A most important event in nursing history in Australia, was the decision to hold the twelfth Quadrennial Congress of the International Council of Nurses in Melbourne in May 1961.[5] The event attracted nurses from all parts of the world and many came through Perth, where they were given hospitality. Some were able to stop over on the return journey and gave their impressions of the congress and its implications for nursing. Royal Perth Hospital inaugurated a plan to attract tutors by offering them their fares and other travelling expenses to the congress in exchange for a year's service in the teaching department. The four who accepted this offer gave valuable service.

One of the far-reaching effects of the congress was the decision that all future nurses should have a broad nursing experience, to include clinical practice in areas outside those of the accepted basic curriculum. These areas must include obstetric experience and additional time to be spent in psychiatric hospitals. Although this was considered desirable, the problem was where such experience could be obtained for the large number requiring it.

This development in nursing education had already been adopted in many of the countries affiliated with the I.C.N. In Western Australia it was certainly desirable because of the huge expansion and development within the state following on the discovery of oil and minerals, notably nickel and iron ore. Referred to as the 'sleeping giant', this state of a million square miles had begun to stir in its sleep. Towns, new and old, were developed along with the deep sea ports in the north, and the pastoralist and grazier gave way to the industrialist. The population growth meant the building of new hospitals and the extension of community health care. Like in the gold-rush days of the turn of the century, there was little difficulty in recruiting nurses to serve in the north, but they needed to be experienced in all clinical areas. Another problem was the care of the Aboriginal population which, deprived of the parental protection of the pastoralist, migrated to the towns where they followed the habits, if not the life style, of their white brothers in a hot and thirsty land.

Exploration in space also came nearer to home, with the installation of a tracking station in Carnarvon, and in February 1962 John Glenn, while orbiting the earth, paid tribute to the lights of Perth, which welcomed him as he spun by, and named Perth as the 'City of Light'.

Although construction companies employed nurses on site, such as at the United States communication base at North West Cape, medical care of the community in such areas was in many cases undertaken by the Australian Inland Mission, which set up small, often convertible, medical posts and hospitals. These were subsequently taken over by the Commonwealth or state governments, either separately or jointly administered. The enormous range of medical services in the state cannot be adequately described and requires a volume of its own, nor can the complexities which arose in each area, which were inevitably linked with the environment and which ranged from the mining of the blue asbestos to the fishing industry. Nature, too, in her savage moods made no exception with hospitals or other agencies caring for the sick when it came to cyclones, bushfires, floods and earthquakes. The action of nursing staffs under these conditions and their devotion to duty can only be described in the annals of heroism.

Following the Congress of the International Council of Nurses in 1961, the Student Nurses' Associations in each state decided to form a National Student Nurses' Unit, within the framework of the R.A.N.F. The First National Student Nurses' Conference was held in Brisbane from 27 November to 2 December 1961.[6] Eight student nurses from Western Australia attended as delegates together with four observers, the delegates being Wendy Fimmell (state president, R.P.H.), Susan Clements (P.M.H.), Robin Miller (R.P.H.) and Jacqueline Fowles (Victoria District Hospital, Geraldton), representing the Government School of Nursing. At the conference a paper was presented by Robin Miller of Western Australia, on the Royal Flying Doctor Service, under the title of 'Conquest of Loneliness'.

Robin, whose name was to become synonymous with the Flying Doctor Service, was one of the pioneers in this field of service which took medical aid to the people of the outback. As nurse and pilot she undertook a programme of immunization which included the administration of the Sabin vaccine against poliomyelitis. This was administered on a cube of sugar, and earned her the name among the native children of 'sugar bird lady'. Her description of the Flying Doctor Service in the Student Nurses' Unit paper clearly outlines the need and emphasizes the loneliness of people in isolated areas. Extracts from the article were printed in the *Journal of the West Australian Nurses*.

> One of the most heartbreaking aspects of our 'Great Australian Loneliness' was always the lonely grave, in many cases that of a young woman and too often little children. What was always described as fever and could have been any one of a great number of things, took a great toll of lives in the outback areas. Almost all these cases would require only routine advice or treatment today but until well into the 1930's were considered part and parcel of bush life, something almost everyone got and of which a number inevitably died . . .
>
> The first Flying Doctor base was established at Cloncurry (Q) in 1928 and during the following years sections were formed in other States, each maintaining and establishing its own base or bases.
>
> Western Australia is served by three sections of the Flying Doctor Service, each being responsible for financing and run-

> ning its own section. In 1935, the Victorian Section undertook the establishment and continued maintenance of a base at Wyndham port for the isolated cattle country of eastern Kimberley (W.A.). This generous gesture on the part of a State that was itself too small to warrant a Flying Doctor Service of its own has been warmly appreciated by the people of the north, who look upon it as one of the most vital aids to development. Other bases at Port Hedland, Meekatharra and Carnarvon were soon afterwards established and financed by West Australian supporters of the scheme and in 1936 a base known as the eastern goldfields section was established privately at Kalgoorlie . . .
>
> In Western Australia, the wireless operator and pilot are employed by the Flying Doctor Service but the doctor unlike in the Eastern States section is employed by the Government and is usually medical officer for the town as well as 'flying doctor' for the outlying districts.
>
> All pilots are pilot engineers and are responsible for the flying and maintenance of his [*sic*] own aircraft. This arrangement drastically reduces running costs.

After graduating from R.P.H. in 1962 Robin Miller qualified as a midwife at St Anne's. As a pilot she joined the Royal Flying Doctor Service in which she continued to serve until illness intervened. In 1971 she published a book, *Flying Nurse*, and following her death in 1975, a plaque was erected to her memory in the seminar room named in her honour in the old Administration Building of R.P.H. A memorial scholarship has also been inaugurated for the purpose of training nurses to be pilots so they can continue her work in the field.[7]

In 1961 Gertrude Siegele retired as matron of Royal Perth Hospital and Kathleen Johnson was appointed in her place. Alice Mattinson relinquished her position as matron of King Edward Memorial Hospital for Women. Dorothy Clarke also resigned as principal tutor of Royal Perth Hospital, and proceeded overseas for further experience. Her place was taken by Merle Parkes. In 1963 the Perth Chest Hospital expanded to become a general hospital and was renamed the Sir Charles Gairdner Hospital in honor of the state governor. It did not immediately become a training school for nurses undertaking the General Certificate, and was staffed mainly by registered nurses.[8]

Changes in medicine invariably caused adjustments in nursing practice and one of the means of coping with the problem was the introduction of refresher courses of a practical nature. Such courses had been introduced by hospitals and other employing agencies over the years, but funding had presented problems as in some quarters there was resistance to allowing staff paid time to attend. Among the first to have such a course were the infant health sisters and those employed in the Public Health Department as schools nurses. Every year the infant health sisters from country and metropolitan areas met for a week for lectures and discussions on the latest trends in their particular field. The Medical Department, too, in conjunction with the W.A. State Committee of the College of Nursing, Australia, introduced what became known as 'Matrons' Week' for matrons of country hospitals and other nursing administrators. Some hospitals, R.P.H. and K.E.M.H., conducted some in-service courses, but these were all in specialist fields and for staff members, or those employed in a specialized area.

Comparatively few nurses did not marry, and those who did were sealed to their environment by home, husband and family. The expansion of the building programme in relation to hospitals by both government and private enterprise was creating job opportunities for nurses living in the vicinity, and many who had not been engaged in practice for a number of years now wished to return for full-time or part-time employment, but found that they had to assure the Nurses' Registration Board of safe practice before they could be re-registered. To meet this need, the W.A. State Committee of the College of Nursing, with the cooperation of the Medical Department and the boards of management of hospitals, decided to introduce a refresher course for non-practising nurses who wished to return to general practice. The venue was the Government School of Nursing in West Perth, the organizer and teaching staff being made available by the Medical Department. A condition of entry was that the participants undertook to give forty hours voluntary service to a selected hospital within a month of completing the course. The hospitals co-operated and treated them as students on a supernumary basis. The cost, which was borne by the participant, provided funds for the W.A. State Committee of the College of Nursing.[9]

The reaction of those undertaking the course depended on what they had decided to do in nursing. Some who had been 'out of nursing' for some fifteen years found the changes hard to accept, and needed assurance to restore self-confidence. Some had envisaged employment in geriatric hospitals and nursing homes and felt that the unfamiliarity with modern drugs was perhaps the greatest hurdle. Looked at in retrospect, it can be seen that there was a lot to catch up with. Patients were still people, but they were becoming better informed and asking for explanations. This, to some extent, could be traced to the influence of the media, and in 1963 everybody was also acquiring a television set.

The metric system, which had become law for use in hospitals and pharmacies, was to many unfamiliar. The fluid balance chart, the centigrade clinical thermometer, the administration of tablets and mixtures all had to be rethought and retranslated. To tell a mother her baby weighed so many grams, and then convert it to the familiar pounds and ounces was an exercise in itself. Medical terminology differed, and the trade names and generic names of the hundreds of new drugs which flooded the market gave rise to indecision which was not helped by the very small print on the containers. There was also the contraceptive pill and its relationship to gynaecology and social problems, for it was the nurse that women invariably turned to for advice and reassurance.

However, the procedures that had been considered the prerogative of the nurse seemed to have gone into reverse, and were the hardest to accept. 'Bedsores' had become 'decubitus ulcers'. Hot water bottles and electric 'cradles' were no longer used in the treatment of patients in 'shock', and in some hospitals the former, because of their misuse, had been banished completely. The evening 'aperient round' had disappeared and was replaced by the 'sedative round'. The observation of signs and symptoms were only accepted as proof of diagnosis when supported by biochemical and pathological tests. Blood-stained and fouled linen was no longer washed by nursing staff at ward level before being sent to the laundry, and the gray army type blanket, so useful in not showing obvious marks, was definitely out. The linen cupboard with its impeccably folded sheets and towels, involving hours of work, and the precise placing of beds, considered to be the hallmark of the efficient ward sister, were no longer a factor in patient care. Perhaps the greatest adjustment that needed to be made by the returning nurses was the introduction of disposable equipment and a Central Sterile Supply Department. 'Waste not, want not' had been the very rock on which the economic and efficient running of hospitals and other nursing agencies had been founded, and having to accept as 'throw away' what appeared to be perfectly good equipment was almost too difficult. There was, too, the inherent fear that 'things' would disappear. That they needed to be counted and locked away or worn on one's person, for safe keeping, along with the keys of the drug cupboard and inevitably a pair of surgical scissors which, because of their misuse in cutting everything from selotape to toenails, formed a significant link in the chain of cross-infection.

A key area which was fast developing in the treatment of the acutely ill person was that of resuscitation, both manually and by means of complicated apparatus which needed the application of scientific principles. The intermittent positive pressure respirator,

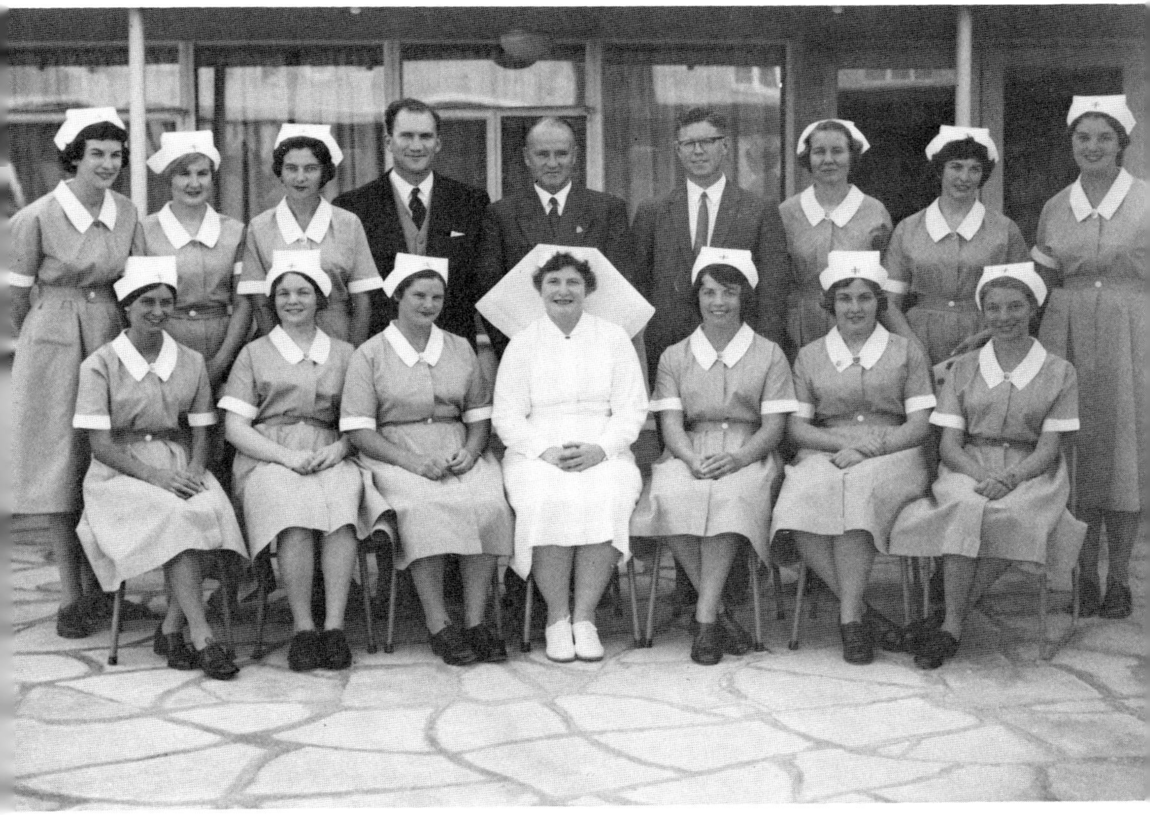

PERTH CHEST HOSPITAL, 1960

First graduates in tuberculosis nursing. *Centre back:* John Brett (tutor), Dr A. King, Dr R. Elphick; *centre front:* O. Anstey (matron)

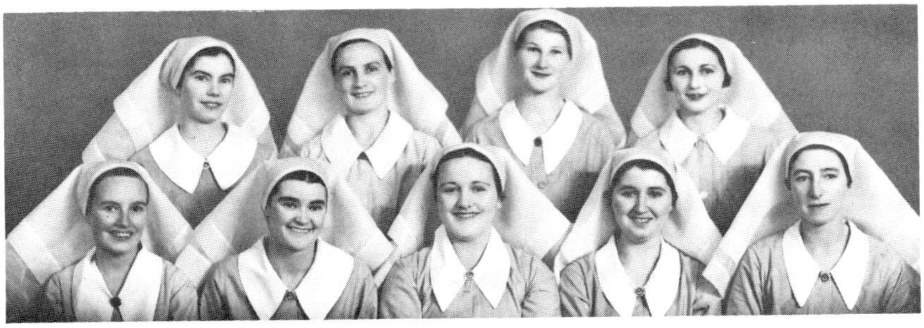

GRADUATES OF GOVERNMENT HOSPITAL, KALGOORLIE, 1937

back row: E. Harler, A. Freeman, —. Johnston, A. Ward; *front row:* J. Winzar, M. Glass, M. Stone, B. Mohen, D. Culmsee.

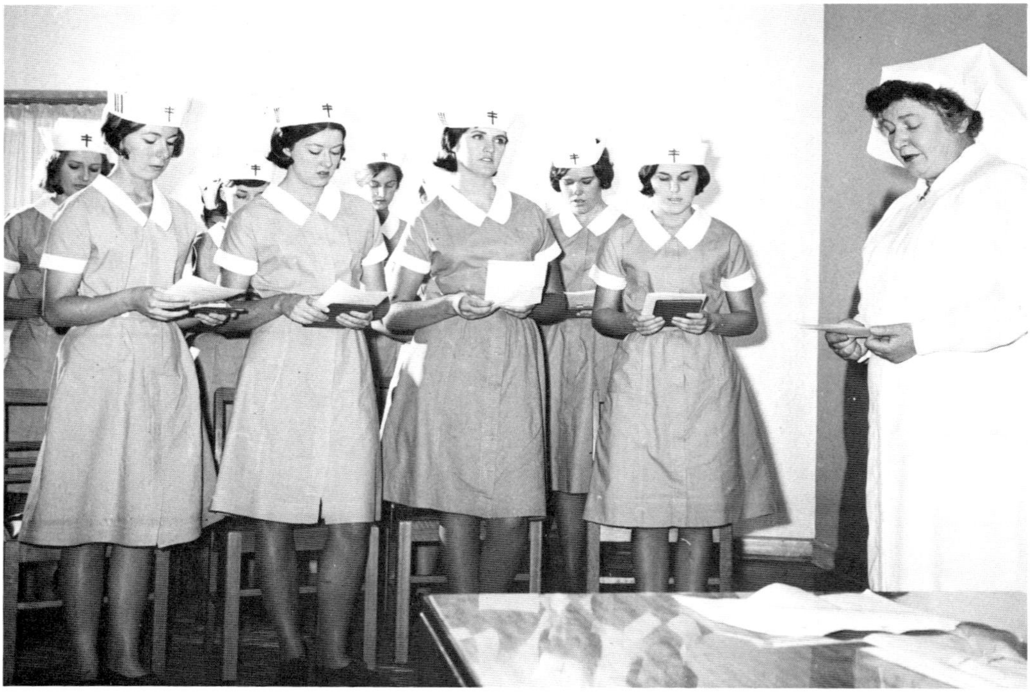

SIR CHARLES GAIRDNER HOSPITAL
formerly Perth Chest Hospital. First General Certificate graduates with O. Anstey (matron).

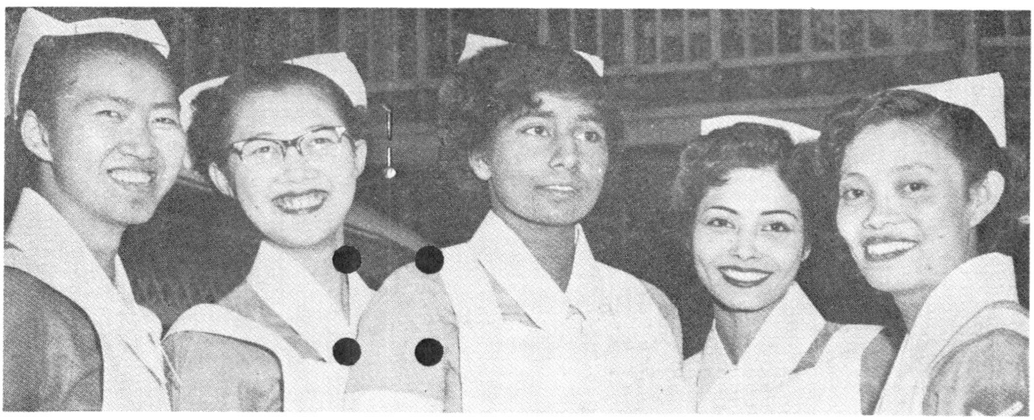

FIRST COLOMBO PLAN NURSING GRADUATES
left to right: I. Oh, of Penang, C. I. Chew, of Kedah, A. Amirthalingam, of Penang, D. Foenander, of Kuala Lumpur, and U. Ali, of Johore, all graduates of Royal Perth Hospital, 1957.

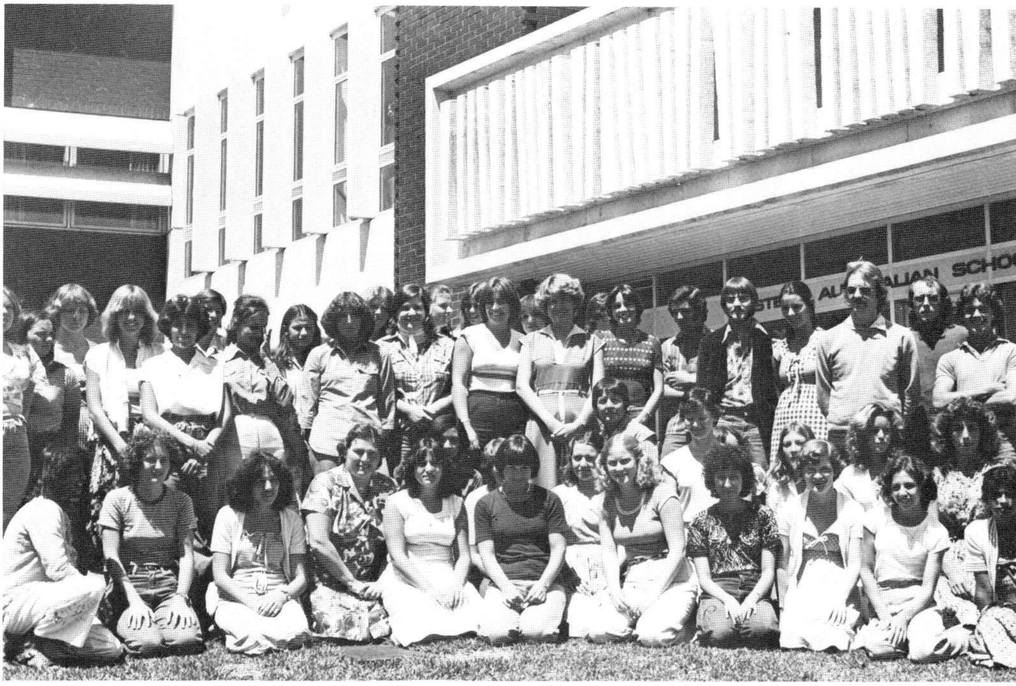

W.A. SCHOOL OF NURSING

above: a group of students, 1977; *below:* the first graduates, 1979.

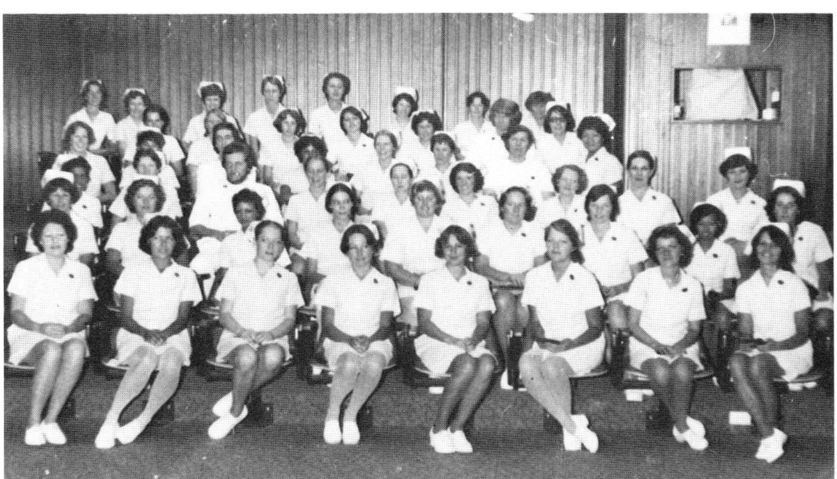

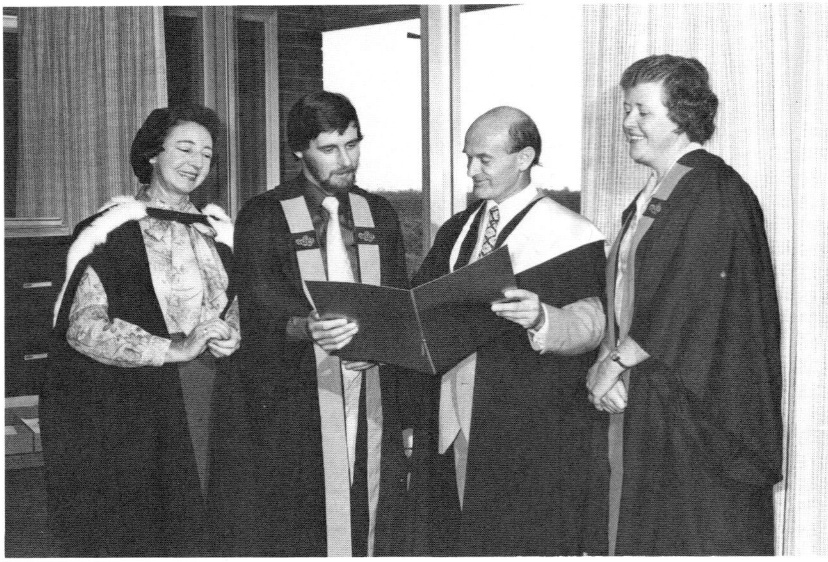

WESTERN AUSTRALIAN INSTITUTE OF TECHNOLOGY

The academic registrar of W.A.I.T. reveals the degree scroll for the degree of Bachelor of Applied Science (Nursing) to some of the people who fought to create it. *Left to right:* M. Parkes (head, Department of Nursing), I. Landsborough (graduant, ex-president of the Nurses' Action Group, 1978), N. Milne (academic registrar), B. Scott (graduant, ex-secretary of the Nurses Action Group, 1977).

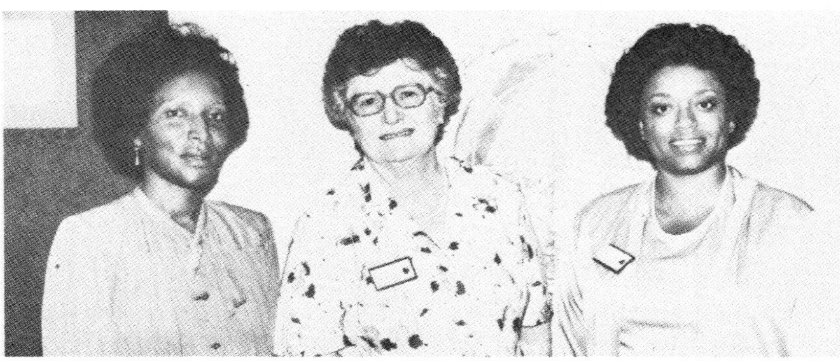

I.C.N. COUNCIL MEETING, 1979

At the biennial meeting of I.C.N.'s governing body, the Council of National Representatives, Nairobi, Kenya, *left to right:* Eunice Muringo Kiereini, president of the National Nurses Association of Kenya; Olive Anstey, president of I.C.N.; and Barbara Nichols, president of the American Nurses Association. Mrs Kiereini gave the Florence Nightingale oration at the WAY 1979 celebrations in Perth.

known more familiarly as the 'bird machine', and the humidicrib were standard equipment and widely distributed throughout all country hospitals. Expertise in their use was essential. The need for such equipment to be centralized had given rise to special units within the hospital structure, notably intensive care units, coronary care units, special nurseries etc. where the staff could be concentrated. In the country such units were provided for in the new regional hospitals, but their use was limited as the regional and outer suburban hospital did not employ resident medical staff. What appeared to be an almost simple task passed on to the nurse was the assessment of the patient's blood pressure by the use of a manometer and a stethescope, but strangely it was one of the areas in which there was less confidence.

Observations of participants of some of the early refresher courses was that they appreciated changes for the better, but that they felt the patient had seemed to disappear and become depersonalized, and that they had lost contact. To some extent this was attributed to 'early ambulation' following surgery and the replacement of the 'sponge' or bedbath, with the shower. There was virtually no preoperative skin preparation and few dressings post-operatively. In actual fact the nursing of a patient had become a shared experience with other members of the health team, the physiotherapist, the occupational therapist, the social worker, the dietician, and others, in a situation where the nurse no longer played the dominant role. However there were areas where ancillary services were not available and even the medical officer was some distance away, and there was still the challenge in having to meet emergencies and be responsible for the total health care of people in the vicinity. For the registered nurse without post-basic educational qualifications, job opportunities were restricted to nursing the terminally ill or to domiciliary care, which was under the control of the Silver Chain and the Bush Nursing Service.

With so many other methods of patient assessment carried out in laboratories, it is curious to find that urine testing was still on the general nursing curriculum. For years, the boiling of specimens with reagents over a spirit lamp or Bunson burner had liberally spattered the walls of the sluice rooms causing almost as much damage to the interior as the boiling water sterilizer. A breakthrough was the introduction of a new method involving the use of tablets and test sticks. Assessment and testing for abnormalities was reduced to a matter of seconds, but as with all 'new' innovations, economy and ability to prove its viability was an early stumbling block in its implementation, as it was not fool proof.

Although the changes in midwifery had been even more radical, they were not so unfamiliar, as most of those undertaking the refresher courses had families and therefore practical experience from the mother's point of view. Those whose children were older found such procedures as the minimal cleansing of infants and the very early ambulation of the mother rather controversial. To quote one lecturer in obstetrics, 'the labor ward scene had changed from masterly inactivity to planned activity'. It was the more sophisticated and technical aspects of the management of midwifery which created some reluctance to return to this type of nursing.

The care of children was also another practical experience which was not new to most mothers, but the progress in genetics and the surgical corrections of abnormalities and social problems such as the 'battered baby' syndrome and other forms of child abuse seemed to have become more accentuated. Rehydration as opposed to dehydration and the unrecognized dangers in many nursing procedures presented a disturbing factor.

The refresher course had come to stay. Fulfilling its purpose of re-education, its image has altered along with its title and venue, which is now the Western Australian Institute of Technology, and the course is conducted through W.A.I.T. Aid.

With the appointment of a nursing education officer, the Nurses' Registration Board was able to extend its function beyond the registration of nurses and plan more effectively how to meet the needs of both nurses and the community in the pattern of health care. A comprehensive survey of the requirements of Western Australia in this field was prepared by Miss H. Bailey, and presented at a joint meeting of hospital administrators, matrons, nurse educators and other interested bodies under the chairmanship of Dr Linley Henzell, commissioner of public health, at Princess Margaret Hospital on 19 October 1962. In his opening remarks, Dr Henzell stated that

> the object of the Board was the revision of the present curriculum and the reconsideration of the training of nurses in toto.
>
> With the emphasis on total health which embraces both its physical and mental aspects, it has been found that nursing training has lagged greatly in respect of the latter, and the Board approves in principle that some steps be taken to amend this.
>
> Nothing concrete has been decided upon and the work to date has been more of a fact finding nature. There will be the appointment of a small working committee and the possibility of 'pilot' courses being undertaken in the near future.

This was the first of several such meetings with hospital administrators and matrons of the main teaching hospitals but measures put forward by the select committee which had been formed did not get wholehearted support, and delaying tactics retarded implementation.

There was a reluctance to accept the disassociation of the hospitals from the particular schools of nursing, and the fear that the necessary raising of the educational standard for entry would mean that fewer would be available for service within the hospital. The Western Australian Institute of Technology expressed willingness to accommodate nursing students with others in the courses dealing with anatomy, physiology and applied science, but such students had to have the requisite educational standard of entry to such courses. Not all those being accepted for nurse training at this time were able to qualify.

The Nurse Aide programme also came up for discussion at this time with a view to increasing the training period and providing an incentive to specialize.

In 1964 Dr W. S. Davidson, commissioner of public health, who succeeded Dr Henzell, proposed the introduction of the health visitor, using the infant health sisters to implement this, together with those giving domiciliary care under the Silver Chain.[10] This plan was ruled out by the infant health sisters as being most unacceptable as they were specialists in their own field, and that to undertake the role of the health visitor would mean further specialized training, which was not available in Western Australia.

An important amendment to the Nurses Registration Act in 1965 was the substitution of 'Nutrition' for 'Invalid Cookery' making it no longer mandatory for the student nurse to pass a practical examination in invalid cookery and produce a certificate of competence in the subject for registration.[11] This applied also to the pupil midwives. A further amendment in 1963 was the substitution of 'student' for 'trainee'. In the same amendment, the minimum educational standard of entry was raised from Second to Third Year High School Certificate with selected subjects.

The registration of St John of God Hospital as a General Certificate training school for students outside the order, in 1962, and the extension of Sir Charles Gairdner Hospital to become a training school for nurses in 1963 had the effect of increasing the competition for students which was already affected by the rise in the educational entry requirement and competition with the Education Department for students for trainee teachers. The salary structure of teachers compared with that of nurses was unrealistic, favouring the former. The absence of a bonding system for nursing students was also one of the contributory factors to what was a very high 'wastage rate' during the first and second years of the training period.

There was, too, the hereditary factor. Mothers who were nurses expected their daughters to be likewise, and expressed hurt, disappointment and even anger when it was suggested that such a student could only be accepted for the Nursing Aide course. For the girl herself, especially if she had been employed as a nursing assistant while waiting to reach the age of entry—17½ years—it was a traumatic experience for which she was not always prepared and a bitter blow to her esteem. The Nursing Aide course only conferred registration in Western Australia. Because of the high wastage rate and the demand for service, schools of nursing accepted a number of intakes of students a year and it was evident that some would be required to work for as much as three extra months while waiting to take their final examinations, which were held twice a year. To overcome this, the Nurses' Registration Board once again introduced a third examination. Although the students welcomed this move, it was not popular with the hospital authorities and the nurse educators in the schools of nursing, the exception being King Edward Memorial Hospital. (Because of the increase of male teachers the term 'sister tutor' had been replaced by that of 'nurse educator' in 1965.) The influence of the university Department of Medicine was being felt particularly in K.E.M.H. where there was keen competition between medical students and pupil midwives for deliveries, as each had to have a requisite number to attain registration in that field. In 1962, with the admission of gynaecological patients, the hospital had fulfilled its intention of becoming a women's hospital. In 1960 a pilot course aimed at giving maternity nursing experience was introduced at the hospital and selected students from all the nurse training centres attended. It sought to fill the gap between general nurses—who needed the experience but did not want necessarily to become practising midwives—and the accredited midwifery nurse, and anticipated the change to a broader general nursing curriculum. The introduction of nursing assistants reduced the intake of pupil midwives, but made the waiting list longer and in some instances nurses married and had families before returning as mature students to undertake the midwifery course.

The fiftieth anniversary of K.E.M.H. was observed in 1966 and a special brochure and a history of the hospital was produced for the occasion.[12] The hospital physically and as a much esteemed institution had come a long way from its humble beginnings as a reformatory and industrial school. The public hospital image had disappeared and its objective as a teaching hospital was the care of all women who required its services. (An interesting point when assessing bed average from the point of view of allotment of staff was whether the baby should be assessed as separate from its mother or not.) The number of establishments for the training of pupil midwives remained at three: St Anne's (Sisters of Mercy), Mount Lawley, St John of God Hospital, Subiaco, and K.E.M.H.

In 1968, due to the efforts of the education officer and other educationalists on the Nurses' Registration Board and with the co-operation of a special committee set up by the state branch of the R.A.N.F., new legislation was introduced and 'an Act to Consolidate and Amend the Law relating to the Nursing Profession was assented to on 25th October 1968. . . . To come into operation on a date to be fixed by proclamation, and the Nurses' Registration Act 1921-59 repealed'. As a result, the Nurses' Registration Board, which had been under the jurisdiction of the commissioner of public health, was replaced by the Nurses Board of Western Australia, which commenced operations as an autonomous body on 1 January 1970 under the authority of the Nurses Act of 1968, and which was subject to the minister for health. The granting of autonomy was unprecedented in Australia and for the nursing profession in this state.

As a corporate body the board was able to acquire property and set up its own establishment outside the framework of the Department of Public Health. The first premises were in Kings Park Road, West Perth, but they were later moved to 1140 Hay Street, West Perth. The building has been named 'Le Soeuf House' in honor of Dr L. E. Le Soeuf, who was appointed chairman under the new regime:

> whilst basically the Board is a registration body, it was established also to consider conditions affecting the education of nurses and research into, and practice of, the nursing profession in this State, with a view to maintaining an efficient, ethical, technical and professional standard,

and with regard to this, works very closely with the Royal Australian Nursing Federation and other nursing bodies. Since its inception there have been three amendments to the Nurses Act: to recognize and control the registration of nursing aides trained in the field of mental health; the inclusion on the Nurses Board of two nursing aide representatives; and an amendment to govern and control property and other assets.

Registration is renewed annually and is reviewed at five yearly intervals. It is compulsory in that a person who is not registered is not allowed to practice for fee or reward or wear the prescribed badge or uniform or any part of it generally worn by a registered nurse in the branch of nursing for which he or she is registered.

Registers kept by the board are as follows: Registers of General Nurses, Midwives, Mental Health Nurses, Mothercraft Nurses, Children's Nurses, Dental Nurses, Infant Health Nurses, Tuberculosis Nurses, Nursing Aides.

The position of secretary to the board, which had been the prerogative of a clerk in the Public Service and was a step in the promotion to a higher position, was abolished and a secretary/registrar was appointed. The first to hold this new appointment is Mr A. L. Cambridge.

The appeal for the Nurses' Memorial Centre had as one of its objectives the provision of premises for a college of nursing in Western Australia, when one was established, for it was recognized that the present system of sending students to colleges on the other side of the continent and overseas was limiting both from an economic and isolationist angle. In the mid-sixties there was an increasing demand for postgraduate education for nurses to be made available in this state, especially in the light of the progress of the teaching hospitals and the expansion of the paramedical services. Government funding for the establishment of a state branch of a college of nursing was promised by the commissioner of public health who was in favour of making it part of a plan to establish a paramedical school at the Shenton Park Annex of Royal Perth Hospital. Formerly the Infectious Diseases Branch, its function had become minimal with the virtual disappearance of infections which required patients being isolated from the community, and the hospital had developed into a unit for the treatment of patients with spinal injuries and neurological conditions resulting in paraplegia, and orthopaedic conditions. At the same time another plan involving the Western Australian Institute of Technology was put forward by the director of the institute. However neither of these plans came to fruition and the founding of the Western Australian branch of the College of Nursing, Australia, was delayed until 1968.

In anticipation, the Nurses' Memorial Centre Committee purchased a small piece of land and commenced building operations. A large lecture hall was erected, with adjoining amenities, and the upper floor of the building comprised a lecture room, offices, common room and library, the latter being made possible by a donation from the War Nurses Memorial Association and one from Sir Thomas Wardle, at that time lord mayor of Perth, who opened the extensions to the centre on Saturday 20 January 1968. Before introducing the lord mayor, the chairman of the Nurses' Memorial Centre, Miss Beryl Grant, gave the audience a detailed analysis of just what nurses had achieved over the past nine years by their own efforts, encouraged and ably assisted by the Lotteries Commission's initial grant of $10 000 to establish the centre and their further grant of $10 000 for extensions for establishment of a Western Australian branch of the College of Nursing, Australia. The War Nurses Memorial Association had contributed $1000 towards the establishment of a library which had been named the War Nurses Memorial Library, available to all nurses in Western Australia, and situated on the first floor of the new building.[13]

Following his opening remarks, the lord mayor also referred to his close connection with nursing and mentioned his aunt, Miss Ann Jewell, ex-trainee of Royal Perth Hospital, who was matron of the *Centaur*. The West Australian Branch of the College of Nursing, Australia, was officially opened on 7 June 1968. The occasion is described in the July issue of *The Journal of the West Australian Nurses*. For Kathleen Yeates, who had given so much of time, money and effort in the pre-war days, it was a dream come true. Also there was Kathleen Reidy, whose hard work and dedication had been a factor in bringing the centre to reality. Missing was Agnes Walsh who had died the previous year.

In December 1966 Kathleen Reidy retired from the position of executive secretary of the R.A.N.F. (W.A. Branch) following fourteen years' service in that capacity. Prior to this she had served on the council of the Australasian Trained Nurses Association (W.A.) and the executive of the Western Australian Nurses' Association for varying periods from 1943, and in 1952 was appointed secretary of the W.A.N.A., continuing that position until the amalgamation of the W.A.N.A. and the A.T.N.A. in 1954 when she then became secretary of this combined association which is now the Royal Australian Nursing Federation, W.A. Branch, Industrial Union of Workers. A tribute to her work was published in the March 1967 issue of the *Journal of the West Australian Nurses* and sums up the achievements of the R.A.N.F. during her term of office.

Speaking to her final annual report in the matter of finance, Miss Reidy stated that for the first few years following the amalgamation great care had to be taken in the spending of any money, 'indeed we often wondered if we would be able to pay the salaries of the book-keeper and myself'.[14] In 1962 the position of assistant secretary was created and Mrs Clare Philpott was appointed. Although Miss Reidy had visited country areas and made personal contact with professional nurses working in these areas, it was now possible to visit them more frequently, and also the rising number employed in C-class hospitals, and in doctors' and dentists' surgeries. When Mrs Philpott resigned to return to 'bedside nursing', and pending the appointment of an industrial officer, Miss Reidy and her small but dedicated staff, which included Mrs Betty King, carried on.

The improvement in salary structure and conditions of employment made for a more realistic membership fee to be levied by the state branch and the federation commitments were able to be met without hardship. Because there were a number of professional nurses who, though willing to accept the benefits were reluctant to join the association, the 'obligatory' clause in the industrial award was made mandatory. All who were employed were required to join within a specified time. Those who objected on grounds of belief or conscience were exempted but required to pay the prescribed membership fee into a nominated charity. The preference clause for those working in hospitals rarely applied as shortage of nurses precluded a rush for positions.

Perth has been described as the most isolated capital city in the world, and time and distance have both been factors which made it impractical for association representatives from Western Australia to be appointed to executive positions on federal bodies such as the National Florence Nightingale Committee of Australia and the National Council of the R.A.N.F. However, the development of an improved jet air service enabled members to leave Perth on a Friday evening and arrive in Melbourne on Saturday morning in time to attend meetings and return on Sunday in time for duty Monday morning. Expense was still a factor in limiting the number of participants. One of the first Western Australians to be elected national president of the National Florence Nightingale Committee in Australia, in 1967, was Miss P. F. Lee, principal matron in the Medical Department.

In the mid-sixties most of the workforce in nursing were employees and therefore eligible for R.A.N.F. membership. The old buildings formerly used as C-class hospitals, and now designated nursing homes, were being upgraded or rebuilt to cater for the ever-increasing numbers of aged persons. They were owned by large groups of business interests, but were under the regulations of the Department of Public Health. These homes also had to meet strict criteria to qualify for Commonwealth government assistance for patients' fees, and the employment of a matron or charge nurse was essential for registration. However there were instances where the matron became a shareholder or part-owner and her position as a member of the association had to be defined. There were also some who had retired from active nursing but were still interested in attending educational seminars and cultural activities. The matter was referred to the membership subcommittee of the branch council, which found that these members could belong to sections and attend conferences under Clause 5a, associate honorary members, and they would have all voting rights other than in arbitration matters. There was some of the older generation of professional nurses who were confused and angry about their membership rights. These were those who had paid a 'life' subscription to the A.T.N.A. and felt that somehow they had been cheated by the amalgamation. They resented the phrase 'industrial union of workers' and refuted any implied connection with the Trades and Labor Council, which was implied in the press statement by the T.L.C. calling a general strike but exempting nurses.

The matter concerned a bill which was brought down by the government on 24 October 1963 and which caused wide publicity throughout the state and concern amongst unions registered in the Arbitration Court. The legislation abolished the Arbitration Court, a three-member body, and replaced it by an Industrial Commission of four. The federation's (W.A.) stand on the matter was clearly defined in a notice in large print appearing in the December 1963 issue of the *Journal of the West Australian Nurses*, as follows:

> *Arbitration Bill—Amendment*
>
> In view of the fact that in the recent General Strike called to protest against the Arbitration Act Amendment Nurses were named by the Trades and Labor Council amongst those exempt and as the Royal Australian Nursing Federation is a non-political Union, and has no affiliation with the Trades and Labor Council, this had no connection with Student Nurses and Nurses registered or eligible to be registered. Other categories of Nurses employed in the State may be members of a Union which is affiliated with the T.L.C. and this would refer to them.[15]

There was also a rising number of professional nurses employed in areas not covered by the R.A.N.F. and whose employment was governed by other industrial awards, such as the Public Service and white-collar workers, but as nurses they did not wish to sever their connections with the R.A.N.F.

With the holding of the Third Biennial Convention of the R.A.N.F. in this state,[16] 1966 could be described as a 'vintage year' for Western Australian nurses, as the mountain had come to Mahomet. The convention drew members from all parts of Australia. It was held in the Subiaco Civic Centre, which was crowded every day. As well as association matters, topics covered a wide selection of subjects dealing with health care. Following the convention a federal council meeting was held, provision being made for observers. Two matters of great importance discussed during the meeting were the complete integration of the R.A.N.F. and the A.N.F.E.S. into one body and how this could finally be achieved, and the function of the R.A.N.F. as presented by the special subcommittee formed for that purpose. The subcommiteee's report was adopted, and published under the heading 'Functions of the Royal Australian Nursing Federation' in the *Journal of the West Australian Nurses*:

1. *To Represent All Nurses Nationally and Internationally*
(a) To maintain standing as a member body of I.C.N.
(b) To act for provision of exchange of privileges for members.
(c) To maintain two-way communications on all matters between the I.C.N. and the member associations of the Royal Australian Nursing Federation.
(d) To associate with other nursing organisations having similar objects for the advancement of nursing service and nursing education.
(e) To provide a common ground for meeting and discussion with member associations.
(f) To provide for discussions with individual nurses.
(g) To make representation to the Commonwealth Government and where desirable to support member associations in approaches to State Governments on matters affecting the health of the community and the nursing profession.
(h) To represent the member associations nationally on Committee or at Conferences.

2. *To Foster Optimal Standards of Nursing Service and Ethics*
(a) To provide information on nursing matters on request.
(b) To co-ordinate and disseminate results of any studies undertaken in this area, including the work of Standing Committees of R.A.N.F.
(c) To arrange professional observation and study programmes nationally and internationally for members of national nursing organisations.
(d) To establish policies which will promote a high status for members of the nursing profession and high standards of ethics as applied to nursing.

3. *To Foster Optimal Standards of Nursing Education*
(a) To make investigations on behalf of member bodies regarding courses of study in Australia and overseas and relevant scholarships and fellowships for members.
(b) To provide information on nursing education on request.

4. *To Foster Economic and Social Welfare of Nurses*
By collecting and making available information on request on ways and means by which satisfactory conditions of employment and equitable remunerations may be obtained.

5. *To Promote and Maintain Public Relations*
(a) By maintaining contact with nurses, nursing organisations and the community generally.

(b) By establishing and producing any publication as may be directed by the Council.[17]

The integration of the Royal Australian Nursing Federation and the Australian Nursing Federation Employees Section was not an instant affair. It involved many meetings and discussions on change of name and constitution of both bodies and although in Western Australia it was unanimous that nursing be presented by one body, this was not the decision of all member states, and it was four years before amalgamation was actually achieved. The suggested relocation of federal headquarters from Melbourne to Canberra was only partially supported.

The Western Australian branch of the federation had been most fortunate in having as legal adviser Mr T. G. Davies who was awarded a M.B.E. in July 1966. Mr Davies was the employee representative in the Court of Arbitration before it was replaced by the Western Australian Industrial Commission. He was well known for his helpful advice to those who sought it, the federation being one of the recipients of his generosity. A good friend and counsellor, his philosophy was that the federation should act for itself and not rely on others. To this end he was a tower of strength to Miss Reidy in arbitration matters.

Miss Reidy's successor as executive secretary of the R.A.N.F. (W.A.) in December 1967 was Rose Broadway. A trainee of R.P.H. Miss Broadway had for a number of years been in charge of the casualty and out-patient departments of that institution. She was an ardent supporter of the Western Australian Nurses' Association and served on its council, holding office as president. She was well versed in industrial matters.

In the mid-sixties there was in the community a rising awareness of the status of women and a movement of equal pay for equal work was gaining momentum. At the same time, the Country Women's Association in Western Australia decided to commemorate the part played by the pioneer women of the state by erecting a memorial fountain in Kings Park in their honour. It was also planned that a record would be kept incorporating the names of as many as possible of these women. Women's organizations as well as individuals were invited to submit names with a donation of $2 for each one. By this means it was hoped to raise sufficient money to finance the project. Being predominantly a women's organization, the R.A.N.F. was approached and invited to submit the names of pioneer nurses. The matter was discussed at the 1966 annual meeting and a small subcommittee appointed to collect data and submit names for selection.[18] The task was much more formidable than would appear and presented the following problems: the difficulty in defining the term 'pioneer nurse'; the criteria which would make any one of a number of nurses an outstanding pioneer in her particular field; the gathering of factual data to support claims. There was practically no documentary evidence of the achievements of early nurses and most of their stories had been passed on by word of mouth, in many cases gaining momentum and losing accuracy in the telling.

A request for information circulated by the Royal Western Australian Historical Society had brought a ready response by relatives and it was evident that nurses were held in the highest regard by the community and people were very proud of their connections with them. The recommendation of the committee was that the task of singling out names would have been impossible and could cause dissension and hurt, therefore it was suggested that a commemorative plaque be placed on the memorial with words to the following effect.

> To the memory of those early nurses and midwives who were pioneers in this State and many of whose names are recorded in the Archives of the Library of the R.A.N.F. You may read their history in a Nation's eyes.

This recommendation was adopted and a donation sent for the project. It did however draw attention to the fact that some means should be taken to have our nursing heritage preserved.

CHAPTER EIGHT

THE SEVENTIES

This was the space age, for in 1969 the first man to set foot on the moon was actually seen by people on earth, an exciting experience which gave a vision of new worlds to conquer. It heralded advances in medical science and technology, so that for nursing the seventies were years of progress and responsibility, not unrelated to concern. Locally, nationally and internationally the three were integrated. However for the purpose of clarification they have been treated individually as far as possible in this narrative.

In Western Australia, one matter of grave concern was the number of back injuries sustained by nurses and those engaged in basic health care. Compensation for this type of injury was costing the authorities dearly and a great deal of research was given to the matter. The high hospital bed was not advantageous to some patients, while the lower bed was not in the best interests of the nurse. The answer to the problem was not at all conclusive but it was found that the situation could be greatly alleviated by having available a second nurse for it was a situation in which two are definitely better than one.

There were new dimensions in surgery and increasing use in diagnosis and treatment with radioactive substances, and the associated problem of the safe disposal of radioactive waste. The use of sophisticated equipment for open-heart surgery and organ transplants all came within the sphere of specialized nursing care. Together with social change, it was becoming more and more imperative that nurses be better equipped to deal with situations involving these, not only in the interests of the person receiving advice and treatment but to lessen the stress and mental trauma which invariably arises from inability to cope.

The expanding role of the nurse in the community was evidenced in the change of name of the area of infant health to maternal and child health, which now included the pre-school child. Problems in this field included help and advice for the rising number of supporting mothers.

In 1970 there occurred an event which is the dread of all who work in places where there are helpless people: a fire broke out in Royal Perth Hospital, but miraculously it was able to be contained and there were no casualties.[1] In coping with the situation, all members of the hospital staff, including the student nurses, acted with courage and fortitude, assuring those in their care and getting them to safety. On hearing the broadcast, nurses returned to duty and from everywhere came offers of help.

In the early 1970s there was a succession of changes in personnel in senior nursing positions as the older members came up for retirement. Most of these had trained in the period prior to the Second World War. They faced a much rosier future than did their predecessors who had not had the benefit of higher salaries, superannuation and social service benefits. Retirement did not mean the end of nursing activities; some elected to continue in part-time capacities, while for others it opened up a new world of fresh interests and travel. This rising affluence of the retired nurse was reflected in the lack of patronage of the Eleanor Harvey Home and the ex-service sisters wing of the War Veterans Home. Unfortunately both these institutions have been superseded by the more acceptable unit in the retirement villages, which allows for ongoing accommodation in the 'Frail and Aged' sections and ultimately the nursing home.

Two important events took place in 1974. One was the amalgamation of the School of Nursing, Royal Perth Hospital, with the Government School of Nursing as an independent school, the Western Australian School of Nursing. Individually the students were not in favour of the venture as they preferred their hospital loyalties and traditions. Functioning independently, the W.A.S.O.N. controls the students who are seconded to the hospitals for practical experience. Royal Perth Hospital had become very specialized and the experience offered in some of the areas was outside the scope of the basic curriculum but maternity and children's nursing was lacking. The country hospitals on the other hand could provide maternity and children's experience but patients needing specialist and intensive care were usually transported to Perth by helicopter. Although the new country hospitals at Geraldton, Northam and Bunbury had been built to cover all aspects of hospitalization, they could not be used to their full potential because of lack of full-time residential medical staff.

The principal of the new school is Richard James of R.P.H., the deputy is Myrtle Underwood of G.S. of N. With the retirement of Edith Harler the position of organizer of nurse training became redundant. The lovely old home in Colin Street, which had been the G.S.N., was handed over to the Department of Mental Health, but most of its garden has been reclaimed for parking. Perhaps one of the people who most regretted the closure of the school at Colin Street was Pam Smart, who had been with it since its inception and who had played a major role in its development. In the first year of completing her training, Pam had become a victim of poliomyelitis which left her confined to a wheel chair. Her courage has given students a very special insight. The new school, which is accommodated in a multi-storeyed building adjacent to Royal Perth Hospital, was opened by the premier of Western Australia, Sir Charles Court, on 24 October 1975. Apart from students who are undertaking basic training, it also includes facilities for the training of nursing aides and students in post-basic courses. Accommodation is provided in the nearby nurses' residence, Jewell House, named in honor of Ann Jewell.

The other event was the transfer of the West Australian Branch of the College of Nursing, Australia, to the Western Australian Institute of Technology in February 1974. The move was motivated by the increased funding and facilities available, and incorporation in the School of Health Science offered opportunities for a degree course. The principal of the W.A. Branch of the college is Merle Parkes. She was appointed when the position became vacant following the resignation of Pauline Lambert, who had accepted the post of education officer to the Nurses Board after Helen Bailey had retired. Miss Parkes was appointed principal of the Department of Nursing (W.A.I.T.), which was to conduct a four year course leading to a Bachelor of Applied Science (Nursing) and which began in February 1975.

The course was accredited but the Commission of Advanced Education which provided the funds advised the institute that it was willing to approve only a three year diploma course for students who wished to become nurses. The commission indicated that it would consider a degree course only for students who had completed their basic nursing training. The institute had planned to provide for this but also considered that there was a vital need for selected students to be able to enter nursing through a bachelor's degree.[2] This in no way conflicted with the traditional nurse education programmes still conducted by the teaching hospitals, i.e. Fremantle, Sir Charles Gairdner and Princess Margaret, and the Western Australian School of Nursing.

When the thirty-six registered nurses who had completed the accredited course at W.A.I.T. in April 1978 were offered a diploma in lieu of a degree, they refused to accept anything less than the degree to which they were entitled and boycotted the graduation ceremony. Supported by the Royal Australian Nursing Federation they staged a peaceful demonstration in the city and held a rally in the Perth Town Hall, the feeling being that they had been singled out for unfair treatment.[3] The following letter from Beryl Grant, state president of the R.A.N.F., in support of the action of the W.A.I.T. students, was sent to each of the students concerned and published in the *Australian Nurses Journal* 11 June 1978.

> The Royal Australian Nursing Federation (Western Australian Branch) recognizes that today was to have been the day when you were to receive the award of Bachelor of Applied Science (Nursing) at the Western Australian Institute of Technology Graduation Ceremony to be held at the Perth Concert Hall.
>
> In recognizing the day we, as members of the national nursing organization pay tribute to the responsible and professional manner in which you have dealt with the delay in the decision regarding the level of the award to be granted.
>
> You are acting on behalf of nurses across Australia and we support you in your actions.
>
> Congratulations on successfully completing the academically accredited degree-level nursing programme.

It was not only the nurses of Western Australia who were struggling for recognition. The College of Nursing, Australia, in Melbourne, which had moved into the Lincoln Institute of Colleges, was facing similar problems. Unfortunately the delay in implementation was resulting in nurses being attracted to other disciplines within the field of health science with the possibility of their being lost to nursing. There was also the problem of nurses needing higher qualifications to enable them to avail themselves of opportunities offering in areas of research overseas.

After an unbelievable amount of hard work on the part of those supporting the W.A.I.T. movement, funding for the degree course was approved, and publicized in the *Australian Nurses Journal*:

> The Western Australian Institute of Technology has received approval for its Degree Course for experienced nurses. This was announced by the Chairman of the Council Mr Justice A. H. J. Barblett.
>
> The approval followed the Report of a National Enquiry into Nurse Education which has resulted in a number of recommendations which are still subject to Commonwealth-State consideration. Mr Barblett said that it was pleasing that early steps had been taken following the publication of the Report, to clarify the situation with respect to the course at W.A.I.T. which had now been the subject of contention for more than 12 months.

> The Commonwealth Tertiary Education Commission has now approved the funding which was previously with held, for the programme and the Western Australian post Secondary Education Commission has reaffirmed the accreditation of the course at degree level. National registration had already been granted by the Australian Council on Awards of Advanced Education.
>
> The first of the students, who successfully completed the course in the 1977 academic year, together with those completing in 1978 will be presented with their degrees at a graduation ceremony of the Institute to be held on Friday March 16 1979.[4]

Thus, Western Australia became the first Australian state to confer a nursing degree. Goals in nursing education have begun to be implemented.

Now it was autonomous the Nurses Board was able to extend its function and play a greater role in nursing education and the assessment of prospective students. The unemployment situation among teenagers and the drop in acceptances for teacher training meant that there was no longer need for recruitment 'for numbers' in those wishing to undertake nurse training as a career. The waiting lists in the teaching hospitals were becoming more extensive. The board is still committed to upholding the nursing curriculum and to applying it to assessment for registration in the various categories, and it employs a full-time staff in this area. The decision of how wide the scope of practice of the registered nurse should be is a continuing difficulty, both legally and for safe practice. Paradoxically a nurse practising in a metropolitan area is limited by the presence and availability of medical practitioners in making a provisional diagnosis and initiating treatment, but in remote areas she is often required to do both, a function for which she is inadequately prepared because of the restrictions imposed by the training curriculum and the reluctance of some members of the medical profession to sanction the initiation of some procedures. The introduction of new categories of registered nurses working in the community in areas such as family planning and family practice was interpreted as 'assuming the role of the doctor', rather than in its right perspective as being part of the team in effecting total health care. Like the infant health sister, family planning and family practice nurses are gaining wider acceptance.

In 1972 the Nurses Board celebrated its golden jubilee and to mark the occasion awarded grants to selected people for the purpose of nursing research and study.[5]

Until the seventies the disciplinary role of the Nurses Board in relation to the large numbers of registered nurses had been exercised infrequently and rarely drastically, but the escalating problems of drug and alcohol abuse within a permissive society have not left nurses untouched. Penalties imposed are for the protection of patients and the rehabilitation rather than punishment of the offender. Difficulties in apprehending offenders are to some extent caused by the fact that each Australian state has its own nurses' board and a nurse has to register in each state if the intention is to practise there. The uniform registration which was so much sought after by the early Western Australian members of the A.T.N.A. is still not a reality, although the rules are accepted in principle, and conferences are held for the discussion of important matters.

It is fortunate that the Nurses Board has retained all its past records including the individual cards, the registers and the minutes books, which yield an enormous amount of information. The yearly publication of registers in the *Government Gazette*, held in the Battye Library, are also a source of information on professional nursing. It is interesting to note that the original registration fee was 7s 6d and included the badge of a black swan at rest. This has been redesigned with the swan in flight.

A unique situation arose in 1975 when the Nurses Board approved of the training of male nurses as midwives and registered the first students for practice. This paved the way for the appointment of male nurses as directors of nursing in establishments which included both general and midwifery patients such as Kalgoorlie Hospital and other regionals.

The implementation of a Nursing Aide Training School at the Derby Hospital where the majority of patients were the indigenous people was planned as a measure to help retrain young girls in the area, many of whom were of Aboriginal descent and were invaluable in bringing community health care to their own people.

In 1969 the amended rules of the constitution of the A.N.F.E.S. were at last approved, and registered on 15 September 1969. In order to put the amalgamation of the two bodies into effect, the Royal Australian Nursing Federation and the Australian Nursing Federation Employees Section were dissolved and integrated into one national nursing organization acceptable to the International Council of Nurses, the Australian Nursing Federation. Later the prefix 'Royal' was restored. The last meetings of the R.A.N.F. and the A.N.F.E.S. took place on 30 June 1970.[6]

In 1971 it was decided that nurses in Australia should have a national journal with sections given to international and state affairs. The venture was costly but did provide an effective means of communication. The *Journal of the West Australian Nurses* was discontinued, the final issue being in June 1971.[7] First published in

1935, the journal had made a significant contribution to Western Australian nursing history. In its early days Kathleen Yeates had produced it on a shoestring budget, selling it at sixpence per copy. The social notes, names of those attending meetings, and even the obituaries brought a personal touch. The fact that much of the news was by word of mouth could account for some of the inaccuracies in names. Following the amalgamation of the A.T.N.A. (W.A.) and the W.A.N.A. in 1954 the journal continued without a break and was compiled by the secretary and staff at the R.A.N.F. office. Like its predecessor, the 'red' journal of the A.T.N.A. in New South Wales, it has provided a continuous record of nurses over the years. Fortunately a full set of journals has been preserved in the office of the R.A.N.F. (W.A. Branch) and there is a further set in the Battye Library. The journals have now been indexed for further research.[8] A journal called *Forward* was published for a short time by the W.A.N.A., but efforts to locate copies have been unsuccessful.

In March 1973 Rose Broadway resigned as executive secretary of the R.A.N.F. and her successor, Netta Yelverton, was appointed in July of the same year. Following the completion of basic training at Royal Perth Hospital Miss Yelverton had been awarded the first Agnes Walsh nursing scholarship by the Florence Nightingale Committee of W.A., and had undertaken a clinical instructors course in Scotland. Attempts to get a similar course established by the College of Nursing, Australia, were unsuccessful. As a graduate of the University of Western Australia, Miss Yelverton spent some time in research before taking up the position of R.A.N.F. secretary. Another change of R.A.N.F. personnel was the appointment of Mr M. Jahn as industrial officer on the resignation of Mr Giles in 1971, and in 1974 Wilma Gardiner was appointed nursing officer. The golden jubilee of the R.A.N.F., 1924-74, was marked by a special issue of the *Australian Nurses Journal*, which covered the years with a history of the organization.

Because of their similar interests and because a growing number of nurses were covered by awards outside the R.A.N.F., the federation considered amalgamation with the Australian Council of Salaried and Professional Associations to be desirable in order to keep in touch with the mainstream of thinking in the white-collar union field. When A.C.S.P.A. gave notice of its intention of becoming a member of the A.C.T.U., the question arose as to the wishes of R.A.N.F. branches on peak affiliations, that is, affiliations with organizations covering a wider field. The decision was based on the following alternatives: to remain with A.C.S.P.A. and through it have affiliation with the A.C.T.U.; to withdraw from

A.C.S.P.A. and seek affiliation with the A.C.T.U. independently—to do this one branch would have had to join the Trades and Labor Council in the state of origin; or to remain completely independent with no peak affiliation. The outcome was based on the number of R.A.N.F. branches in favour of such a move.

This was a contentious issue and members were greatly divided. There was a school of thought that a non-militant nursing federation with its no-strike philosophy could by gaining affiliation with A.C.T.U. act as a 'little leaven leavening the whole'. However this view was certainly not shared by nurses in Western Australia, who after showing little interest in the industrial side of nursing suddenly realized the implications of change. After an historic meeting in 1977, which because of the numbers attending had to be moved from the Nurses' Memorial Centre to the Subiaco Civic Centre, a referendum was demanded with all financial members being contacted and given the opportunity of a postal vote, and the result was the decision to withdraw from A.C.S.P.A. and remain independent. However, at the national level, the majority of state branches voted to affiliate with the A.C.T.U., with at least one branch seeking T.L.C. membership. Conditions of affiliation were as follows: that the no-strike clause in the federation's rules remain unchanged; that A.N.F. funds would not be channelled to any political association; that the federation could disaffiliate at any time.[9]

In Western Australia, the present position is that in order to comply with technicalities in industrial legislation, the nursing organization has two councils, one governing the Royal Australian Nursing Federation (W.A. Branch) and the second legislation for the R.A.N.F. Industrial Union of Workers, Perth. The office bearers for both councils, including the secretaries, are elected and serve in an honorary capacity.

Following the resignation of Netta Yelverton as executive secretary in 1977, a further appointment was not made, the duties being carried out by Wilma Gardiner in an acting capacity. From 1978 the 'office' position became that of principal nursing officer, a full-time paid appointment. Miss Gardiner is the first to hold this office.

The Nurses' Memorial Centre had fulfilled its earlier promise in providing a venue for nursing organizations and in housing the Western Australian branch of the College of Nursing, Australia, and had been used extensively for the refresher groups which had increased in numbers in the depression of the agricultural areas, when many of the married nurses on farming properties, like the school teachers in these areas, returned to their former professions and were employed in the local hospitals and schools.

When the college students moved to W.A.I.T. the premises

vacated were re-let to the W.A. Nurses' Credit Society. Formed in 1972, the Credit Society started in a small way in one room in what is now Kathleen Reidy House, but its popularity and rapid expansion necessitated new premises, which became available in 1974. One of the chief advocates of its founding was Harry Harris, a nurse educator, now with the W.A.S.O.N. and chairman of the society's board of directors. The manager is Tony Bishop, appointed in 1974. The venture has proved most profitable and an enormous help to nurses, giving them an incentive to save and enabling them to borrow with a sense of security. Through its liaison with authorized travel agents, it also offers opportunities for travel. The depressed economic climate has made it imperative that nurses do not resign their positions to travel overseas and now with faster air travel and longer leave periods they can achieve their travel ambitions, especially to the nearby Asian countries, without resigning. The W.A. Nurses' Credit Society extends its services to all accredited nurses and their families.

In 1976 it was announced that the property at 34 Kings Park Road was now freehold, and because it belonged to the nurses of Western Australia, it was felt that to protect their interests it was necessary to have the Nurses' Memorial Centre incorporated as an association. On 6 September 1976 a certificate of incorporation was issued and the inaugural meeting of the new association took place on the 17 November of the same year. In her address the chairman, Miss J. Butt, paid tribute to those who had by their foresight and endeavour made the project possible. Special mention was made of the part played by the dedicated group of women, mostly retired nurses, who under the leadership of Greta Harris, undertook the catering for functions which resulted in considerable financial support. The centre is administered by an elected committee and membership of the association has been set down at £20 for life membership and £5 per year for annual membership. It is available to nurses and approved applicants with similar interests. It is hoped that every nurse will become a member.

It was a proud moment for Australia and Western Australia in particular when Olive Anstey, M.B.E., was elected president of the International Council of Nurses at the council's 16th Quadrennial Congress in Tokyo in May 1977.[10] As one of Australia's most notable nurses Miss Anstey has served nursing at state, national and international levels. A key member of the R.A.N.F. (W.A. Branch) Council, she has been involved in most of the nursing activities in the state. In 1971 she became the first Western Australian representative to be elected president of the R.A.N.F. at national level. Internationally she served on the key membership committee of

I.C.N. in 1969 before becoming a member of the board of directors in 1973. Her dedication to her profession has been a driving force in the progress of professional nurses in Western Australia, and an inspiration to the student nurses who are to follow.

Since its inception in 1899 the retiring president of the I.C.N. at each Congress has given a 'watchword'. When Susan McGahey, representing Australia, was elected president in 1904, the 'watchword' was 'courage'. Miss McGahey was secretary of the newly formed Australasian Trained Nurses Association and it was certainly a courageous undertaking to press towards the goal of creating and upholding a standard of nursing care by uniting nurses in a professional organization. In Tokyo in 1977 the 'watchword' given by the outgoing president for the next quadrennium was 'accountability'. To the nurses of the eighty-eight affiliated national associations this has brought the realization that they are bound to be responsible and be called to account for their actions as they affect all persons within the sphere of their professional involvement.

In this country, the R.A.N.F., the College of Nursing, Australia, and the National Florence Nightingale Committee have accepted this challenge and have combined in a programme which will enable them through nursing service and nursing education to reach their goals in providing quality health care.[11]

History is on-going. It does not stop with an event or a celebration. The incidents of one hundred and fifty years only serve as signposts for the W.A.Y. ahead.

> Whatever makes the past distant or the future predominate over the present advances us in the dignity of thinking beings
>
> [Dr Johnson]

APPENDIX I

LIST OF NURSES
1896-1922

The lists in Appendix I include all those who trained as nurses in Western Australia from 1896 to 1922, as well as some of those, trained and untrained, who came from interstate and overseas and nursed. The majority were accepted for membership of the Australasian Trained Nurses Association.

There are two lists. First there are extracts reproduced directly from the *Blue Books* of the period, and from the *Perth Public Hospital Annual Report* for the year ended 30 June 1916. Following these are lists which have been compiled from incomplete registers and hand-written reports, so it is possible that there are errors in the spelling of names, and omissions.

After 1922, when state registration was achieved, registers were kept by the Nurses' Registration Board, and published annually in the *Government Gazette*. A complete set is held in the Battye Library.

(1) No. (consecutive).	(2) Designation of Office.	(3) Name.	(4) Date of Appointment.	(5) Rate of Annual Salary. To 30th June, 1899.	(5) Rate of Annual Salary. From 1st July, 1899.	(6) First Appointment under the Government.
				£ s. d.	£ s. d.	
1899	*Perth Public Hospital*					
8	Matron	Wemyss, Eliz. G. G. ...	March, 1899	120 0 0	120 0 0	March, 1899
9	Nurse	Hurnall, Jessie	October, 1893	70 0 0	70 0 0	October, 1893
10	Do.	Marrett, Florence... ..	April, 1897	52 0 0	52 0 0	April, 1897
11	Do.	Marrett, Annie	April, 1897	52 0 0	52 0 0	April, 1897
12	Do.	Arstall, Ada *d*	April, 1897	52 0 0	...	April, 1897
13	Do.	Broomhall, Florence *e* ...	April, 1897	52 0 0	52 0 0	April, 1897
14	Do.	Timmins, Edith M. *f* ...	May, 1897	52 0 0	...	May, 1897
15	Do.	Culley, Florence	December, 1897	52 0 0	52 0 0	December, 1897
16	Do.	Milne, Bessie	December, 1897	52 0 0	52 0 0	December, 1897
17	Do.	Wincey, Minnie *d* ...	January, 1898	52 0 0	...	January, 1898
18	Do.	Moody, Edith *g*	February, 1898	70 0 0	...	February, 1898
19	Do.	Kirkman, Annie *h* ...	January, 1896	52 0 0	...	January, 1896
20	Do.	Rogers, Laura	February, 1899	70 0 0	70 0 0	February, 1899
21	Do.	Techow, Ulla Eliz. *i* ...	July, 1896	30 0 0	52 0 0	July, 1896
22	Probationer Nurse...	Blain, Sarah Mary *h* ...	May, 1896	30 0 0	...	May, 1896
23	Do.	Collier, May *i*	December, 1896	30 0 0	30 0 0	December, 1896
24	Do.	Shaw, Ellie *i*	January, 1897	30 0 0	30 0 0	January, 1897
25	Do.	Hodgson, Grace A. ...	March, 1897	30 0 0	30 0 0	March, 1897
26	Do.	Bole, Eliza	April, 1897	30 0 0	30 0 0	April, 1897
27	Do.	Power, Marie	May, 1897	30 0 0	30 0 0	May, 1897
28	Do.	Rose, Alice Emily ...	December, 1897	20 0 0	20 0 0	December, 1897
29	Do.	Minchin, Lucy	January, 1898	20 0 0	20 0 0	January, 1898
30	Do.	Quinn, Ellen *j*	February, 1898	12 0 0	...	February, 1898
31	Do.	Ward, Kate	February, 1898	20 0 0	20 0 0	February, 1898
32	Do.	Wilson, Constance C. ...	March, 1898	20 0 0	20 0 0	March, 1898
33	Do.	Atcheson, Jeannie ...	April, 1898	20 0 0	20 0 0	April, 1898
34	Do.	Hicks, Annie D.	April, 1898	20 0 0	20 0 0	April, 1898
35	Do.	Lee, Lulu	May, 1898	20 0 0	20 0 0	May, 1898
36	Do.	Bridges, Annie Maria *h* ...	June, 1898	12 0 0	...	June, 1898
37	Do.	McMahon, Hannah *f* ...	June, 1898	12 0 0	...	June, 1898
38	Do.	Tindall, Eleanor F. ...	June, 1898	12 0 0	20 0 0	June, 1898
39	Do.	Dunne, M. H. *j*	June, 1898	12 0 0	...	June, 1898
40	Do.	Balding, Maida Florence	February, 1899	12 0 0	12 0 0	February, 1899
41	Do.	Orchard, Annie M. ...	February, 1899	12 0 0	12 0 0	February, 1899
42	Do.	Shapcott, Florence Maud	February, 1899	12 0 0	12 0 0	February, 1899
43	Do.	Butler, Leah F.	February, 1899	12 0 0	12 0 0	February, 1899
44	Do.	Hitches, Ada *k*	May, 1899	12 0 0	12 0 0	May, 1899
45	Do.	O'Callaghan, Annie ...	August, 1899	...	12 0 0	August, 1899

46	Do.	Cordingley, Daisy Edith	November, 1899	...	12 0 0	November, 1899
47	Do.	Aithbert, Mildred G. ...	November, 1899	...	12 0 0	November, 1899
48	Do.	Goldman, Violet	December, 1899	...	12 0 0	December, 1899
49	Do.	Fry, Ruby Frances ...	December, 1899	...	12 0 0	December, 1899
	Coolgardie.					
1	District Medical Officer	Seed, W. P. *a*	August, 1898	250 0 0	250 0 0	February, 1896
2	Resident Physician	Leschen, H. A. *b*	August, 1898	350 0 0	350 0 0	August, 1898
3	Matron	Snodgrass, R. *c*	August, 1897	150 0 0	150 0 0	May, 1897
4	Charge Nurse	Fraser, M. *c*	February, 1897	75 0 0	70 0 0	February 1897
5	Do.	Steers, M. *c f*	February, 1897	75 0 0	...	February 1897
		succeeded by				
6	Do.	Combley, E. *c*	February, 1899	75 0 0	...	February, 1899
7	Do.	Scales, M. *c*	March, 1897	75 0 0	70 0 0	March, 1897
8	Do.	O'Callaghan, B *c f* ...	December, 1897	75 0 0	70 0 0	December, 1897
		succeeded by				
9	Do.	O'Keefe, M. *c*	October, 1899	...	70 0 0	March, 1897
10	Do.	Abernethy, A. E. *c e* ...	July, 1899	...	70 0 0	October, 1897
11	Nurse	Abernethy, A. E. *c* ...	January, 1899	60 0 0	...	October, 1897
12	Do.	O'Keefe, M. *c*	March, 1897	60 0 0	60 0 0	March, 1897
13	Do.	Fitzsimons, H. J. *c* ...	February, 1899	60 0 0	60 0 0	March, 1897
14	Do.	Bird, N. *c d*	February, 1898	60 0 0	...	February, 1898
		succeeded by				
15	Do.	Grover, M. *c e*	February, 1899	60 0 0	60 0 0	November, 1897
16	Do.	Pledge, E. *c*	August, 1898	60 0 0	60 0 0	February, 1897
17	Do.	Duncan, E. *c*	January, 1898	60 0 0	60 0 0	January, 1898
18	Charge Nurse	Varian, N. *c d*	May, 1898	70 0 0	...	May, 1897
		succeeded by				
19	Nurse	Mann, E. *c*	May, 1899	60 0 0	60 0 0	May, 1899
20	Do.	Daw, F. A. *c d*	August, 1898	60 0 0	...	August, 1898
		succeeded by				
21	Do.	Kirkman, A. *c*	May, 1898	60 0 0	60 0 0	May, 1898
22	Do.	Smith, B. *c d*	February, 1899	60 0 0	...	December, 1897
23	Do.					
		succeeded by				
		Blain, S. *c*	June, 1899	60 0 0	60 0 0	June, 1899
24	Do.	Reid, M. C. *c*	March, 1897	60 0 0	...	March, 1897
25	Junior Nurse	Grover, M. *c*	November, 1897	46 0 0	...	November, 1897
26	Probationer...	Farnsworth, E. *c*	August, 1897	36 0 0	...	May, 1897
27	Do.	Mildred, G. M. *c d* ...	October, 1898	18 0 0	...	October, 1898
		succeeded by				
28	Do.	McCarthy, J. *c*	March, 1899	18 0 0	18 0 0	March, 1899
29	Do.	King, O. *c*	January, 1899	24 0 0	24 0 0	January, 1899
30	Do.	Dowson, A. *c*	November, 1898	18 0 0	24 0 0	November, 1898
31	Do.	Tucker, M. *c*	November, 1898	18 0 0	24 0 0	November, 1898
32	Do.	Rose, M. *c d*	January, 1899	18 0 0	18 0 0	January, 1899
		succeeded by				
33	Do.	Walker, A. *c*	November, 1899	...	18 0 0	November, 1899
34	Do.	Barker, M. *c*	January, 1899	18 0 0	18 0 0	January, 1899

(1) No. (consecutive).	(2) Designation of Office.	(3) Name.	(4) Date of Appointment.	(5) Rate of Annual Salary. To 30th June, 1899. £	s.	d.	From 1st July, 1899. £	s.	d.	(6) First Appointment under the Government.
	Kalgoorlie.									
8	District Medical Officer	O'Meehan, J. A.	February, 1896	250	0	0	250	0	0	September, 1877
9	Resident Physician	Love, A. A. *a*	November, 1897	350	0	0	350	0	0	November, 1897
10	Matron	Harvey, B. *a*	December, 1898	130	0	0	150	0	0	October, 1896
11	Night Superintendent	Sadler, M. *a*	January, 1899	75	0	0	75	0	0	February, 1896
12	Charge Nurse	Jenkins, M. E. *a*	February, 1896	70	0	0	70	0	0	February, 1896
13	Do. do.	Herbert, E. *a*	January, 1897	70	0	0	70	0	0	January, 1897
14	Do. do.	Newland, T. *a*	February, 1899	70	0	0	70	0	0	September, 1896
15	Do. do.	Siekmann, F. B. *a* ...	December, 1898	70	0	0	70	0	0	January, 1897
16	Nurse	Kirchner, M. P. *a*	March, 1897	60	0	0	60	0	0	March, 1897
17	Do.	Richardson, J. *a*	March, 1898	60	0	0	60	0	0	March, 1898
18	Do.	O'Callaghan, M. *a* ...	March, 1897	60	0	0	60	0	0	March, 1897
19	Do.	O'Callaghan, E. M. *a* ...	September, 1897	60	0	0	60	0	0	September, 1897
20	Do.	Bruton, K. *a*	October, 1899	...			60	0	0	October, 1899
21	Do.	Tucker, E. *a c*	October, 1897	50	0	0	50	0	0	October, 1897
		succeeded by								
22	Do.	Hopkins, L. *a*	October, 1899	...			60	0	0	October, 1899
23	Do.	Hutton, H. *a*	May, 1899	50	0	0	50	0	0	April, 1897
24	Probationer Nurse...	Bromilow, C. A. *a*... ...	November, 1898	18	0	0	18	0	0	November, 1898
25	Do. do.	Smythe, M. *a*	December, 1898	18	0	0	18	0	0	December, 1898
26	Do. do.	McCarthy, J. *a*	August, 1899...	18	0	0	18	0	0	August, 1899
	Fremantle Public Hospital									
3	Matron	Warden, Jessie	April, 1898 ...	125	0	0				April, 1898
4	Nurse	Birt, Margaret	February, 1898	60	0	0				February, 1898
5	Do.	Emmics, Annabella. ...	February, 1898	60	0	0				February, 1898
6	Do.	Powell, Mary	July, 1898 ...	48	0	0				July, 1898
7	Do.	Mortimer, Mary	June, 1896 ...	48	0	0				June, 1896
8	Do.	Dixon, Alice	June, 1898 ...	60	0	0				June, 1898
9	Do.	Broomhall, Florence ...	August, 1899...	60	0	0				August, 1899
10	Do.	Kerr, Hannah	July, 1899 ...	48	0	0				July, 1899
11	Probationer Nurse	Dingle, Rebecca *a* ...	November, 1897	40	0	0				November, 1897
12	Do.	Crudden, Rebecca *b* ...	February, 1897	40	0	0				February, 1897
13	Do.	Webb, Lillian	January, 1897	40	0	0				January, 1897
14	Do.	McLaren, Lily	December, 1897	30	0	0				December, 1897
15	Do.	McLeod, Catherine *c* ...	January, 1899	20	0	0				January, 1899
16	Do.	Anthony, Isabella ...	May, 1899 ...	20	0	0				May, 1899
17	Do.	Broomhall, Annie ...	July, 1899 ...	20	0	0				July, 1899
18	Do.	Lowrie, Jean	July, 1899 ...	20	0	0				July, 1899

1900

				To 30th June, 1900.	From 1st July, 1900.	
	Coolgardie.					
30	District Medical Officer	Seed, W. P. *f*	August, 1898	250 0 0	250 0 0	**February**, 1896
31	Resident Physician	Leschen, H. A. *g*	August, 1898	350 0 0	...	**August**, 1898
		succeeded by				
32	Do	Miskin, L. J. *a*	February, 1900	350 0 0	350 0 0	**February**, 1900
33	Matron	Snodgrass, R. *a*	August, 1897	150 0 0	150 0 0	**May**, 1897
34	Secretary	Peart, R.	July, 1898	208 0 0	208 0 0	**July**, 1898
35	Dispenser	Bennett, W. *a*	July, 1898	160 0 0	160 0 0	**July**, 1898
36	Night Superintendent	Abernethy, A. E. *a b* ...	February, 1900	75 0 0	...	October, 1897
		succeeded by				
37	Do do	Fitzsimmons, H. J. *a b* ...	April, 1900	75 0 0	75 0 0	**March**, 1897
		succeeded by				
38	Do do	Birt, Margaret *a b* ...	August, 1900	...	75 0 0	**April**, 1900
		succeeded by				
39	Do do	Blain, S. *a*	November, 1900	...	75 0 0	**June**, 1899
40	Charge Nurse	Fraser, M. *a b*	February, 1897	70 0 0	...	**February**, 1897
		succeeded by				
41	Do do	Birt, M. *a b*	April, 1900	70 0 0	70 0 0	**April**. 1900
		succeeded by				
42	Do do	Grover, M. *a*	August, 1900	...	70 0 0	**November**, 1897
43	Do do	O'Keefe, N. *a h*	March, 1897	60 0 0	...	**March**, 1897
		succeeded by				
44	Do do	Fitzsimmons, H. J. *a* ...	August, 1900	...	70 0 0	**March**, 1897
1	Charge Nurse	Abernethy, A. E. *a b* ...	July, 1899	70 0 0	...	October, 1897
		succeeded by				
2	Do do	Grover, M. *a b*	July, 1900	...	70 0 0	November, 1897
		succeeded by				
3	Do do	Blain, S. *a b*	August, 1900	...	70 0 0	June, 1899
		succeeded by				
4	Do do	Birt, Margaret *a*	November, 1900	...	70 0 0	April, 1900
5	Do do	Scales, M. *a c*	January, 1900	70 0 0	...	March, 1897
6	Nurse	Mortimer, M. *a*	April, 1900	60 0 0	60 0 0	April, 1900
7	Do	Grover, M. *a b*	February, 1899	60 0 0	...	November, 1897
		succeeded by				
8	Do	Kirkman, Annie *a* ...	July, 1900	...	60 0 0	May, 1898
9	Do	Fitzsimmons, H. T. *a c* ...	February, 1899	60 0 0	...	March, 1897
10	Do	Pledge, E. *a d*	August, 1898	60 0 0	...	February, 1897
11	Do	Duncan, E. *a d*	January, 1898	60 0 0	...	January, 1898
12	Do	Kirkman, A. *a c*	May, 1898	60 0 0	60 0 0	May, 1898
13	Do	Blain, S. *a*	June, 1899	60 0 0	60 0 0	June, 1899
14	Do	Fraser, Annie *a*	June, 1900	60 0 0	60 0 0	June, 1900
15	Probationer Nurse...	King, Olive *a*	January, 1899	30 0 0	30 0 0	January, 1899
16	Do	Dowson, A. *a*	November, 1898	24 0 0	36 0 0	November, 1898
17	Do	Tucker, M. *a*	November, 1898	24 0 0	36 0 0	November, 1898
18	Do	Walker, A. *a*	November, 1899	18 0 0	24 0 0	November, 1899
19	Do	Barker, M. *a g*	January, 1899	24 0 0	...	January, 1899
20	Do	Thompson, E. *a*	April, 1900	18 0 0	18 0 0	April, 1900

(1) No. (consecutive).	(2) Designation of Office.	(3) Name.	(4) Date of Appointment.	(5) Rate of Annual Salary. To 30th June, 1900. £	s.	d.	From 1st July, 1900. £	s.	d.	(6) First Appointment under the Government.
	Kalgoorlie.									
16	District Medical Officer	O'Meehan, J. A.	February, 1896	250	0	0	250	0	0	September, 1877
17	Resident Physician	Love, A. *a*	November, 1897	350	0	0	350	0	0	November, 1897
18	Matron	Harvey, B. *a*	December, 1898	150	0	0	150	0	0	October, 1896
19	Secretary and Dispenser	Tratman, C. S. *a*	May, 1899	200	0	0	208	0	0	May, 1899
20	Charge Nurse	Herbert, E. *a*	January, 1897	70	0	0	70	0	0	January, 1897
21	Do do	Jenkins, M. E. *a*	February, 1896	70	0	0	70	0	0	February, 1896
22	Do do	Sickmann, F. B. *a* ...	December, 1898	70	0	0	70	0	0	January, 1897
23	Do do	Newland, T. *a*	February, 1899	70	0	0	70	0	0	September, 1896
24	Nurse	O'Callaghan, M. *a b* ...	March, 1897	60	0	0	60	0	0	March, 1897
		succeeded by								
25	Do	Kirkman, Annie *a* ...	November, 1900	...			60	0	0	May, 1898
26	Do	O'Callaghan, E. M. *a f* ...	February, 1898	60	0	0	60	0	0	February, 1898
27	Do	Kirchner, M. P. *a b* ...	March, 1897	60	0	0	...			March, 1897
		succeeded by								
28	Do	Stables, J. *a c*	January, 1900	60	0	0	...			July, 1900
		succeeded by								
29	Do	Dellow, J. *a g*	February, 1900	60	0	0	...			February, 1900
30	Do	Richardson, J. *a*	March, 1898	60	0	0	60	0	0	March, 1898
31	Do	Bruton, K. *a c*	October, 1899	60	0	0	...			October, 1899
		succeeded by								
32	Do	Fyfe, J. *a b*	February, 1900	60	0	0	...			February, 1900
		succeeded by								
33	Do	O'Keefe, N. *a*	April, 1900	60	0	0	60	0	0	March, 1897
34	Do	Hopkins, L. *a c*	October, 1899	60	0	0	...			October, 1899
		succeeded by								
35	Do	Crump, E. *a c*	April, 1900	60	0	0	60	0	0	March, 1899
		succeeded by								
36	Do	Fraser, Annie *a*	November, 1900	...			60	0	0	June, 1900
37	Do	McLeod, C. *a*	February, 1900	60	0	0	60	0	0	February, 1900
38	Do	Hutton, H. *a*	May, 1899	50	0	0	50	0	0	April, 1897
39	Do	Hodgson, G. A. *a*	April, 1900	60	0	0	60	0	0	April, 1900
40	Do	Brooks, Nancy, *a*	June, 1900	60	0	0	60	0	0	July, 1898
41	Do	Scales, M. *a*	December, 1900	...			60	0	0	March, 1897
42	Probationer Nurse	Smythe, M. *a*	December, 1898	24	0	0	36	0	0	December, 1898
43	Do do	McCarthy, Ivy *a h* ...	August, 1899	24	0	0	...			August, 1899

Fremantle Public Hospital

5	Matron	Warden, J. *a*	April, 1898	125 0 0	...	April, 1898
6	Do	Dixon, A. T.	June, 1898	60 0 0	125 0 0	June, 1898
7	Nurse	Birt, M. C. *a*	February, 1898	60 0 0	...	February, 1898
8	Do	Broomhall, F.	August, 1899	60 0 0	60 0 0	August, 1899
9	Do	Smith, M.	April, 1900	52 0 0	52 0 0	January, 1900
10	Do	Abernethy, A. E.	April, 1900	52 0 0	52 0 0	February, 1897
11	Do	Powell, M. *a*	July, 1898	48 0 0	...	July, 1898
12	Do	Mortimer, M. *a*	June, 1896	48 0 0	...	June, 1896
13	Do	Kerr, H. *c*	July, 1899	48 0 0	48 0 0	July, 1899
14	Do	Dingle, R. J.	June, 1900	48 0 0	48 0 0	November, 1897
15	Do	Nickolls, N. S.	April, 1900	48 0 0	48 0 0	April, 1900
16	Probationer Nurse	Webb, L. *d*	January, 1897	40 0 0	...	January, 1897
17	Do	McLaren, L.	December, 1897	40 0 0	48 0 0	December, 1897
18	Do	McLeod, C. *d*	January, 1899	30 0 0	...	January, 1899
19	Do	Anthony, J.	May, 1899	20 0 0	30 0 0	May, 1899
20	Do	Broomhall, Annie	July, 1899	20 0 0	30 0 0	July, 1899
21	Do	Lowrie, J.	July, 1899	20 0 0	30 0 0	July, 1899
22	Do	Connolly, A.	January, 1900	20 0 0	30 0 0	April, 1899
23	Do	Rossiter, M.	April, 1900	20 0 0	20 0 0	April, 1900
24	Do	Hayes, L. *d*	April, 1900	20 0 0	...	April, 1900
25	Do	Turner, E.	May, 1900	20 0 0	20 0 0	May, 1900
26	Do	Gardiner, H.	June, 1900	20 0 0	20 0 0	June, 1900

1901

				To 30th June, 1901.	From 1st July, 1901.	
	Coolgardie.					
1	Nurse	Kirkman, Annie *a b*	July, 1900	60 0 0	...	May, 1898
		succeeded by				
2	Do	Tucker, Ella *b*	May, 1901	60 0 0	...	October, 1897
		succeeded by				
3	Do	Mundy, Rachael *a*	July, 1901	...	60 0 0	July, 1901
4	Do	Futton, Maude F. *a b*	June, 1899	60 0 0	...	January, 1899
5	Do	Fraser, Annie *a d*	June, 1900	60 0 0	...	June, 1900
6	Probationer Nurse	King, Olive *a d*	January, 1899	30 0 0	...	January, 1899
7	Do	Dowson, A. *d*	November, 1898	36 0 0	...	November, 1898
		succeeded by				
8	Do	Walker, A. *a*	May, 1901	24 0 0	36 0 0	November, 1899
9	Do	Tucker, Mary *a*	November, 1898	36 0 0	36 0 0	November, 1898
		succeeded by				
10	Do	White, Alice M. *a*	December, 1901	...	36 0 0	May, 1901
11	Do	Walker, A. *d*	November, 1899	24 0 0	...	November, 1899
		succeeded by				
12	Do	Foley, J. A. *a*	April, 1901	18 0 0	24 0 0	March, 1901
13	Do	Thompson, E. *a*	April, 1900	18 0 0	24 0 0	April, 1900

(1) No. (consecutive).	(2) Designation of Office.	(3) Name.	(4) Date of Appointment.	(5) Rate of Annual Salary. To 30th June, 1901.	(5) Rate of Annual Salary. From 1st July, 1901.	(6) First Appointment under the Government, followed by continuous service.
				£ s. d.	£ s. d.	
	Kalgoorlie.					
1	Nurse	Hutton, H. *a*	May, 1899	50 0 0	50 0 0	April, 1897
2	Do	Hodgson, G. A. *b*	April, 1900	60 0 0	...	April, 1900
		succeeded by				
3	Do	Edwards, B. *a b*	February, 1901	36 0 0	...	February, 1901
4	Do	Brooks, Nancy *a*	June, 1900	60 0 0	60 0 0	July, 1898
5	Do	Scales, M. *a b*	December, 1900	60 0 0	...	March, 1897
6	Do	Smyth, M. T. *a*	December, 1898	36 0 0	42 0 0	December, 1898
7	Do	Hamilton, C. *b*.	April, 1900	36 0 0	...	April, 1900
		succeeded by				
8	Do	Futton, F. M. *a*	January, 1901	36 0 0	36 0 0	January, 1899
9	Nurse Probationer...	Scott, Edith *c*	January, 1901	18 0 0	24 0 0	January, 1901
10	Do do	Wilson, May *a*	July, 1901	...	18 0 0	July, 1901
	Fremantle Public Hospital					
3	Matron	Dixon, A. T.	June, 1898	125 0 0	125 0 0	June, 1898
4	Nurse	Broomhall, F. *m*	August, 1899	60 0 0	60 0 0	August, 1899
5	Do	Smith, M. *k*	April, 1900	52 0 0	...	January, 1900
6	Do	Abernethy, A. E. *l* ...	April, 1900	52 0 0	...	February, 1897
7	Do	Dingle, R. J.	June, 1900	48 0 0	48 0 0	November, 1897
8	Do	Nickolls, N. S. *n*	April, 1900	48 0 0	...	April, 1900
9	Do	Nickolls, Christina *k* ...	January 11, 1901	48 0 0	...	January 11, 1901
10	Do	McCulloch, Elizabeth ...	June 1, 1901	52 0 0	52 0 0	June 1, 1901
11	Do	Sturman, Agnes	June 15, 1901	52 0 0	52 0 0	June 15, 1901
12	Do	Corrigan, Mary *q*	July, 1901	...	52 0 0	July, 1901
13	Do	Brown, Mary	July 2, 1901	...	48 0 0	July, 1901
14	Probationer Nurse	McLaren, L. *k*	December, 1897	48 0 0	...	December, 1897
15	Do	Anthony, J.	May, 1899	30 0 0	30 0 0	May, 1899
16	Do	Broomhall, Annie ...	July, 1899	30 0 0	30 0 0	July, 1899
17	Do	Lowrie, J.	July, 1899	30 0 0	30 0 0	July, 1899
18	Do	Connolly, A.	January, 1900	30 0 0	30 0 0	April, 1899
19	Do	Rossiter, M.	April, 1900	20 0 0	20 0 0	April, 1900
20	Do	Turner, E....	May, 1900	20 0 0	20 0 0	May, 1900
21	Do	Gardiner, H.	June, 1900	20 0 0	20 0 0	June, 1900
22	Do	Kerr, Ellen	June, 1901	20 0 0	20 0 0	June, 1901
23	Do	Callaghan, Vera	June, 1901	20 0 0	20 0 0	June, 1901
24	Do	Howarth, Bertha ...	December, 1901	...	20 0 0	December, 1901
25	Do	Claire, Muriel *q*	June, 1901	20 0 0	20 0 0	June, 1901

				To 30th June, 1902.	From 1st July, 1902.	
1902						
	Coolgardie.					
9	District Medical Officer	Seed, William Pope *e*	Aug., 1898	250	250	Feb., 1896
10	Resident Physician	Miskin, Leonard John *d l*	Oct., 1901	350	...	Feb., 1900
		succeeded by				
11	Do	Thompson, James *d l*	April, 1902	350	350	July, 1899
		succeeded by				
12	Do	Miskin, Leonard John *d l*	Sept., 1902	...	350	Feb., 1900
13	Secretary and Dispenser	Bennett, William *m*	April, 1901	225	225	July, 1898
14	Matron	Hewton, Theresa *b*	March, 1901	150	150	Feb., 1897
15	Night Superintendent	Birt, M. C. *b d*	Nov., 1902	75	...	April, 1900
		succeeded by				
16	Do	Grover, Margaret Martha *b d*	Jan., 1902	75	...	Nov., 1897
		succeeded by				
17	Do	Blain, Sarah Mary *b d*	March, 1902	75	...	June, 1898
		succeeded by				
18	Do	Sturman, Agnes *b d*	May, 1902	75	...	March, 1902
		succeeded by				
19	Do	Grover, Margaret Martha *b d f*	July, 1902	...	75	Nov., 1897
20	Charge Nurse	Grover, Margaret Martha *b d*	Aug., 1901	70	...	Nov., 1897
		succeeded by				
21	Do	Birt, M. C. *b c*	Jan., 1902	70	...	April, 1900
		succeeded by				
22	Do	Sturman, Agnes *c b*	July, 1902	...	70	March, 1902
23	Do	Sturman, Agnes *b d*	March, 1902	70	...	March, 1902
		succeeded by				
24	Do	Blain, S. M. *b*	May, 1902	70	70	June, 1898
25	Do	Blain, S. M. *b d*	March, 1901	70	...	June, 1898
		succeeded by				
26	Do	Grover, Margaret A. *b*	March, 1902	70	70	Nov., 1897
27	Nurse	Mundy, Rachael *b c*	July, 1901	60	60	July, 1901
		succeeded by				
28	Do	Dowson, Amy *b*	Nov., 1902	...	50	Nov., 1898
29	Do	Pingelly, Ethel *b g*	Jan., 1902	50	60	April, 1896
30	Probationer Nurse	Pizey, Mary Hanfield Ellen *b*	May, 1902	18	18	May, 1902
31	Do	Thompson, Emily *b h*	April, 1900	24	36	April, 1900
32	Do	White, Alice Miriam *b*	Dec., 1901	36	36	April, 1901
33	Do	Walker, Annie M. *b*	Nov., 1899	36	36	Nov., 1899
34	Do	Foley, Josephine Bernardette *b d*	March, 1901	24	...	March, 1901
	Kalgoorlie.					
3	District Medical Officer	O'Meehan, John Albert *b*	Feb., 1896	250	250	Sept., 1877
4	Resident Physician	Love, Archibald A. *c d*	Nov., 1897	350	350	Nov., 1897
		succeeded by				
5	Do do	Lewis, John Brook *c d*	July, 1902	...	350	July, 1902
		succeeded by				
6	Do do	Thompson, James *c d*	Nov., 1902	...	350	July, 1899

(1) No. (consecutive).	(2) Designation of Office.	(3) Name.	(4) Date of Appointment.	(5) Rate of Annual Salary. To 30th June, 1902.	From 1st July, 1902.	(6) First Appointment under the Government, followed by continuous service.
				£	£	
7	Secretary and Dispenser	Tratman, Charles Stanley *c*	May, 1899	258	258	May, 1899
8	Matron	Harvey, Florence Jane Elizabeth *c* ...	Dec., 1898	150	150	Oct., 1896
9	Charge Nurse	Jenkins, Mary Eleanor *c e*	Feb., 1896	70	...	Feb., 1896
		succeeded by				
10	Do do	Fraser, Annie Mackenzie *c*	March, 1902	70	70	June, 1900
11	Do do	McLeod, Catherine *c f*	March, 1901	70	...	Feb., 1900
		succeeded by				
12	Do do	O'Callaghan, Mary *c*	March, 1902	70	70	March, 1897
13	Do do	Siekmann, Franziska Brinkworth *c* ...	Dec., 1898	70	70	Sept., 1896
14	Do do	Newland, Teresa *c*	Feb., 1899	70	70	Sept., 1896
15	Nurse	O'Keefe, Mary Geneviève *c e*	April, 1900	60	...	March, 1897
		succeeded by				
16	Do	Tucker, Ella Jane *c g*	March, 1902	60	60	Oct., 1897
		succeeded by				
17	Do	Lowrie, Jean E. *c*	Dec., 1902	...	60	Dec., 1902
18	Do	Fraser, Annie Mackenzie *c h*	Nov., 1900	60	...	June, 1900
		succeeded by				
19	Do	Foley, Josephine Bernardette *c*	May, 1902	24	24	March, 1901
20	Do	Brooks, Nancy *c g*	June, 1900	60	60	July, 1898
21	Do	Griggs, May *c*	June, 1902	60	60	June, 1902
22	Do	Hutton, Helena *c g*	May, 1899	50	...	April, 1897
		succeeded by				
23	Do	Wilson, C. C. *c g*	Jan., 1902	55	...	Jan., 1902
		succeeded by				
24	Do	Foreman, Eliza *c i*	May, 1902	36	36	May, 1902
		succeeded by				
25	Do	Daw, Francis E. *c j*	Sept., 1902	...	60	May, 1902
		succeeded by				
26	Do	Wray, Ernestine *c*	Dec., 1902	...	18	Dec., 1902
27	Do	DeLeon, J. *c k*	March, 1902	60	...	March, 1902
		succeeded by				
28	Do	McMahon, Ellen *c l*	April, 1902	36	36	April, 1902
		succeeded by				
29	Do	Ormiston, Agnes Campbell *c*	Oct., 1902	...	60	Oct., 1902

30	Do	Dowson, Amy *c g*	Jan., 1901	36	42	Nov., 1898
		succeeded by				
31	Do	Smith, Barbara *c*	Dec., 1902	...	60	Jan., 1902
32	Do	King, Olive *c m*	March, 1902	44	...	Jan., 1899
33	Do	Thompson, Emily *c*	Sept., 1902	...	36	April, 1900
34	Do	Smyth, M. T. *c n*	Dec., 1898	42	...	Dec., 1898
		succeeded by				
35	Do	Byfield, Alice E. *c*	Feb., 1902	36	36	Feb., 1902
36	Do	Futton, F. M. *c g*	Jan., 1901	36	...	Jan., 1899
		succeeded by				
37	Probationer Nurse	Graham, Elizabeth *c*	Feb., 1902	18	18	Feb., 1902
38	Do do	Scott, Edith Grace *c o*	Jan., 1901	24	...	Jan., 1901
		succeeded by				
39	Do do	Hutchinson, Anne *c*	Jan., 1902	18	24	Jan., 1902
40	Do do	Wilson, May *c*	July, 1901	18	24	July, 1901
	Fremantle Public Hospital					
3	Matron	Dixon, Alice	June, 1898	125	125	June, 1898
4	Nurse	Dingle, Rebecca H. *a j*	June, 1901	52	60	Nov., 1897
5	Do	Sturman, Agnes *b*	June, 1901	52	...	June, 1901
6	Probationer Nurse	Lowrie, Jean *c*	July, 1899	40	...	July, 1899
7	Do	Connolly, Annie *d*	Jan., 1900	40	40	April, 1899
8	Do	Howarth, Bertha *e*	Dec., 1901	20	...	Dec., 1901
9	Nurse	Cameron, Dolinda	Oct., 1902	...	52	Oct., 1902
10	Probationer Nurse	Poole, Christina	Jan., 1902	20	20	Jan., 1902
11	Do	Collins, Helena	June, 1902	20	20	June, 1902
12	Do	McKenna, Veotti	June, 1902	20	20	June, 1902
13	Do	Cottell, Daisy	July, 1902	...	20	July, 1902
14	Do	McDonald, Mary	Nov., 1902	...	20	Nov., 1902
				To 30th June, 1903.	From 1st July, 1903.	
1903						
	Claremont Asylum.					
4	Chief Attendant	Gallagher, William *a*	Aug., 1903	...	200	May, 1897
5	Attendant	Bolger, Thomas Joseph *a*	Aug., 1903	...	130	Jan., 1895
6	Do	Lyons, James *a*	Aug., 1903	...	90	Feb., 1903
7	Do	House, Herbert John *a f*	Aug., 1903	...	90	April, 1903
		succeeded by				
8	Do	Berry, William *a*	Dec., 1903	...	90	Aug., 1903

No. (consecutive).	Designation of Office.	Name.	Date of present Appointment.	Rate of Annual Salary. To 30th June, 1903.	Rate of Annual Salary. From 1st July, 1903.	Date of First Appointment under the Government, followed by continuous service.
				£	£	
	Coolgardie.					
21	District Medical Officer	Seed, William Pope *h*	Aug., 1898	250	350	Feb., 1896
22	Secretary and Dispenser	Bennett, William *i b*	April, 1901	225	...	July, 1898
		succeeded by				
23	Do	Loveley, William John Quarrier *i* ...	June, 1903	225	264	June, 1903
24	Matron	Hewton, Theresa *a*	March, 1901	150	150	Feb., 1897
25	Charge Nurse	Blain, Sarah Mary *a b*	March, 1902	70	70	June, 1898
		succeeded by				
26	Do	Hicks, Annie Bennett *a*	Dec., 1903	...	70	April, 1898
27	Do	Grover, Margaret Martha *a b*	July, 1902	70	...	Nov., 1897
		succeeded by				
28	Do	Pengelly, Ethel May *a b*	March, 1903	65	65	April, 1896
29	Do	Grover, Margaret Martha *a b*	July, 1903	...	70	Nov., 1897
		succeeded by				
30	Do	Pengelly, Ethel May *a*	Dec., 1903	...	70	April, 1896
31	Nurse	Dowson Amy	Nov., 1902	50	50	Nov., 1898
		succeeded by				
32	Do	Stewart, Kathleen *a g*	Nov., 1903	...	60	Nov., 1903
33	Do	Pengelly, Ethel May *a b*	Jan., 1903	60	60	April, 1896
34	Do	Pengelly, Ethel May *a j*	Aug., 1903	...	60	April, 1896
35	Junior Nurse	Pizey, Mary Hanfield Ellen *a*	May, 1902	18	24	May, 1902
36	Do	Shapira, Elsie Violet *a b*...	March, 1903	18	18	March, 1903
		succeeded by				
37	Do	Shapira, Dorothy Emily *a*	Nov., 1903	...	18	March, 1903
38	Probationer Nurse...	Walker, Annie M. *a b*	Nov., 1899	36	...	Nov., 1899
		succeeded by				
39	Do	Glentworth, Clarrie *a*	Jan., 1903	18	18	Jan., 1903
40	Do	White, Alice Mirian *a*	July, 1902	36	36	March, 1901
	Kalgoorlie.					
22	District Medical Officer	O'Meehan, John Albert	Feb., 1896	250	250	Sept., 1877
23	Resident Physician	Thompson, James *a b d*	Nov., 1902	350	...	July, 1899
		succeeded by				
24	Do do	Forshaw, William Joseph *a*	June, 1903	350	350	June, 1903
25	Secretary and Dispenser	Tratman, Charles Stanley *a*	May, 1899	258	258	May, 1899
26	Matron	Harvey, Florence Jane Elizabeth *a* ...	Dec., 1898	150	150	Oct., 1896
27	Charge Nurse	Fraser, Annie McKenzie *a*	March, 1902	70	70	June, 1900
28	Do	O'Callaghan, Mary *a*	March, 1902	70	70	March, 1897

29	Do	Siekmann, Franziska Brinkworth *a*	Dec., 1898	70	70	Sept., 1896
30	Do	Newland, Teresa *a*	Feb., 1899	70	70	Sept., 1896
31	Nurse	Lowrie, Jean E. *a c*	Jan., 1903	60	...	Dec., 1902
32	Do	Hopkins, Lulu Gabrielle *a d*	Jan., 1903	60	60	Aug., 1900
		succeeded by				
33	Do	Tucker, Ella *a*	Dec., 1903	...	60	April, 1897
34	Do	Griggs, May *a*	June, 1902	60	60	June, 1902
35	Do Probationer	Wray, Ernestine *a*	Dec., 1902	18	24	Dec., 1902
36	Do	Ormiston, Agnes Campbell *a c*	Oct., 1902	60	...	Oct., 1902
		succeeded by				
37	Do	Duncan, Emma *a d*	March, 1903	60	...	Jan., 1898
		succeeded by				
38	Do Probationer	Scott, Edith *a*	June, 1903	36	36	Jan., 1901
39	Do	Smith, Barbara *a b*	Dec., 1902	60	...	Jan., 1902
		succeeded by				
40	Do	Webb, Agnes Phœbe *a*	Feb., 1903	60	60	Feb., 1903
41	Do	Moore, Alice Mary *a b*	Jan., 1903	50	60	Jan., 1903
		succeeded by				
42	Do	Balding, Maida *a*	Dec., 1903	...	60	April, 1902
43	Do Junior	Thompson, Emily *a d*	Sept., 1902	42	42	April, 1900
44	Probationer Nurse	Foley, Josephine Bernardette *a b*	May, 1902	36	...	March, 1901
1	**Probationer Nurse**	**Byfield, Alice E. *a b***	Feb., 1902	36	...	**Feb., 1902**
		succeeded by				
2	**Do do**	**Wilson, Mary *a***	**April, 1903**	**24**	**36**	**April, 190**
3	**Do do**	**Graham, Elizabeth *a***	**Feb., 1902**	**24**	**24**	**Feb., 1902**
4	**Do do**	**Hutchinson, Anne *a***	**Jan., 1902**	**24**	**36**	**Jan., 1902**
5	**Do do**	**Wilson, Mary *a c***	**July, 1901**	**24**	...	**July, 1901**
		succeeded by				
6	**Do do**	**Shapira, Dorothy Emily *a c***	**March, 1903**	**18**	18	**March, 19**
		succeeded by				
7	**Do**	**Shapira, Elsie Violet *a***	**Nov., 1903**	...	**18**	**March, 190**
8	**Nurse**	**McDaniel, Charlotte *a d***	**July, 1903**	...	40	**July, 1903**

Fremantle Public Hospital

4	Matron	Dixon, Alice	April, 1901	125	125	June, 1898
5	Charge Nurse	McCulloch, Elizabeth	July, 1901	60	60	Nov., 1897
6	Do	Anthony, Isabel	May, 1899	52	...	May, 1899
7	Do	Cameron, Dolinda	Oct., 1902	52	...	Oct., 1902
8	Nurse	Rossiter, Maude	March, 1903	48	...	March, 1900
9	Do	Browne, Mary	July, 1901	48	...	July, 1901
10	Do	Gardiner, Hettie	May, 1903	48	...	May, 1900
11	Do	Sadlier, Nancy	Jan., 1903	48	...	Jan., 1903
12	Probationer Nurse	Brownhall, Annie *b*	July, 1899	48	...	July, 1899
13	Do	Turner, Emily *c*	March, 1900	40	...	March, 1900

No. (consecutive).	Designation of Office.	Name.	Date of present Appointment.	Rate of Annual Salary. To 30th June, 1903.	Rate of Annual Salary. From 1st July, 1903.	Date of First Appointment under the Government, followed by continuous service.
				£	£	
14	Do	Kerr, Ellen	June, 1901	40	...	June, 1901
15	Do	Callaghan, Veva	June, 1901	40	...	June, 1901
16	Do	Poole, Christina	Jan., 1902	30	...	Jan., 1902
17	Do	Collins, Helena	June, 1902	30	...	June, 1902
18	Do	McKenna, Veotti	June, 1902	20	...	June, 1902
19	Do	Cottell, Daisie	July, 1902	20	...	July, 1902
20	Do	McDonald, Mary	Nov., 1902	20	...	Nov., 1902
21	Do	Marie, Josephine	March, 1903	20	...	March, 1903
22	Do	Bellamy, Amy	May, 1903	20	...	May, 1903

1904

No.	Designation of Office.	Name.	Date of present Appointment.	To 30th June, 1904.	From 1st July, 1904.	Date of First Appointment
	Coolgardie.					
11	District Medical Officer	Seed, William Pope *b*	Aug., 1898	350	...	Feb., 1896
		succeeded by				
12	Acting District Medical Officer	Webster, Alfred	April, 1904	350	350	April, 1904
13	Secretary and Dispenser	Lovely, William John Quarrier	June, 1903	264	264	June, 1903
14	Matron	Hewton, Teresa *c*	March, 1901	150	150	Feb., 1897
		succeeded by				
15	Acting Matron	Sadler, Margaret	Dec., 1904	...	150	Feb., 1896
16	Charge Nurse	Hicks, Anne Bennett *d*	Dec., 1903	70	70	April, 1898
		succeeded by				
17	Do	Stevenson, Bertha	Nov., 1904	...	70	April, 1904
18	Do	Pengelly, Ethel May *d*	Dec., 1903	70	70	April, 1896
19	Nurse	Balding, Maida	Jan., 1904	60	60	April, 1902
20	Do	Lee, Lulu *d*	Feb., 1904	60	60	Feb., 1904
		succeeded by				
21	Do	King, Olive *d*	Oct., 1904	...	60	Jan., 1899
		succeeded by				
22	Do	Hopkins, Lulu	Dec., 1904	...	60	Aug., 1900
23	Junior Nurse	White, Alice Miriam *b*	July, 1902	36	...	March, 1901
24	Do	Pizey, Ellen Mary Handfred *d*	May, 1902	36	...	May, 1902
25	Do	Glentworth, Clarrie *d*	Jan., 1903	24	...	Jan., 1903
26	Do	Shapira, Dorothy Emily	Nov., 1903	24	24	March, 1903
27	Nurse	Brown, Eva Mary	May, 1904	60	60	May, 1904
37	Nurse	Barclay, Edith *h*	Oct., 1904	...	109/10/0	Oct., 1904

	Kalgoorlie.					
16	District Medical Officer	O'Meehan, John Albert	Feb., 1896	250	250	Sept., 1877
17	Resident Medical Officer	Forshaw, William Joseph	June, 1903	350	350	June, 1903
18	Secretary and Dispenser	Tratman, Charles Stanley	May, 1899	258	258	May, 1899
19	Matron	Harvey, Florence Jane Elizabeth	Dec., 1898	150	150	Oct., 1896
20	Charge Nurse	Fraser, Annie McKenzie	March, 1902	70	70	June, 1900
21	Do do	Tucker, Ella	June, 1904	70	70	April, 1897
22	Do do	Griggs, May	Jan., 1904	70	70	June, 1902
23	Do do	Newland, Teresa *d*	Feb., 1899	70	70	Sept., 1896
24	Probationary Nurse	McCully, Nance Ashton	April, 1904	18	18	April, 1904
25	Do do	Glentworth, Clarrie *e*	March, 1904	24	24	Jan., 1903
26	Do do	Scott, Edith Grace *d*	June, 1903	36	...	Jan., 1901
		succeeded by				
27	Do do	Balfour, Mary Russell	Jan., 1904	18	18	Dec., 1903
28	Do do	Youl, Alice Miriam	Jan., 1904	18	18	Jan., 1904
29	Do do	Day, Kate Jane Maud	Jan., 1904	18	18	Jan., 1904
30	Do do	Blake, Henrietta Eyre Mannsell	3rd Jan., 1904	18	18	3rd Jan., 1904
31	Junior Nurse	Wilson, May *d*	April, 1904	42	42	April, 1901
32	Probationary Nurse	Graham, Elizabeth	Feb., 1904	36	36	Feb., 1902
33	Do do	Hutchinson, Annie	Dec., 1903	36	36	Jan., 1902
34	Do do	Wray, Ernestine	Dec., 1903	24	24	Dec., 1902
35	Do do	Shapira, Elsie Violet	Nov., 1903	24	24	March, 1903
36	Do do	Selk, Grace	Nov., 1904	...	18	Nov., 1904
37	Do do	Pizey, Ellen Mary	June, 1904	36	36	May, 1902
38	Do do	Sutton, Mary E. M.	Nov., 1904	...	18	Nov., 1904
39	Do do	Perry, Isabel	Nov., 1904	...	18	Nov., 1904
40	Do do	Dobbie, Ethel M.	Oct., 1904	...	18	Jan., 1904
	Fremantle Public Hospital					
3	Matron	Dixon, Alice	April, 1901	125	125	June, 1898
4	Charge Nurse	McCulloch, Elizabeth	July, 1901	60	60	Nov., 1897
5	Do	Anthony, Isabel	May, 1899	60	60	May, 1899
6	Do	Cameron, Dolina	Oct., 1902	60	60	Oct., 1902
7	Nurse	Rossiter, Maude	Mar., 1903	48	48	Mar., 1900
8	Do	Browne, Mary	July, 1901	48	48	July, 1901
9	Do	Gardiner, Hettie *a*	May, 1903	48	...	May, 1900
10	Do	Sadlier, Nancy	Jan., 1903	48	48	Jan., 1903
11	Do	Kerr, Ellen *b*	June, 1901	40	40	June, 1901
12	Do (Probationer)	Callaghan, Vera	June, 1901	40	40	June, 1901
13	Do do	Poole, Christina *c*	Jan., 1902	40	40	Jan., 1902
14	Do do	Collins, Helena	June, 1902	30	40	June, 1902
15	Do do	McKenna, Veotti	June, 1902	30	40	June, 1902
16	Do do	Cottell, Daisie	July, 1902	30	30	July, 1902
17	Do do	McDonald, Mary	Nov., 1902	30	30	Nov., 1902
18	Do do	Marie, Josephine	Mar., 1903	30	30	Mar., 1903
19	Do do	Bellamy, Amy	May, 1903	30	30	May, 1903
20	Do do	McMahon, Ellen	June, 1904	20	20	June, 1904
21	Do do	Kelleher, Mary Frances	June, 1904	20	20	June, 1904
22	Do do	Phillips, Kate Douglas	Nov., 1904	...	20	Nov., 1904

No. (consecutive.)	Designation of Office.	Name.	Date of present Appointment.	Rate of Annual Salary. To 30th June, 1905.	Rate of Annual Salary. From 1st July, 1905.	Date of First Appointment under the Government, followed by continuous service.
				£	£	
1905						
	Coolgardie.					
32	Acting District Medical Officer ...	Webster, Alfred	April, 1904	350	350	April, 1904
33	Secretary and Dispenser	Lovely, William John Quarrier	June, 1903	264	264	June, 1903
34	Matron	Hewton, Theresa *h*	March, 1901	150	150	Feb., 1897
		succeeded by				
35	Do	Sadler, Margaret	Dec., 1904	150	150	Feb., 1896
36	Nurse-in-Charge	Stevenson, Bertha	Dec., 1904	70	70	April, 1904
37	Nurse	Rogers, Elizabeth	Jan., 1905	60	60	Jan., 1905
38	Do	Balding, Maida	Jan., 1904	60	60	April, 1902
39	Do	Hopkins, Lulu	Dec , 1904	60	60	Aug., 1900
40	Do	Brown, Eva Mary *i*	May, 1904	60	60	May, 1904
41	Do	Shapira, Dorothy M.	Nov., 1903	24	...	March, 1903
42	Do	Shapira, Dorothy M.	1st Mar., 1905	36	36	March, 1903
43	Do	Pizey, Ellen Mary Hanfred	April, 1905	42	...	May, 1902
44	Do	Pizey, Ellen Mary Hanfred *j*	June, 1905	60	...	May, 1902
45	Do	Pizey, Ellen Mary Hanfred	Aug., 1905	...	60	May, 1902
46	Do	Hart, Sophey *k*	Jan., 1905	60	60	Nov., 1903
47	Do	Ballan, Ethel	Nov., 1905	...	36	Nov., 1905
48	Do	Sutcliffe, Ethel	June, 1905	18	18	June, 1905
	Kalgoorlie.					
2	District Medical Officer	O'Meehan, John Albert *a*	Feb., 1896	250	...	Sept., 1877
		succeeded by				
3	Acting District Medical Officer ...	Barber, George Walter *b*	Nov., 1904	£1 1s. a day	...	Nov., 1904
		succeeded by				
4	District Medical Officer	Miskin, Leonard John	June, 1905	250	250	Feb., 1900
5	Resident Physician	Forshaw, William Joseph *c*	June, 1903	350	...	June, 1903
		succeeded by				
6	Acting Resident Physician ...	Thomson, John Erskine *d*	Feb., 1905	250	...	Feb., 1905
		succeeded by				
7	Resident Physician	Beadel, Algernon James	May, 1905	250	250	May, 1905
8	Secretary and Dispenser	Tratman, Charles Stanley	May, 1899	258	258	May, 1899
9	Matron	Harvey, Florence Jane Elizabeth ...	Dec., 1898	150	150	Oct., 1896
10	Nurse	Fraser, Annie McKenzie *e*	March, 1902	70	70	June, 1900
11	Do	Newland, Theresa *f*	April, 1905	70	70	Sept., 1896
12	Do	Hicks, Annie Bennett	Oct., 1904	70	70	April, 1898
13	Do	Griggs, May *g*	Jan., 1904	70	70	June, 1902
14	Do	Tucker, Ella	June, 1904	70	70	April, 1897
15	Do	Wilson, May	Sept., 1905	...	70	April, 1901

16	Do	Graham, Elizabeth *h*	Feb., 1904	36	...	Feb., 1902
17	Do	Sievers, Christina	Feb., 1905	36	36	July, 1904
18	Do	Hutchinson, Annie *i*	Dec., 1904	42	...	Dec., 1901
19	Do	Foreman, Eliza	March, 1905	36	36	May, 1902
20	Do	Pizey, Ellen Mary *j*	June, 1904	36	...	May, 1902
21	Do	Pizey, Ellen Mary *k*	March, 1905	42	...	May, 1902
22	Do	Selk, Grace *l*	Nov., 1904	18	18	Nov., 1904
23	Do	Selk, Grace	23 Nov., 1905	...	24	Nov., 1904
24	Do	Sutton, Mary E. M. *m*	Nov., 1904	18	18	Nov., 1904
25	Do	Perry, Isabel *n*	Nov., 1904	18	18	Nov., 1904
26	Do	Perry, Isabel	10 Nov., 1905	...	24	Nov., 1904
27	Do	McLeod, Annie	Feb., 1905	18	18	Feb., 1905
28	Do	Wray, Ernestine	Dec., 1903	36	36	Dec., 1902
29	Do	Shapira, Elsie Violet *o*	Nov., 1903	24	36	March, 1903
30	Do	Shapira, Elsie Violet	March, 1905	36	36	March, 1903
31	Do	Youl, Alice Miriam *p*	Jan., 1904	18	24	Jan., 1904
32	Do	Youl, Alice Miriam *q*	Jan., 1905	24	24	Jan., 1904
33	Do	Balfour, Mary Russell	Jan., 1904	24	24	Dec., 1903
34	Do	Dobbie, Ethel M. *r*	Oct., 1904	18	24	Jan., 1904
35	Do	Dobbie, Ethel M. *s*	Jan., 1905	24	...	Jan., 1904
36	Do	Davoren, Margaret F.	Dec., 1904	18	18	Dec., 1904
37	Do	Blake, Henrietta Eyre Maunsell *t*	Jan., 1904	18	24	Jan., 1904
38	Do	Blake, Henrietta Eyre Maunsell	Jan., 1905	24	24	Jan., 1904
39	Do	Day, Kate J. M. *u*	July, 1905	...	18	Jan., 1904
40	Do	Shapira, Dorothy Emily	Aug., 1905	...	36	March, 1903

Fremantle Public Hospital

3	Matron	Dixon, Alice	April, 1901	125	125	June, 1898
4	Charge Nurse	McCulloch, Elizabeth	July, 1901	60	60	Nov., 1897
5	Do	Anthony, Isabel *a*	May, 1899	60	60	May, 1899
6	Do	Cameron, Dolina	Oct., 1902	60	60	Oct., 1902
7	Nurse	Rossiter, Maude *b*	March, 1903	48	48	March, 1900
8	Do	Browne, Mary	July, 1901	48	48	July, 1901
9	Do	Sadlier, Nancy	Jan., 1903	48	48	Jan., 1903
10	Do	Callaghan, Viva	June, 1904	48	48	June, 1901
11	Do (Probationer)	Collins, Helena *c*	June, 1902	40	...	June, 1902
12	Do do	McKenna, Viotta *d*	June, 1902	40	...	June, 1902
13	Do do	Cottell, Daisie *e*	July, 1902	40	48	July, 1902
14	Do do	McDonald, Mary	Nov., 1902	40	40	Nov., 1902
15	Do do	Marie, Josephine	March, 1903	40	40	March, 1903
16	Do do	Bellamy, Amy	May, 1903	40	40	May, 1903
17	Do do	McMahon, Ellen	June, 1904	30	30	June, 1904
18	Do do	Kellcher, Mary Frances	June, 1904	30	30	June, 1904
19	Do do	Phillips, Kate Douglas	Nov., 1904	20	20	Nov., 1904
20	Do do	Lee, Jessie	Jan., 1905	20	20	Jan., 1905
21	Do do	Waller, Mary	June, 1905	20	20	June, 1905
22	Do do	Davey, Olive	July, 1905	...	20	July, 1905
23	Do do	Kestel, Rose	Oct., 1905	...	20	Oct., 1905

LIST OF NURSES TRAINED AT THE PERTH PUBLIC HOSPITAL.

Name.	Date of Certificate.	Name.	Date of Certificate.
1. Kirkman, Annie	19th December, 1899	30. White, Emily	17th January, 1904
2. Blain, Sarah Mary	19th December, 1899	31. Brown, Eva Mary	19th January, 1904
3. Techow, Una Elizabeth ..	19th December, 1899	32. Tildesley, Ella Longmore ..	6th February, 1904
4. Collier, May	19th December, 1899	33. Knight, Margaret Helen ..	19th March, 1904
5. Shaw, Ellie	29th December, 1899	34. Mann, Alice Gertrude	21st March, 1904
6. Bole, Elizabeth	11th March, 1900	35. Chapman, Agnes Craig ..	27th March, 1904
7. Hodgson, Grace A.	11th March, 1900	36. Kingerley, Jessie Mary ..	16th April, 1904
8. Power, Marie	25th May, 1900	37. Arnott, Anna Carter	19th April, 1904
9. Rose, Alice Emily	15th November, 1900	38. McNeil, Emily Louisa ..	24th April, 1904
10. Minchin, Lucy	30th November, 1900	39. Mackintosh, Arabella Cecilia ..	18th June, 1904
11. Ward, Kate	26th January, 1901	40. Reynolds, Ethel Maud ..	17th July, 1904
12. Wilson, Clare Constance ..	6th February, 1901	41. Alexander, Evelyn	14th October, 1904
13. Lee, Lulu	4th April, 1901	42. Foley, Nora	15th February, 1905
14. Tindale, Eleanor F.	9th May, 1901	43. Goodwin, Florence Ida ..	28th February, 1905
15. Hicks, Annie Bennett	10th June, 1901	44. Ashton, May	24th April, 1905
16. Atcheson, Jean	14th June, 1901	45. Austin, Sydney Marion ..	27th May, 1905
17. Balding, Maida Florence ..	2nd February, 1902	46. Johnstone, Marian Glenfield ..	10th June, 1905
18. Shapcott, Florence Maud ..	14th February, 1902	47. Lawrence, Mabel Gertrude ..	9th October, 1905
19. O'Callaghan, Annie	1st August, 1902	48. Cooper, Violet Mary	12th October, 1905
20. Cordingley, Daisy Edith ..	13th November, 1902	49. Kuehn, Mary Gertrude ..	6th December, 1905
21. Buchanan, Muriel Mildred ..	30th November, 1902	50. Buckland, Sarah Hilda ..	18th December, 1905
22. Goldman, Violet Amy	4th December, 1902	51. Ashton, Lucy	5th February, 1906
23. Fry, Ruby Frances	11th December, 1902	52. Prince, Ethel Rose	6th February, 1906
24. Walker, Ada Lucy	26th February, 1903	53. Anderson, Emily Blanche ..	1st March, 1906
25. Johnstone, Margaret Hope ..	22nd March, 1903	54. De Mole, Fannie	19th April, 1906
26. Wright, Evangeline Helen Meddens	11th April, 1903	55. Field, Laura	8th May, 1906
		56. Peile, Mary Isabel	28th May, 1906
27. Parkes, Isabel Matheson ..	15th May, 1903	57. Parsons, Isabel Charlotte ..	8th June, 1906
28. Brown, Grace Emily	9th June, 1903	58. Spaven, Marion Hay	4th July, 1906
29. Phillips, Frances Annie ..	3rd August, 1903	59. Cooke, Ada Maude	7th November, 1906

60. Gjedsted, Eleanor Dagmar	1st March, 1907
61. Fanning, Christina	6th March, 1907
62. Tucker, Dora Constance	23rd March, 1907
63. Monkhouse, Helen May	23rd April, 1907
64. Wilson, Alice Maude	28th April, 1907
65. Wheeler, Katherine Florence	2nd May, 1907
66. Ellis, Ellen Marie	26th May, 1907
67. Tatlow, Flora Amelia	8th June, 1907
68. Potten, Frances Elizabeth	27th June, 1907
69. Weston, Mary Ethel	7th December, 1905
70. Allen, Elizabeth	25th December, 1907
71. Lord, Hilda	30th January, 1908
72. Begg, Elsie	7th February, 1908
73. Hillman, Jessie Elizabeth Agnes	7th February, 1908
74. Ranford, Sarah Agnes	13th February, 1908
75. James, Alice Maud	14th February, 1908
76. Lee, Susie Rosie	14th March, 1908
77. Anderson, Beatrice Victoria	2nd July, 1908
78. Scharer, Alice Hilda	23rd October, 1908
79. Newnham, Alice Maud	14th December, 1908
80. Ellis, Dora	8th January, 1909
81. Bromley, Phyllis	15th January, 1909
82. Palfreyman, Martha Lovedy	15th January, 1909
83. Yelland, Effie	2nd March, 1909
84. Cassell, Jessie Ann	5th May, 1909
85. Jenkinson, Nancy	14th May, 1909
86. Donnell, Annie	23rd May, 1909
87. Grover, Elizabeth	17th July, 1909
88. Loxton, Isabel Edith	30th July, 1909
89. Walsh, Nance	15th December, 1909
90. Jeffrey, Lilian Clarice	2nd January, 1910
91. Moore, Clarice Evylin	17th January, 1910
92. Cox, Elizabeth	17th January, 1910
93. Kiss, Ethel Avina Mary	24th January, 1910
94. Spaven, Florence Ethel	1st April, 1910
95. Burt, Margaret	14th April, 1910
96. Skinner, Alicia May Victoria	26th April, 1910
97. Burnett, Cecilia Edith	26th May, 1910
98. McNeill, Margaret	4th June, 1910
99. Thompson, Ruby Mary	12th June, 1910
100. Ross, Angela Mary	26th June, 1910
101. Phillips, Miriam	6th July, 1910
102. Saw, Lily Hilda	12th August, 1910
103. Hedges, Alice Ada	13th August, 1910
104. Wood, Laura Florence	22nd August, 1910
105. Gibson, Jessie	29th August, 1910
106. Inglis, Daisy	30th September, 1910
107. Davidson, Kathleen	3rd October, 1910
108. Phipps, Emily Beatrice	8th October, 1910
109. Scott, Margaret Ann	10th November, 1910
110. Bickford, Ellen Mary	17th November, 1910
111. Murray, Ada	16th December, 1910
112. Sprahan, Catherine Josephine	28th December, 1910
113. Harvey, Eleanor Alice	7th January, 1911
114. Lewis, Ethel Daisy	23rd February, 1911
115. Trotter, Pauline Rosalie	8th March, 1911
116. Dawson, Amy Jesica	8th March, 1911
117. Johnson, Muriel Norgrove	13th March, 1911
118. Hallion, Jennie	15th May, 1911
119. Latta, Charlotte Ellen	2nd June, 1911
120. Solomon, Carrie Adele	19th June, 1911
121. Hutchinson, Harriett Mary	27th June, 1911
122. Ashworth, Helen	7th August, 1911
123. Stanbrook, Lottie Evelina	16th August, 1911
124. Stubbs, Annie	4th November, 1911
125. Luyer, Ethel May	29th November, 1911
126. Smith, Emilie Hildred	2nd February, 1912
127. Baker, Maud Isabel	9th February, 1912
128. Jackson, Maggie Dinah	23rd February, 1912
129. Peate, Lena Eva	29th March, 1912
130. Bennett, Ruby Olive	12th June, 1912
131. Cheatley, Elizabeth Mary	22nd July, 1912.
132. Mearns, Dora	14th August, 1912
133. Hicks, Clarice	23rd September, 1912
134. Spring, Elsie Maud	25th December, 1912
135. Ward, Mary Ann	28th February, 1913

List of Nurses Trained at the Perth Public Hospital—*continued*

Name.	Date of Certificate.
136. Doherty, Gertrude Marion ..	11th May, 1913
137. Carey, Mary Veronica	30th May, 1913
138. Manning, Florence Agnes ..	7th July, 1913
139. Martin, Alice Maud	4th August, 1913
140. Krakouer, Elizabeth Mary ..	14th August, 1913
141. Middleton, Jean	16th August, 1913
142. Hopkins, Olive Irene	21st August, 1913
143. Robertson, Christina Florence ..	21st August, 1913
144. Hambley, Helena Beatrice ..	23rd October, 1913
145. Hudson, Florence May ..	10th November, 1913
146. Scanlan, Mary	7th December, 1913
147. Brown, Mary Dorothy ..	12th December, 1913
148. Crohan, Eugenie	15th December, 1913
149. Craike, Dorothy May	15th December, 1913
150. Sampson, Clara	11th January, 1914
151. D'Arcy, Ruby Gertrude ..	23rd January, 1914
152. Lappin, Margaret Frances ..	6th February, 1914
153. Parker, Patricia Mary Catherine	6th February, 1914
154. Smith, Vera Winifred	6th February, 1914
155. Hall, Olive Goldridge	16th March, 1914
156. Rowan, Eliza	16th March, 1914
157. Herrmann, Linda Leonora Zenghan	22nd March, 1914
158. Ryan, Kathleen Emily Margaret	25th March, 1914
159. Denson, Irene May	31st March, 1914
160. Smith, Dora Handron	4th May, 1914
161. Simpson, Jean Florence ..	4th May, 1914
162. Sharpe, Grace May	29th May, 1914
163. Whitelaw, Frances Maud ..	7th July, 1914
164. Lightbody, Minnie Jane ..	19th July, 1914
165. Croni, Inez Clare	7th December, 1914
166. Parish, Emily Cornelia ..	22nd September, 1914
167. Shadforth, Annie	9th October, 1914
168. Wignall, Catherine Helen ..	20th February, 1915
169. Bridgeman, Kate	26th October, 1914
170. Gibbs, Phoebe Jane	7th December, 1914
171. Squires, Violet Maud	16th December, 1914
172. McGillivray, Catherine Ann ..	27th January, 1915
173. Huffam, Dorothy	10th February, 1915
174. Cowcher, Alma Eliza	24th February, 1915
175. Monger, Ethel Susanna ..	29th April, 1914
176. Bartlett, May	10th March, 1915
177. Tait, Agnes Mary	10th April, 1915
178. Coomer, Lillian	8th May, 1915
179. Negus, Alice Eliza	3rd March, 1915
180. Cook, Florence Beatrice ..	11th July, 1915
181. Stubbs, Mary Jane	15th July, 1915.
182. Lauritz, Grace Lauritta ..	20th May, 1915
183. Cobley, Catherine	8th August, 1915.
184. Ryan, Bridget Frances ..	19th August, 1915.
185. Brownfield, Constance	20th August, 1915.
186. Dugdale, Mary Dorothy ..	29th September, 1915
187. O'Brien, Margaret	1st June, 1915
188. Tuckey, Bertha Amelia Grace	11th September, 1915
189. Saw, Nellie Mabel	12th December, 1915
190. Astley, Hilda May	6th January, 1916
191. Clapp, Hilda Winifred ..	2nd January, 1916
192. Leishman, Doreen Elsie ..	1st February, 1916
193. Doherty, Winifred Eleanor ..	29th February, 1916
194. Lane, Rita Constance	25th March, 1916
195. Simpson, Ethel Frances Mary	27th May, 1916
196. Spring, Elizabeth	22nd January, 1916
197. Paisley, Vera Agnes Margaret	20th April, 1916
198. Bradshaw, Ivy Corinella ..	9th June, 1916.

PERTH PUBLIC HOSPITAL
(nurses who completed training)

From June 1916
Nicholson, Robina
Berthold, Pauline Hilda
Williamson, Alexandra Love
Baxter, Violet Phoebe
Moyle, Zetta
Jones, Ruth Victoria
Bradshaw, Ivy C.
Paisley, Vera Agnes

December 1916
Wintle, Clarice Evalyn Alice
Delaney, Eily Beatrice
Thompson, Isabella M.
Watts, Ada
Jeffrey, Edith Olive
Johns, Ellen
Perkins, Edythe
Pickells, Amelia M.
Phipps, Miriam B.
Larsen, Flora
Connor, Elva Agnes
McAleer, Kathleen
Gibson-White, Ina
Reidy, Elizabeth

June 1917
Donaldson, M. Olive
Aquilar, Teresa
Seldon, Hazel
Shepherd, D. F.
Scown, B. M.
Dobrigh, M. Frances
Lacey, M. G.
Hyde, Hilda
Schlaker, Lily
Paterson, Kathleen
Powell Muriel
Williams, Florence

November 1917
Leeds, Enid
Bovell, Lily
Simpson, Rita
Davies, Avonia
Peat, Bessie
Hart, Pearl
Stuchbury, Adela M.
Waghorn, Olive M.
Taylor, Vera E. W.
Cox, Eugenie
Muirson, Eleanor G.

June 1918
Prosser, E.
Stroschen, A.
Stuchbury, I.
George, Enid
Burke, M.
Muir, Kitty
Steedman, D.
Broadhurst, Hazel
Burton, Mary
Curwood, Eileen Ivy
Piesse, Ivy
Stokes, L.
Field, Ethel
Rodriquez, Elsie
Doherty, Emily

December 1918
Ottaway, Gladys
Pearson, Amy
Farrow, Ellen
McKenzie-Murray, Jeannie

June 1919
Saw, Lily H.
Brockman, Amy V.
Mannion, Cecile
Fowlie, May E.
Hungerford, Mabel
McBurney, Zilla

December 1919
Parker, Ivy M.
Verney, E. M.
Walsh, Agnes Marion McLean
Bruce, M. A.
Knight, Adele L.
Mulgrave, Adelaide
Blechynden, Gertrude A.
Martin, Ida J.
Jones, Elise I.
Kiernan, Florence
Beere, Leah
Harvey, Ina
Mansbridge, Wurdell Olive
Hollywell, Amy E.
Brown, Agnes Mary

June 1920
Solomon, Stella
Cronin, Winifred
McGillivray, Mamie
Halvorsen, Gladys
Richardson, Kathleen
Cadden, Pearl
Whiteside, Harriett
Mouchmore, Estelle
Seldon, Doris

December 1920
Noak, Clarice
Wait, Lillian Maude
Blomfield, Eva Florence
Stradwick, Viginia
Donaldson, Doris Jane
Hayes, Ida
Darch, Muriel Hope
Lawson, Alice Irene
Moorhouse, Vera Mabel
Carne, Eva Kathleen
Ormiston, Annie
Craig, Bessie Neves
McCracken, Jean
Joy, Marguerite
Hunter, Margaret J.
Currie, May Couper

June 1921
Richardson, Doris E.
Gilbert, W. M.
Saw, A. L.
Karnaghan, F. E.
Hunter, C. A.
Darling, M. H.
Mortiboys, N. C.
McDonald, J. S.
Bruce, F. E.
Candy, R. G.
Harris, G. E. M.

December 1921
Purkiss, Gladys
Jefferies, Kathleen M.
Geddes, Ivy
Coombe, Ada
Parker, Alberta
Broomhall, Beryl
Stuchbury, Myra
Strom, Nellie

May 1922
Irwin, Eva J.
Boland, Naomi
Ward, Margaret
Snell, Olive
Miller, Esmeralda
Williams, Edna
Lowe, Beatrice
Spears, Ruby
Armstrong, Laura
Hadley, Gertrude
O'Toole, Beryl
Sandilands, Edith
Lukin, Gladys

THE GOVERNMENT HOSPITALS
(Coolgardie, Kalgoorlie, and associated country hospitals)

December 1909
Graham, Lavinia
Lynch, Nellie U.
Coleman, K.
Laurence, Lydia

December 1910
Fallon, A. (Bunbury)
Fleming, J.
Hall, M. E.
Perry, I.

June 1911
Hamersley, Florence
Nicholls, Florence A.

December 1911
Gibbings, B. M.
Tuckey, Ella
Whitely, I.

December 1912
Cadlolo, Mary Ann
Doyle, Helen Grace
Friedman, M. B.
Gladwin, M.A.
Leahey, Alice Evelyn

December 1913
Beaden, Annetta
Graham, Lily J.
Basejou, Gwendoline Constance

June 1914
Horswill, Valetta
Hunter, Margaret

December 1914
Edis, Dorothy Margaret
England, Elvera Constance

June 1915
Bailey, Grace Agnes
Faram, Lizzie
Grigg, Bessie
Liddell, Nellie Mary

McBride, Gretta
Maley, Grace Kismet
Mellowship, Chloride Mary
White, Erica Virginia

December 1915
Alfred, Ellen
Nicholas, Shirley
Cave, Elva Jessie
Lowe, Florence

June 1916
Allen, Minnie
Boardman, —
Bradshaw, Dorothy
Dudley, Adelaide Roseanna
Fogarty, Margaret E.

December 1916
Begley, Eleanor
Brockman, Clare
Donovan, Alice
Livesey, Jennie
Jackson, Kathleen
Mulgrue, Eleanor
Ryan, Dorothea

June 1917
Naylor, Mildred
Taylor, Cecilia

December 1917
Easterbrook, Lily
McLean, Perth L.
Sticpwich, Clarice E.
Tweddle, Annie Elizabeth
Stafford, Isabel

June 1918
Arthur, G.
McRohan, M.
O'Byrne, Kathleen
O'Byrne, M.
Pringle, M.
Saint, M.

December 1918
Attwood, M.
Connolly, M.
Fisher, Alice
Judge, E.
McWhinney, Vera K.
Parker, Jane
Shields, Sarah
Newman, Lillian Ellen
Juleff, Dorothea
O'Byrne, Josephine

June 1919
Bridge, Gwendoline
Campbell, Daisy
Kendrick, Doreen
Pugh, Pearl Lois
Raines, Dorothea
Rose, Margaret E.
James, Amy Millicent
Shaw, Lily R.
Sparks, Edith
Stewart, Florence H.
Taylor, Mary
Tourney, Henrietta
Cor, Mary Ivy
Thompson, Margaret

December 1919
Cartwright, Marjorie
Hansen, Matilda C.
Jenner, Dorothy
Lewis, Doris F.
McNally, Eileen
Mills, Helen
Moore-Smith, Phyllis
Moore, Gladys
Morrel, Stella D.
Morrow, Millicent
Trigg, Jessie
Linthorne, Winnie
Fraser, Elizabeth
Cowcher, Ivy Adelaide
Rohan, Aileen
Stanton, Ethel
Gannaway, Dorothy Ellen

June 1920
Humphrey, Lucy
Reid, Clarice

December 1920
Briggs, Ida
Cornwall, Gladys
Delaney, Kathleen
Doust, Laura
Kendrick, Ethel
Smith, Ellen
Smith, Jessie H.
Sticpwich, Hilda
Williams, Helen

June 1921
Bennett, M.
Colson, I. M.
Culleton, M.
Franklin, D. E.
Hillman, R. V.

McSherry, E. M.
Mulvay, D.
Watts, E.
Youd, E.

December 1921
Delamotte, Shirley
Doig, Dorothy
Doig, Mary
Fowler, Elsie
Fullarton, Eliza Jane
Mulvae, Federal

Parker, Frances Amy
Quinn, Elsie

May 1922
Baston, Ethel
English, Mary
Furze, Edith
Muldoon, Mabel
Nicholls, Rose
Peat, Nellie
Thompson, Elizabeth
Wilkinson, Ivy

FREMANTLE PUBLIC HOSPITAL

1908
Anderson, Florence
Main, Isabella
Waller, May Isabelle

June 1909
Grey, Annie
Haines, Myrtle

December 1909
Edsall, Florence
Kimber, Alice M.
Crombie, Alice M.

December 1910
Callaghan, O. L.

December 1911
Giles, B.
Cardow, S.
Haines, M.
Hicks, M. H.

June 1912
Hayes, M. E.

June 1913
Bottle, Ruby (Ruth)
Carson, Mary Catherine

December 1913
Lyons, Lena G.
McGurk, Lillie
Wilson, Edith M.

December 1914
Baillie, Lavinia
Blain, Maud
Kiernan, Irene
Kirkham, Sarah Alice

June 1915
Roche, Fanny

June 1916
Butterley, Ellen
Wood, Blanche Eleanor

December 1916
Mollan, Frances
Waters, Annie M.
Wilkins, Maud

June 1917
Cauward, Mary
Leeds, Dorothy

December 1917
Cowcher, Emmiline Jane
Doherty, Abigail
O'Shanassy, Mary C.
Quealy, Catherine
Taylor, Rose

June 1918
Elphick, E.

December 1919
Couper, May
Donnelly, Clarice
Draper, Mabel A.
Eley, Ethel D.
Grono, Florence
Livermore, Alice
Mercer, Kathleen

June 1920
Bell, Edith
Evans, Eileen
Lacy, Jean
Jouning, Louisa
Kimber, — (Mrs)
Riley, Iris

December 1920
Bell, Mabel Edith
Leo, Rene Marion
Gill, Vera
Kiernan, Florence
Smith, Mary A.

December 1921
Coram, Isabell Annie
Matthews, Ivy
Morrison, Alice
Munro, Alexandrina
Smith, Mary

PERTH CHILDREN'S HOSPITAL

June 1912
Miller, Mona
Williams, Alice Beatrice
Waterhouse, Olive
Hamersley, Eulalie Margaret

December 1912
Bailey, May
Hunt, Mildred
Cook, Gertrude Grace
Pustkuchen, Paula Erna F.

June 1913
Fitzpatrick, Stella

December 1913
White, A. Muriel
Williams, Hilda
England, Doris

June 1914
Still, Georgina M.

December 1914
Graham, Hilda May
Vickery, Rhoda

June 1915
Brown, Elizabeth
Deakin, Cecile Esther
Eastwood, Doris
Prowse, Elizabeth
Fleming, Pearl
Follington, Emily
Hopwood, Dorothy
Sprigg, Ivy

December 1915
Bailey, Muriel
Fitzpatrick, Clare
Hogan, Mabel
Hough, Edith
Nicholas, Shirley
Preston, Gladys
Roberts, Evelyn
Yeldon, Bessie

June 1916
Symonds, Faith
Sinclair, Frances
Piesse, Geraldine
Holiday, Evelyn

December 1916
Pittman, Winnie Eulalie
Proudfood, Bessie
Dennehy, Frances
Cowcher, Ruby
Doherty, Constance
Gray, Allana
Neate, Mercy

June 1917
Thomas, Irene
Courthope, Dorothy
Nickoll, Emily Mary (Mollie)
Kott, Pauline
Preston, Ethel

December 1917
Barclay, Aimee H.
Freeman, Elizabeth
Morrison, Ailsa

June 1918
Bennett, M.
Goldstein, R.
James, G.
Taylor, A.

December 1918
Bell, Hylda
Creagh, G.
Fitzpatrick, Josephine
Kidston-Hunter, Bessie
McMurtle, Beatrice
Piesse, Alberta

June 1919
Brown, Eva
Holland, Constance
Nickoll, Gwendoline
Parker, Margaret

December 1919
Carmichael, Ida
Glover, Mavis
Hayman, Bina

Philipson, Evelyn
Piesse, Dorothy E.
Simpson, Jean
Stokes, Eileen
Russell, Enid
Taylor, Bernice
Munro, S.
Humble, Maud

June 1920
Carlisle, Phyllis
Clifton, Tita

December 1920
Eastwood, Florence
Guy, Gladys
Howes, Kathleen
Kelly, Dorothea
McEvoy, Kathleen
Moseley, Elsie
Hayes, Kathleen
Phillips, Millie
Throssell, Evelyn Crystal
Timmings, Gladys

June 1921
Cornwall, L. F.
Luton, I.
Molloy, K.
Turner, M. A.

December 1921
Field, Veronica
Foster, Dorothy
Newman, Alice
Paynter, Margaret
Reardon, Hilda
Russell, Eleanor
Rust, Myrtle
Williams, Irene

May 1922
Allen, Gwenyth
Browne, Dorothy
Rodriquez, Muriel
Glasson, Rita
Levy, Lionette
Simms, Doris

ST JOHN OF GOD HOSPITAL

December 1913
Brennan, Sister M. Angela
Kenny, Sister M. Alacoque
Mullaly, Sister M. Patrick

December 1914
Grogan, Sister M. Gertrude
Heenan, Sister M. Phillip
Keating, Sister M. Aloysius
Grogan, Sister M. Gabrielle
Greene, Sister M. Gertrude

June 1915
McDonnell, Sister M. Conception
Murphy, Sister M. Aidan
O'Driscoll, Sister M. Carmel
Kennedy, Sister M. Scholastica

December 1917
Cressy, Sister M. Aquinas
Hanrahan, Sister M. Immaculate

June 1919
Bock, Sister M. Imelda
Corbett, Sister M. de Lellis
Earle, Sister M. Philomena
Tuttle, Sister M. Raphael

December 1919
Boyce, Sister M. Agatha
Boyce, Sister M. Antonia
De Sales, Sister M. Rouche

December 1920
Kissane, Sister M. Baptist
Noonan, Sister M. Teresa

June 1921
McCarthy, Sister M. Augustine

May 1922
Comyn, Sister M. Rosarii
Costello, Sister M. Consilli
McNamara, Sister M. Borgia
O'Brien, Sister M. of the Cross

APPENDIX II

FIRST REGISTER OF MIDWIVES
1913

Supplement to Government Gazette

OF

WESTERN AUSTRALIA.

[Published by Authority.]

[REGISTERED AT THE GENERAL POST OFFICE, PERTH, FOR TRANSMISSION BY POST AS A NEWSPAPER.]

PERTH: FRIDAY, FEBRUARY 7. [1913

THE HEALTH ACT, 1911.

MIDWIVES' REGISTRATION BOARD.

REGISTER OF MIDWIVES

THE HEALTH ACT, 1911.

MIDWIVES' REGISTRATION BOARD.

IN accordance with the provisions of "The Health Act, 1911," the following copy of the Register of Midwives as at the 31st December, 1912, is hereby published.

2nd January, 1913.

F. J. HUELIN,
Clerk to the Midwives' Registration Board.

Registration No.	Name.	Address.	Date of Registration.	Section of Act under which Registration was effected.	Qualification.
136	ABBOTT, Ellen	"Salvan," Palmerston Street, Perth	8th Nov., 1911	255 (2)	In practice, June, 1909.
330	AITKEN, Mary Agnes	3 Harvest Terrace, Perth	8th Dec., 1911	255 (1)	London Obstetrical Society.
391	ALCOCK, Elizabeth	Kanowna	8th Dec., 1911	255 (2)	In practice, June, 1909.
641	ALDERDICE, Margaret	Gwalia	5th Jan., 1912	255 (2)	In practice, June, 1909.
453	ALLEN, Caroline Mary	Brookman Street, Kalgoorlie	20th Dec., 1911	255 (1)	Women's Hospital, Melbourne.
207	ALLEN, Elizabeth Ann	Brookman Street, Kalgoorlie	22nd Nov., 1911	255 (2)	In practice, June, 1909.
491	ALLEN, Mary	Princess Road, Claremont	20th Dec., 1911	255 (2)	In practice, June, 1909.
464	ANDERSON, Adelaide Mary	Middleton Road, Albany	20th Dec., 1911	255 (2)	In practice, June, 1909.
648	ANDERSON, Mary Ann	Hopkins Street, Boulder	5th Jan., 1912	255 (2)	In practice, June, 1909.
477	ANDERSON, Sarah Jane	Golden Gate, Kalgoorlie	20th Dec., 1911	255 (2)	In practice, June, 1909.
51	ANDREWS, Annie Elizabeth	Worsley	10th Oct., 1911	255 (2)	In practice, June, 1909.
842	ANGEL, Cordelia Emma	Ravensthorpe	9th Aug., 1912	255 (2)	In practice, June, 1909.
329	ANGUS, Janet White	3 Harvest Terrace, Perth	8th Dec., 1911	255 (1)	Glasgow Maternity Hospital.
539	ANNELLS, Louisa Harriet	194 Stirling Street, Perth	29th Dec., 1911	255 (1)	Queen's Home, Adelaide.
827	ARBON, Emma	Warne Street, Maylands	9th Aug., 1912	255 (2)	In practice, June, 1909.
82	ARMSTRONG, Julia	109 Hampton Road, Fremantle	25th Oct., 1911	255 (2)	In practice, June, 1909.
603	ARMSTRONG, Lillian Margaret	Merredin	29th Dec., 1911	255 (2)	In practice, June, 1909.
819	ARNOLD, Clara Helena	603 Murray Street, West Perth	9th Aug., 1912	255 (2)	In practice, June, 1909.
262	ARNOLD, Kate Harriette	14 Charles Street, North Perth	29th Nov., 1911	255 (2)	In practice, June, 1909.
54	ARNOLD, Mary	Aberdeen Street, Katanning	10th Oct., 1911	255 (2)	In practice, June, 1909.
335	ARUNDALE, Henrietta Helena	Grosvenor Hospital, Fremantle	8th Dec., 1911	255 (2)	In practice, June, 1909.
564	ASH, Sarah	437 William Street, Perth	29th Dec., 1911	255 (2)	In practice, June, 1909.
164	ASHTON, May	"Haddon," Almondbury Road, Mt. Lawley, Perth	15th Nov., 1911	255 (1)	Women's Hospital, Melbourne.
2	ASHWORTH, Helen	59 Canning Road, East Fremantle	13th Sept., 1911	255 (1)	Home Training School, Newtown, Sydney.
304	ATKINSON, Louisa	10 Park Street, North Perth	29th Nov., 1911	255 (2)	In practice, June, 1909.
753	AUSTIN, Elizabeth Emma	Marine Terrace, Geraldton	19th April, 1912	261 (1)	Central Midwives' Board, England.
383	AYLETT, Caroline Florence	17 Wallcott Street, North Perth	8th Dec., 1911	255 (2)	In practice, June, 1909.
199	AYTON, Eva Elizabeth Jane	32 Hampton Road, Fremantle	22nd Nov., 1911	255 (1)	Fremantle Midwifery Training School.
400	BACK, Mary	Public Hospital, Wagin	13th Dec., 1911	255 (1)	London Obstetrical Society.
746	BACKMAN, Clara Jane	73 Leviathan Street, Boulder	15th Mar., 1912	255 (2)	In practice, June, 1909.
223	BAILEY, Emma	Wagin	22nd Nov., 1911	255 (2)	In practice, June, 1909.
242	BAILLIE, Elizabeth	Victoria Park	22nd Nov., 1911	255 (1)	Sefton Hospital, Melbourne.
412	BALDWIN, Ellen	55 Walker Street, South Fremantle	13th Dec., 1911	255 (2)	In practice, June, 1909.
852	BALDWIN, Mary Jane	Public Hospital, Wagin	25th Oct., 1912	255 (2)	In practice, June, 1909.
312	BALMER, Catherine	Stanmore Street, Subiaco	29th Nov., 1911	255 (2)	In practice, June, 1909.
815	BARKER, Ada	Garland Estate, Russell Street, Victoria Park	9th Aug., 1912	255 (2)	In practice, June, 1909.

494	BARKER, Lilian	Lockridge Hospital, West Guildford	20th Dec., 1911	255	(2)	In practice, June, 1909.
846	BARKER, Sarah Ann	35 Marlborough Street, Perth	5th Sept., 1912	255	(2)	In practice, June, 1909.
69	BARLOW, Mary Ann	C/o Tullock & Co., Leonora	10th Oct., 1911	255	(2)	In practice, June, 1909.
80	BARNES, Elizabeth	Wittenoom Street, Collie	25th Oct., 1911	255	(2)	In practice, June, 1909.
163	BARNES, Ellen Price	Trent Street, Wagin	15th Nov., 1911	255	(1)	St. Margaret's Hospital, Sydney.
289	BARNES, Frances Catherine	Cecilia Street, Subiaco	29th Nov., 1911	255	(2)	In practice, June, 1909.
419	BARNES, Rebecca	Mount Pleasant, Bridgetown	13th Dec., 1911	255	(2)	In practice, June, 1909.
428	BARRASS, Mary Jane	Hewitt Street, Kalgoorlie	13th Dec., 1911	255	(2)	In practice, June, 1909.
803	BARRON, May	White Feather Hospital, Kanowna	7th June, 1912	261	(1)	Central Midwives' Board, England.
421	BASTEN, Jane Ann	50 King Street, Boulder	13th Dec., 1911	255	(2)	In practice, June, 1909.
146	BAUER, Elizabeth	65 Hill Street, Perth	8th Nov., 1911	255	(2)	In practice, June, 1909.
420	BAWDEN, Lucy Ann	25 Chatsworth Road, Highgate Hill, Perth	13th Dec., 1911	255	(2)	In practice, June, 1909.
645	BAXTER, Annie	56 George Street, Kalgoorlie	5th Jan., 1912	255	(2)	In practice, June, 1909.
143	BAXTER, Phoebe Charlotte	Eastbourne Street, Cottesloe Beach	8th Nov., 1911	255	(2)	In practice, June, 1909.
325	BEADEN, Annie	387 Beaufort Street, Perth	8th Dec., 1911	255	(1)	St. Margaret's Hospital, Sydney.
17	BEATTY, Mary Ann Jane	47 Howard Street, Fremantle	27th Sept., 1911	255	(2)	In practice, June, 1909.
140	BEECK, Dorothy Johanna	"Villa Nova," Railway Terrace, W. Guildford	8th Nov., 1911	255	(2)	In practice, June, 1909.
687	BEER, Lily	Bunbury	26th Jan., 1912	255	(2)	In practice, June, 1909.
166	BEHRENDT, Johanna	Trained Nurses' Home, 65 Hill Street, Perth	15th Nov., 1911	255	(1)	Women's Hospital, Sydney.
83	BELL, Bessie Caroline	Busselton	25th Oct., 1911	255	(2)	In practice, June, 1909.
439	BELL, Elizabeth Alice	71 Churchill Avenue, Subiaco	13th Dec., 1911	255	(2)	In practice, June, 1909.
122	BELL, Jane	Norseman	8th Nov., 1911	255	(2)	In practice, June, 1909.
126	BENNETT, Annie Elsie	Dwellingup	8th Nov., 1911	255	(2)	In practice, June, 1909.
41	BENNETT, Sarah Eleanor	Harvey Street, Collie	10th Oct., 1911	255	(2)	In practice, June, 1909.
156	BENTLEY, Edith	29 Attfield Street, Fremantle	15th Nov., 1911	255	(1)	Fremantle Midwifery Training School.
314	BERGIN, Sarah Ann	Victoria Avenue, North Fremantle	29th Nov., 1911	255	(2)	In practice, June, 1909.
283	BEVAN, Louise	122 Aberdeen Street, Perth	29th Nov., 1911	255	(2)	In practice, June, 1909.
458	BILLETT, Dora Maria	Perth Road, West Guildford	20th Dec., 1911	255	(2)	In practice, June, 1909.
286	BIRCH, Elizabeth Ellen	195 Lord Street, Perth	29th Nov., 1911	255	(2)	In practice, June, 1909.
315	BIRT, Alice Rachel	Southern Cross	[illegible]	255	(2)	In practice, June, 1909.
341	BIRT, Margaret Coombe	Tambellup	8th Dec., 1911	255	(2)	In practice, June, 1909.
837	BISHOP, Henrietta	Thompson Road, Rocky Bay, North Fremantle	9th Aug., 1912	255	(2)	In practice, June, 1909.
820	BISHOP, Ruth Alice	Karri Street, South Bunbury	9th Aug., 1912	255	(2)	In practice, June, 1909.
218	BLACK, Allice	C/o Dr. Wilbe, Kalgoorlie	22nd Nov., 1911	255	(2)	In practice, June, 1909.
40	BLACKBURNE, Nellie	Prince Street, Busselton	10th Oct., 1911	255	(1)	Central Midwives' Board, England.
538	BLACKMORE, Minnie	56 Kimberley Street, Leederville	29th Dec., 1911	255	(1)	Women's Hospital, Sydney.
99	BLAKE, Ada Elizabeth	50 Nelson Crescent, East Perth	25th Oct., 1911	255	(2)	In practice, June, 1909.
673	BLAKE, Charlotte Catherine	Aroha Whare, 267 Egan Street, Kalgoorlie	12th Jan., 1912	255	(2)	In practice, June, 1909.
113	BLAKE, Henrietta Eyre Maunsell	180 St. George's Terrace, Perth	8th Nov., 1911	255	(1)	Queen's Home, Adelaide, South Australia.
197	BOEHM, Esther Augusta	"St. Anne's," Williams	22nd Nov., 1911	255	(2)	In practice, June, 1909.
386	BOEHM, Selma Augusta	Lion Mill	8th Dec., 1911	255	(2)	In practice, June, 1909.
606	BOHAN, Lucy	Sandstone	29th Dec., 1911	255	(2)	In practice, June, 1909.
322	BOLE, Eliza Amelia	Claisebrook Road, Perth	8th Dec., 1911	255	(1)	London Obstetrical Society.
287	BOND, Annie	Melba Buildings, Hay Street, Perth	29th Nov., 1911	255	(2)	In practice, June, 1909.
520	BOOTH, Margaret	Moora	20th Dec., 1911	255	(2)	In practice, June, 1909.
636	BORWICK, Isabella Tait	Public Hospital, Sandstone	30th Dec., 1911	255	(1)	Queen's Home, Adelaide.
530	BOURKE, Eileen Mary	Harvest Road, North Fremantle	29th Dec., 1911	255	(1)	Fremantle Midwifery Training School.
408	BOURKE, Margaret Georgina	86 Dugan Street, Kalgoorlie	13th Dec., 1911	255	(2)	In practice, June, 1909.
720	BOWEN, Mary May Elizabeth	"Latona," cr. Langsford Street and Claremont avenue, Claremont	16th Feb., 1912	255	(2)	In practice, June, 1909.
549	BOWEN, Sarah Ann	Boulder	29th Dec., 1911	255	(2)	In practice, June, 1909.

Registration No.	Name.	Address.	Date of Registration.	Section of Act under which Registration was effected.	Qualification.
521	BRADBURY, Kathleen	179 Lake Street, Perth	20th Dec., 1911	255 (2)	In practice, June, 1909.
204	BRADSHAW, May	113 Moran Street, Boulder	22nd Nov., 1911	255 (2)	In practice, June, 1909.
206	BREHENY, Sarah	Charles Street, Maylands	22nd Nov., 1911	255 (2)	In practice, June, 1909.
582	BRIDGE, Elizabeth	Menzies	29th Dec., 1911	255 (2)	In practice, June, 1909.
362	BRIGHT, Jessie Emily Jane	Cookernup	8th Dec., 1911	255 (2)	In practice, June, 1909.
96	BROAD, Minnie Elizabeth	221 Havelock Street, West Perth	25th Oct., 1911	255 (2)	In practice, June, 1909.
691	BRODIE, Emma	White Road, Bunbury	26th Jan., 1912	255 (2)	In practice, June, 1909.
486	BROOKS, Sophia	Pirie Street, Boulder	20th Dec., 1911	255 (2)	In practice, June, 1909.
328	BROOMHALL, Annie Eliza	"Kareenya," St. George's Terrace, Perth	8th Dec., 1911	255 (1)	Women's Hospital, Melbourne.
352	BROTHERIDGE, Amy Elizabeth	64 Grosvenor Road, North Perth	8th Dec., 1911	255 (2)	In practice, June, 1909.
350	BROWN, Catherine Jeanetta	Coolgardie	8th Dec., 1911	255 (2)	In practice, June, 1909.
476	BROWN, Elizabeth	Gwalia	20th Dec., 1911	255 (2)	In practice, June, 1909.
579	BROWN, Emily	Melville House, Albany	29th Dec., 1911	255 (2)	In practice, June, 1909.
492	BROWN, Eva Julia	Cornwall Street, Trafalgar, Kalgoorlie	20th Dec., 1911	255 (2)	In practice, June, 1909.
595	BROWN, Frances Margaret	26 Saunders Street, Perth	29th Dec., 1911	255 (2)	In practice, June, 1909.
853	BROWN, Jane	324 Lord Street, East Perth	25th Oct., 1912	255 (2)	In practice, June, 1909.
751	BROWN, Maud Mary	Cavendish Street, Victoria Park	15th Mar., 1912	255 (2)	In practice, June, 1909.
247	BROWNE, Ellen	Sunbeam Lease, Kanowna	22nd Nov., 1911	255 (2)	In practice, June, 1909.
110	BROWNE, Matilda	Guy's Maternity Hospital, Donnybrook	8th Nov., 1911	255 (1)	Fremantle Midwifery Training School.
288	BRYANT, Emily	36 Vivian Street, Boulder	29th Nov., 1911	255 (2)	In practice, June, 1909.
399	BURKE, Christina	Hines Hill	13th Dec., 1911	255 (1)	Women's Hospital, Sydney.
50	BURT, Hannah	4 Ethel Street, North Perth	10th Oct., 1911	255 (2)	In practice, June, 1909.
460	BURTON, Kate	Zoe Street, Bunbury	20th Dec., 1911	255 (2)	In practice, June, 1909.
228	BYGRAVE, Sarah	Beverley Road, York	22nd Nov., 1911	255 (2)	In practice, June, 1909.
429	BYRNES, Emma	Mount Morgans	13th Dec., 1911	255 (2)	In practice, June, 1909.
565	BYRNES, Harriett Ann Elizabeth	Packenham Street, Mount Lawley, Perth	29th Dec., 1911	255 (2)	In practice, June, 1909.
87	BYTHELL, Sarah Frances	Marmion Street, Cottesloe	25th Oct., 1911	255 (2)	In practice, June, 1909.
885	CADLOLO, Emma	123 Charles Street, West Perth	20th Dec., 1912	255 (2)	In practice, June, 1909.
59	CAHILL, Mary Anne	1852 Boundary Street, Kalgoorlie	10th Oct., 1911	255 (2)	In practice, June, 1909.
630	CAIRNES, Alice Duncan	12 Hamilton Street, Subiaco	29th Dec., 1911	255 (2)	In practice, June, 1909.
185	CALLAGHAN, Annie	North Fremantle	15th Nov., 1911	255 (2)	In practice, June, 1909.
580	CALLAN, Ellen	26 Mary Street, Highgate Hill, Perth	29th Dec., 1911	255 (2)	In practice, June, 1909.
192	CAMPBELL, Mary	Meckering	15th Nov., 1911	255 (2)	In practice, June, 1909.
542	CAMPBELL, Rosanna	126 Aberdeen Street, Perth	29th Dec., 1911	255 (1)	Glasgow Maternity, and Lying-in Hospital.
869	CANNON, Mary Agnes	65 Hill Street, Perth	22nd Nov., 1912	261 (1)	St. Margaret's Hospital, Sydney.
657	CARPENTER, Elizabeth	Augustus Street, Geraldton	5th Jan, 1912	255 (2)	In practice, June, 1909.
818	CARR, Mary	Menzies	9th Aug., 1912	255 (2)	In practice, June, 1909.
187	CARROLL, Annie Jane	Tammin	15th Nov., 1911	255 (2)	In practice, June, 1909.
845	CARSLAW, Catherine Henderson	241 Charles Street, Perth	5th Sept., 1912	255 (2)	In practice, June, 1909.
273	CARTER, Martha Susana	Carey Street, Bunbury	29th Nov., 1911	255 (2)	In practice, June, 1909.
600	CATCHPOLE, Catherine	Gwalia	29th Dec., 1911	255 (2)	In practice, June, 1909.
224	CAVE, Jessie Ethel Olive	75 Dwyer Street, Boulder	22nd Nov., 1911	255 (2)	In practice, June, 1909.
556	CHAMBERS, Mary Anne	Bayswater	29th Dec., 1911	255 (2)	In practice, June, 1909.

451	CHAMPION, Elizabeth Lorna	37 Malcolm Street, Perth	20th Dec., 1911	255	(2)	In practice, June, 1909.
24	CHAPMAN, Mary	Geraldton	27th Sept., 1911	255	(2)	In practice, June, 1909.
292	CHARLES, Louisa	79 Padbury Street, Perth	29th Nov., 1911	255	(2)	In practice, June, 1909.
868	CHATFIELD, Norah Alicia	Caversham, Guildford	25th Oct., 1912	255	(2)	In practice, June, 1909.
291	CHEATLEY, Alice	65 Hill Street, Perth	29th Nov., 1911	255	(2)	In practice, June, 1909.
290	CHEATLEY, Rebecca	65 Hill Street, Perth	29th Nov., 1911	255	(2)	In practice, June, 1909.
18	CHINNERY, Alice Mary	Copley Street, Bayswater	27th Sept., 1911	255	(2)	In practice, June, 1909.
683	CHITTY, Martha	Jumperding, Toodyay	26th Jan., 1912	255	(2)	In practice, June, 1909.
599	CHRISTMAS, Mary Jane	Grass Valley	29th Dec., 1911	255	(2)	In practice, June, 1909.
774	CLARK, Charlotte	Kingston Road, Victoria Park	17th May, 1912	255	(2)	In practice, June, 1909.
232	CLARK, Margaret	149 Beaufort Street, Perth	22nd Nov., 1911	255	(2)	In practice, June, 1909.
870	CLARKE, Elizabeth Darley	"Beaulieu," Robinson Estate, Albany	22nd Nov., 1912	255	(2)	In practice, June, 1909.
727	CLARKE, Eva	141 King Street Boulder	16th Feb., 1912	255	(2)	In practice, June, 1909.
854	CLARKE, Gertrude	Hospital for Insane, Claremont	25th Oct., 1912	255	(2)	In practice, June, 1909.
608	CLARKE, Margaret	Geraldton	29th Dec., 1911	255	(2)	In practice, June, 1909.
251	CLARKSON, Sarah	Eleanor Street, Geraldton	22nd Nov., 1911	255	(2)	In practice, June, 1909.
568	CLATWORTHY, Emily Elizabeth	Smith's Mill	29th Dec., 1911	255	(2)	In practice, June, 1909.
296	CLAYDON, Eleanor	192 York Street, Subiaco	29th Nov., 1911	255	(2)	In practice, June, 1909.
613	CLAYTON, Elizabeth Mary	28 Nairn Street, Fremantle	29th Dec., 1911	255	(2)	In practice, June, 1909.
483	CLEARY, Jean	16 Brookman Street, Perth	20th Dec., 1911	255	(2)	In practice, June, 1909.
550	COATES, Alice	Shaw Street, Coolgardie	29th Dec., 1911	255	(2)	In practice, June, 1909.
250	COLINS, Sarah Ann	Geraldton	22nd Nov., 1911	255	(2)	In practice, June, 1909.
276	COLK, Eleanor	137A Richardson Street, Boulder	29th Nov., 1911	255	(2)	In practice, June, 1909.
379	COLL, Catherine	150 Hopkins Street, Boulder	8th Dec., 1911	255	(2)	In practice, June, 1909.
749	COLLETT, Edith	Boulder	15th Mar., 1912	255	(2)	In practice, June, 1909.
149	COLLINS, Amelia	94 John Street, Perth	8th Nov., 1911	255	(2)	In practice, June, 1909.
778	COLLINS, Beatrice Anne	Lister Private Hospital, Shenton Road, Claremont	17th May, 1911	255	(2)	In practice, June, 1909.
553	COLLINS, Helena Mary	Addis Street, Kalgoorlie	29th Dec., 1911	255	(2)	In practice, June, 1909.
791	COLLINS, Mary Louisa	Edgar Street, South Kalgoorlie	7th June, 1912	255	(2)	In practice, June, 1909.
724	COLTON, Mary Ann	Roelands	16th Feb., 1912	255	(2)	In practice, June, 1909.
535	CONDON, Eliza	194 Stirling Street, Perth	29th Dec., 1911	255	(1)	Women's Hospital, Melbourne.
56	CONN, Margaret	Lawley Avenue, Northam	10th Oct., 1911	255	(2)	In practice, June, 1909.
95	CONNELL, Annie Brown	Bridgetown	25th Oct., 1911	255	(2)	In practice, June, 1909.
573	CONNORS, Sarah Jane	104 Havelock Street, Perth	29th Dec., 1911	255	(2)	In practice, June, 1909.
871	COOK, Elsie	30 King William Street, South Fremantle	22nd Nov., 1912	255	(2)	In practice, June, 1909.
723	COOK, Rose Jane	Habgood Street, Northam	16th Feb., 1912	255	(2)	In practice, June, 1909.
427	COOKE, Fredericka Georgina Elizabeth	Boulder	13th Dec., 1911	255	(2)	In practice, June, 1909.
785	COONAN, Annie	Waterloo	17th May, 1912	255	(2)	In practice, June, 1909.
632	CORBITT, Catherine	Swan Street, Guildford	29th Dec., 1911	255	(2)	In practice, June, 1909.
462	COWLING, Edith	Eagle Street, Trafalgar, Kalgoorlie	20th Dec., 1911	255	(2)	In practice, June, 1909.
656	COX, Mary	Eleanor Street, Geraldton	5th Jan., 1912	255	(2)	In practice, June, 1909.
436	COX, Mary Ann	30 Ruby Street, Leederville	13th Dec., 1911	255	(2)	In practice, June, 1909.
756	COX, Rose Darlington	C/o Mr. Stewart Jones, Fitzgerald Street, Geraldton	19th April, 1912	255	(2)	In practice, June, 1909.
742	CRAGGS, Beatrice	The Rectory, Subiaco	15th Mar., 1912	261	(1)	Central Midwives' Board, England; Newcastle-on-Tyne Maternity Hospital.
872	CRITCHLEY, Winifred Ursula	St. John's Lodge, Hanbury Street, Kalgoorlie	22nd Nov., 1912	255	(2)	In practice, June, 1909.
398	CROSS, Evaline	Kelmscott	8th Dec., 1911	255	(2)	In practice, June, 1909.
130	CROWE, Annie Ursula	121 Aberdeen Street, Perth	8th Nov., 1911	255	(2)	In practice, June, 1909.
572	CRUDACE, Clara	Burbanks	29th Dec., 1911	255	(2)	In practice, June, 1909.
78	CUMING, Hannah	Stuart Street, Cottesloe Beach	25th Oct., 1911	255	(2)	In practice, June, 1909.
551	CUNDILL, Matilda Esther	108 Hay Street, Subiaco	29th Dec., 1911	255	(2)	In practice, June, 1909.

Registration No.	Name.	Address.	Date of Registration.	Section of Act under which Registration was effected.	Qualification.
102	CUNNING, Emily	55 Lord Street, Perth	25th Oct., 1911	255 (2)	In practice, June, 1909.
697	CUNNINGHAM, Emma Maria	Duke Street, West Northam	26th Jan., 1912	255 (2)	In practice, June, 1909.
497	CUTHBERT, Mildred Stanley	Merredin	20th Dec., 1911	255 (2)	In practice, June, 1909.
849	DALZIELL, Margaret	28 Alfred Street, Leederville	5th Sept., 1912	255 (2)	In practice, June, 1909.
873	DAMYON, Ellen Mary	Perth Road, Albany	22nd Nov., 1912	261 (1)	South Sydney Women's Hospital.
725	DANES, Rebecca	Bellevue	16th Feb., 1912	255 (2)	In practice, June, 1909.
789	DANIELS, Mary	194 Stirling Street, Perth	7th June, 1912	255 (2)	In practice, June, 1909.
591	DART, Sadie	17 John Street, West Perth	29th Dec., 1911	255 (2)	In practice, June, 1909.
397	DAVERN, Susannah	St. Helen's Hospital, 241 Stirling Street, Perth	8th Dec., 1911	255 (1)	Fremantle Midwifery Training School.
430	DAVEY, Alice Maud Mary	Hopkins Street, Boulder	13th Dec., 1911	255 (2)	In practice, June, 1909.
765	DAVIDSON, Sarah	Station Street, Gwalia	19th April, 1912	255 (2)	In practice, June, 1909.
509	DAVIES, Isabella	Kanowna	20th Dec., 1911	255 (2)	In practice, June, 1909.
222	DAVIES, Martha	Sydney Street, North Perth	22nd Nov., 1911	255 (2)	In practice, June, 1909.
500	DAVIS, Catherine	Guildford Road, Maylands	20th Dec., 1911	255 (2)	In practice, June, 1909.
529	DAVIS, Janet	Bay View Terrace, Claremont	29th Dec., 1911	255 (1)	Fremantle Midwifery Training School.
824	DAVIS, Jean	Kirupp	9th Aug., 1912	255 (2)	In practice, June, 1909.
316	DAVIS, Mary Ann	Kulyaling	29th Nov., 1911	255 (2)	In practice, June, 1909.
506	DAVIS, Sarah	Hanson's Cottage, White Road, Bunbury	20th Dec., 1911	255 (2)	In practice, June, 1909.
162	DAWSON, Alice Frances	Public Hospital, Greenbushes	15th Nov., 1911	255 (2)	In practice, June, 1909.
42	DAY, Ann Caroline	Crawford Road, Maylands	10th Oct., 1911	255 (2)	In practice, June, 1909.
505	DAY, Jessie Yeldham	Preston Point Road, East Fremantle	20th Dec., 1911	255 (2)	In practice, June, 1909.
874	DAY, Mary Jane	Sewell Street, East Fremantle	22nd Nov., 1912	255 (2)	In practice, June, 1909.
157	DEANS, May	25 Victoria Road, Fremantle	15th Nov., 1911	255 (1)	Fremantle Midwifery Training School.
374	DELANEY, Bridget Mary	Bunbury	8th Dec., 1911	255 (2)	In practice, June, 1909.
855	DELANEY, Ida Agnes	C/o Miss O'Connor, Douglas Street, West Perth	25th Oct., 1912	255 (2)	In practice, June, 1909.
524	DESPARD, Charlotte Letitia	Public Hospital, Beverley	20th Dec., 1911	255 (2)	In practice, June, 1909.
875	DEUTSCHER, Bertha Christina	194 Stirling Street, Perth	22nd Nov., 1912	261 (1)	Women's Hospital, Melbourne.
886	D'EVELYNES, Flora	896 Wellington Street, West Perth	20th Dec., 1912	255 (2)	In practice, June, 1909.
378	DHU, Esther Ann	126 Harold Street, Perth	8th Dec., 1911	255 (2)	In practice, June, 1909.
480	DICK, Eleanor	60 Pirie Street, Boulder	20th Dec., 1911	255 (2)	In practice, June, 1909.
561	DILLON, Lydia	Smyth Road, West Subiaco	29th Dec., 1911	255 (2)	In practice, June, 1909.
108	DIXON, Catherine	53 Woolwich Street, Leederville	8th Nov., 1911	255 (1)	Fremantle Midwifery Training School.
351	DIXON, Grace	10 Brookman Street, Perth	8th Dec., 1911	255 (2)	In practice, June, 1909.
867	DODD, Emma	Arrino	25th Oct., 1912	255 (2)	In practice, June, 1909.
672	DONALDSON, Catherine	1022 Hay Street, West Perth	12th Jan., 1912	255 (2)	In practice, June, 1909.
20	DONALDSON, Maria	Bay Road, Claremont	27th Sept., 1911	255 (2)	In practice, June, 1909.
361	DONNELLY, Elizabeth	Waverley Hospital, Adelaide Terrace, Perth	8th Dec., 1911	255 (2)	In practice, June, 1909.
694	DONNELLY, Margaret	Narrogin	26th Jan., 1912	255 (2)	In practice, June, 1909.
338	DONOHOE, Ellen	100 Dwyer Street, Boulder	8th Dec., 1911	255 (2)	In practice, June, 1909.
253	DONOVAN, Alice Maud Mary	Grosvenor Hospital, Fremantle	29th Nov., 1911	255 (1)	Fremantle Midwifery Training School.
830	DONOVAN, Katherine	South Bunbury	9th Aug., 1912	255 (2)	In practice, June, 1909.
629	DORAN, Agnes	407 William Street, Perth	29th Dec., 1911	255 (2)	In practice, June, 1909.
515	DORE, Margaretta	Venn Street Cottesloe	20th Dec., 1911	255 (2)	In practice, June, 1909.

348	DORRATT, Sarah	Forrest Street, Northam	8th Dec., 1911	255 (2)	In practice, June, 1909.
488	DORRINGTON, Louise	Shenton Road Claremont	20th Dec., 1911	255 (2)	In practice, June, 1909.
394	DOUGLAS, Fanny Marion	Albany	8th Dec., 1911	255 (2)	In practice, June, 1909.
590	DOULEAVY, Louisa Mary Liza Blanche	Carnarvon	29th Dec., 1911	255 (2)	In practice, June, 1909.
734	DOWN, Mary Ann	Wickepin	15th Mar., 1912	255 (2)	In practice, June, 1909.
22	DOWNEY, Ellen	Hamilton Street, Boulder	27th Sept., 1911	255 (2)	In practice, June, 1909.
584	DOWNEY, Hariett Maud	Rosella Private Hospital, Geraldton	29th Dec., 1911	255 (2)	In practice, June, 1909.
456	DOYLE, Annie	Wickepin	20th Dec., 1911	255 (1)	St. Margaret's Hospital, Sydney.
856	DOYLE, Winifred Elfredith	55 Leviathan Street, Boulder	25th Oct., 1912	255 (2)	In practice, June, 1909.
649	DRAFFIN, Janet	34 Dwyer Street, Boulder City	5th Jan., 1912	255 (2)	In practice, June, 1909.
857	DRAKEFORD, Julia	W.C.T.U. Perth	25th Oct., 1912	261 (1)	Central Midwives' Board and L.O.S., England.
320	DRANSFIELD, Dora	Wagin	8th Dec., 1911	255 (1)	Central Midwives' Board, England.
382	DRISCOLL, Mary Ann	Dongara	8th Dec., 1911	255 (2)	In practice, June, 1909.
533	DUCHATEL, Marie	65 Hill Street, Perth	29th Dec., 1911	255 (1)	Women's Hospital, Melbourne.
612	DUCKHAM, Mary Ann	York	29th Dec., 1911	255 (2)	In practice, June, 1909.
555	DUGDALE, Mary Alice	Duchess Street, Busselton	29th Dec., 1911	255 (2)	In practice, June, 1909.
353	DUNN, Lily Elizabeth	20 McCourt Street, Perth	8th Dec., 1911	255 (2)	In practice, June, 1909.
887	DUNNE, Irene Hilda Agnes	C/o Dr. Birmingham, Fremantle	20th Dec., 1912	255 (2)	In practice, June, 1909.
177	DU RIEU, Bertha	292 William Street, Perth	15th Nov., 1911	255 (2)	In practice, June, 1909.
12	DURLACHER, Miriam Dorothy	Toodyay	13th Sept., 1911	255 (2)	In practice, June, 1909.
445	DWYER, Catherine Beatrice	Swan Street, Bayswater	13th Dec., 1911	255 (2)	In practice, June, 1909.
570	DYE, Martha	Reading Street, South Bunbury	29th Dec., 1911	255 (2)	In practice, June, 1909.
620	EADIE, Ellen	Gregory Street Geraldton	29th Dec., 1911	255 (2)	In practice, June, 1909.
704	EAGLES, Emily	Newcastle Road, Midland Junction	26th Jan., 1912	255 (2)	In practice, June, 1909.
597	EAMER, Mary	Meekatharra	29th Dec., 1911	255 (2)	In practice, June, 1909.
581	EDESON, Eleanor	30 Opal Street, Leederville	29th Dec., 1911	255 (2)	In practice, June, 1909.
888	EDMONDSON, Letitia	Kodj Kodjin	20th Dec., 1912	255 (2)	In practice, June, 1909.
731	EDWARDS, Ellen	Silas Street, East Fremantle	16th Feb., 1912	255 (2)	In practice, June, 1909.
787	EDWARDS, Grace	Barrabup	17th May, 1912	255 (2)	In practice, June, 1909.
67	EDWARDS, Mary Ann	6 Gallop Street, Perth	10th Oct., 1911	255 (2)	In practice, June, 1909.
6	EDWARDS, Mary Mervyn	Vincent Street, Beverley	13th Sept., 1911	255 (2)	In practice, June, 1909.
876	EGAN, Alice	Private Hospital, Boulder	22nd Nov., 1912	255 (2)	In practice, June, 1909.
586	EGAN, Hanora	96 Richardson Street, Boulder	29th Dec., 1911	255 (2)	In practice, June, 1909.
255	EHRLICH, Dora	104 Brown Street, East Perth	29th Nov., 1911	255 (1)	Fremantle Midwifery Training School.
732	ELLERBY, Sarah Ann	Gibney Street, Cottesloe Beach	16th Feb., 1912	255 (2)	In practice, June, 1909.
489	ELLIOTT, Lucy Ruble	Boulder	20th Dec., 1911	255 (2)	In practice, June, 1909.
662	ELLIS, Mary	Cowell Street, West Perth	5th Jan., 1912	255 (2)	In practice, June, 1909.
479	ENGLET, Mary	Falkirk Avenue, Maylands	20th Dec., 1911	255 (2)	In practice, June, 1909.
155	ETHELL, Rose	Marine Terrace, Geraldton	8th Nov., 1911	255 (2)	In practice, June, 1909.
475	EVANS, Sophia	Victoria Park	20th Dec., 1911	255 (2)	In practice, June, 1909.
380	FARQUHARSON, Marie	48 Ventnor Avenue, Perth	8th Dec., 1911	255 (2)	In practice, June, 1909.
366	FAZEY, Harriet Leah	Burgoyne Street, Northam	8th Dec., 1911	255 (2)	In practice, June, 1909.
518	FELL, Elizabeth	24 Attfield Street, Fremantle	20th Dec., 1911	255 (2)	In practice, June, 1909.
45	FENN, Elizabeth Ann	162 Wittenoom Street, Perth	10th Oct., 1911	255 (2)	In practice, June, 1909.
306	FERGUSON, Christina Anne	C/o Mrs. Whiteman, Amherst Road, West Midland	29th Nov., 1911	255 (2)	In practice, June, 1909.
719	FERGUSON, Martha	Meekatharra	16th Feb., 1912	255 (2)	In practice, June, 1909.
652	FEWINGS, Annie	30 Marquis Street, West Perth	5th Jan., 1912	255 (2)	In practice, June, 1909.
274	FIDDES, Emma Jane	Boulder	29th Nov., 1911	255 (2)	In practice, June, 1909.
252	FIELD, Selina Tryphena	"Rothesay," Claremont Avenue, Claremont	29th Nov., 1911	255 (1)	Fremantle Midwifery Training School.

Registration No.	Name.	Address.	Date of Registration.	Section of Act under which Registration was effected.	Qualification.
332	FISHER, Margaret	Trafalgar Street, Trafalgar	8th Dec., 1911	255 (2)	In practice, June, 1909.
806	FITZGERALD, Elizabeth Charlotte Ann	108 Cornwall Street, Trafalgar	5th July, 1912	255 (2)	In practice, June, 1909.
417	FITZGERALD, Margaret Frances	"Victoria House, Hay Street, Perth	13th Dec., 1911	255 (2)	In practice, June, 1909.
234	FITZSIMONS, Agens Helena Jane	Bridge Street, Guildford	22nd Nov., 1911	255 (2)	In practice, June, 1909.
31	FLAWS, Rose	Broome Street, North Fremantle	27th Sep., 1911	255 (2)	In practice, June, 1909.
214	FLAXMAN, Louisa McGregor Jane	"Allir," Market Street, Guildford	22nd Nov., 1911	255 (2)	In practice, June, 1909.
433	FLINN, Emily Sarah	132 Charles Street, Perth	13th Dec., 1911	255 (2)	In practice, June, 1909.
523	FOAT, Sarah Ann	Infectious Diseases Hospital, Kalgoorlie	20th Dec., 1911	255 (1)	London Obstetrical Society.
342	FOGARTY, Ipsa Mary	Harold Street, West Leederville	8th Dec., 1911	255 (2)	In practice, June, 1909.
646	FORSTER, Isabella	John Street, Cottesloe	5th Jan., 1912	255 (2)	In practice, June, 1909.
877	FORTINGTON, Ada Jemima	Public Hospital, Broad Arrow	22nd Nov., 1912	255 (2)	In practice, June, 1909.
468	FOWLES, Sophia Elizabeth	Albany	20th Dec., 1911	255 (2)	In practice, June, 1909.
46	FOYEL, Emily Jane	Rowley Road, off Middleton Road, Albany	10th Oct., 1911	255 (2)	In practice, June, 1909.
112	FRASER, Mary	Women's Home, Fremantle	8th Nov., 1911	255 (1)	Fremantle Midwifery Training School.
396	FREDBERG, Sarah Anne	186 Newcastle Street, Perth	8th Dec., 1911	255 (2)	In practice, June, 1909.
889	FRENCH, Anne Elizabeth	Gosnells	20th Dec., 1912	255 (2)	In practice, June, 1909.
145	FULLERTON, Ellen	Weld Street, Northam	8th Nov., 1911	255 (2)	In practice, June, 1909.
514	GANNAWAY, Charlotte May	Williamstown, Kalgoorlie	20th Dec., 1911	255 (2)	In practice, June, 1909.
84	GARBUTT, Mary Jane	169 Sewell Street, East Fremantle	25th Oct., 1911	255 (2)	In practice, June, 1909.
799	GARD, Ruth Yennings	49 Millen Street, Boulder	7th July, 1912	255 (2)	In practice, June, 1909.
703	GARTRELL, Susan Jane	South Greenbushes	26th Jan., 1912	255 (2)	In practice, June, 1909.
302	GAWTHORP, Elizabeth Evena	Mason Street, North Fremantle	29th Nov, 1911	255 (2)	In practice, June, 1909.
741	GIBSON, Mary Anne	Claremont	15th Mar., 1912	255 (2)	In practice, June, 1909.
481	GIDDENS, Adelaide Mayston	Beach Road, South Bunbury	20th Dec., 1911	255 (2)	In practice, June, 1909.
537	GILBERT, Hannah Maria	Women's Home, Fremantle	29th Dec., 1911	255 (1)	London Obstetrical Society.
752	GILL, Maud	Denmark	19th April, 1912	261 (1)	Central Midwives' Board, England.
624	GILMOUR, Elizabeth	194 Stirling Street, Perth	29th Dec., 1911	255 (1)	St. Margaret's Hospital, Sydney.
786	GLASGOW, Louisa Mary Josephine	Carnarvon	17th May, 1912	255 (2)	In practice, June, 1909.
392	GLASKIN, Laura Annie	136 Charles Street, West Perth	8th Dec., 1911	255 (2)	In practice, June, 1909.
767	GLASS, Beatrice	Narrogin	19th Apr., 1912	255 (2)	In practice, June, 1909.
834	GOLDING, Emily	Queen Victoria Street, Leonora	9th Aug., 1912	255 (2)	In practice, June, 1909.
812	GOODALL, Elke Zelde	194 Stirling Street, Perth	5th July, 1912	261 (1)	Central Midwives' Board, England.
766	GOODE, Edith Ellen	35 Hesperus Street, South Boulder	19th Apr., 1912	255 (2)	In practice, June, 1909.
343	GOODLET, Ettie	Seventh Avenue, Maylands	8th Dec., 1911	255 (2)	In practice, June, 1909.
77	GOSSAGE, Maria	14 Axon Street, Subiaco	25th Oct., 1911	255 (2)	In practice, June, 1909.
390	GOULD, Flora Ann	Narrogin	8th Dec., 1911	255 (2)	In practice, June, 1909.
903	GOULD, Elsie Gertrude	Ensor Hospital, Stirling Street, Perth	20th Dec., 1912	261 (1)	Central Midwives' Board, England.
331	GRAHAM, Augusta Carlotta	Sayer Street, Midland Junction	8th Dec., 1911	255 (2)	In practice, June, 1909.
761	GRANGER, Lily Rosa	Cuballing	19th Apr., 1912	255 (2)	In practice, June, 1909.
825	GRAY, Emily	Meekatharra	9th Aug., 1912	255 (2)	In practice, June, 1909.
295	GREEN, Eliza Thomas	Preston House, Johnston Street, Collie	29th Nov., 1911	255 (2)	In practice, June, 1909.
485	GREEN, Emily	Eggleston Street, South Bunbury	20th Dec., 1911	255 (2)	In practice, June, 1909.
548	GREENALL, Annie	148 Barker Road, Subiaco	29th Dec., 1911	255 (1)	London Obstetrical Society.

63	GREENALSH, Kate Mary	Burnside Street, Bayswater	10th Oct., 1911	255 (2)	In practice, June, 1909.
240	GREGG, Margaret	Wood Street, Fremantle	22nd Nov., 1911	255 (2)	In practice, June, 1909.
543	GRIFFITH, Charlotte Magdalena	Bunbury	29th Dec., 1911	255 (1)	St. Margaret's Hospital, Sydney.
810	GROVER, Elizabeth Bridget	Indinup, Katanning	5th July, 1912	261 (1)	Central Midwives' Board, England.
210	GROVES, Bella	Boulder Road, Kalgoorlie	22nd Nov., 1911	255 (2)	In practice, June, 1909.
534	GRUENERT, Myra	"Eltrym," Swanbourne Terrace and North Street, Cottesloe North	29th Dec., 1911	255 (1)	Sefton Hospital, Melbourne.
142	GUNST, Emily Lydia Elizabeth	Carey Street, Bunbury	8th Nov., 1911	255 (2)	In practice, June, 1909.
245	HAGUE, Millington May	Bunbury Post Office	22nd Nov., 1911	255 (2)	In practice, June, 1909.
748	HAINING, Minna Mary Frances	The Rectory, Southern Cross	15th Mar., 1912	255 (2)	In practice, June, 1909.
750	HALL, Caroline	Oberthur Street, Kalgoorlie	15th Mar., 1912	255 (2)	In practice, June, 1909.
779	HALL, Mary Elizabeth	Claremont	17th May, 1912	255 (2)	In practice, June, 1909.
121	HALL, Sarah Elizabeth	44 Milligan Street, Perth	8th Nov., 1911	255 (2)	In practice, June, 1909.
220	HALLYBURTON, Jeanet	23 Walcott Street, Mount Lawley, Perth	22nd Nov., 1911	255 (2)	In practice, June, 1909.
567	HAMILTON, Catherine	C/c E. Willmott, Isabella Street, Kanowna	20th Dec., 1911	255 (2)	In practice, June, 1909.
301	HAMILTON, Martha Jane	42 Charles Street, Perth	29th Nov., 1911	255 (2)	In practice, June, 1909.
248	HAMPSHIRE, Mary Josephine	Public Hospital, Toodyay	22nd Nov., 1911	255 (2)	In practice, June, 1909.
202	HAMPSON, Elizabeth	Woodbridge Terrace, Midland Junction	22nd Nov., 1911	255 (2)	In practice, June, 1909.
681	HANCOCK, Mary	43 Bourke Street, Kalgoorlie	12th Jan., 1912	255 (2)	In practice, June, 1909.
478	HANCOCK, May	887 Outram Street, Boulder	20th Dec., 1911	255 (2)	In practice, June, 1909.
890	HANNAH, Helena Longmore	c/o Mrs. Deas, 98 Piesse Street, Boulder	20th Dec., 1912	255 (2)	In practice, June, 1909.
115	HANNAH, Margaret	194 Stirling Street, Perth	8th Nov., 1911	255 (1)	Liverpool Maternity Hospital; Central Midwives' Board, England.
381	HANSEN, Alice Maud	Wroxton Street, Midland Junction	8th Dec., 1911	255 (2)	In practice, June, 1909.
769	HANSON, Mary Ann	Burt Street, Cottesloe	19th Apr., 1912	255 (2)	In practice, June, 1909.
847	HARMAN, Frances	Anstey Road, West Guildford	5th Sep., 1912	255 (2)	In practice, June, 1909.
743	HARPER, Hannah Norah	Prospect Street, Armadale	15th Mar., 1912	255 (2)	In practice, June, 1909.
688	HARRINGTON, Mary	2031 Wilson Street, South Kalgoorlie	26th Jan., 1912	255 (2)	In practice, June, 1909.
74	HARRIS, Antoinette	Lincoln Street, Perth'	25th Oct., 1911	255 (1)	Women's Hospital, Melbourne.
425	HARRIS, Margaret Gertrude	Gosnells	13th Dec., 1911	255 (2)	In practice, June, 1909.
663	HARRIS, Martha	75 Hubble Street, Fremantle	5th Jan., 1912	255 (2)	In practice, June, 1909.
605	HARRIS, Nellie	Laverton	29th Dec., 1911	255 (2)	In practice, June, 1909.
809	HARRISON, Ellen Theresa	Karridale, *via* Busselton	5th July, 1912	255 (2)	In practice, June, 1909.
360	HARRISON, Jemima	Albert Street, Victoria Park	8th Dec., 1911	255 (2)	In practice, June, 1909.
438	HARTMANN, Pauline Anna	60 Davis Street, Boulder	13th Dec., 1911	255 (2)	In practice, June, 1909.
607	HARTNUP, Emma Jane	Vancouver Street, Albany	29th Dec., 1911	255 (2)	In practice, June, 1909.
676	HARTSHORN, Vergena	Wickepin	12th Jan., 1912	255 (2)	In practice, June, 1909.
628	HATTON, Mary	13 Robertson Street, Perth	29th Dec., 1911	255 (2)	In practice, June, 1909.
640	HAUB, Auguste	Waroona	5th Jan., 1912	255 (2)	In practice, June, 1909.
575	HAYES, Lucretia Jane	65 Hill Street, Perth	29th Dec., 1911	255 (2)	In practice, June, 1909.
513	HEAD, Fanny	Nannine	20th Dec., 1911	255 (2)	In practice, June, 1909.
470	HEANEY, Sarah	Morrell Street, Northam	20th Dec., 1911	255 (2)	In practice, June, 1909.
839	HEAP, Florence	Government Hospital, Coolgardie	9th Aug., 1912	261 (1)	Central Midwives' Board, England.
840	HEAP, Mary Clarkson	Government Hospital, Kalgoorlie	9th Aug., 1912	261 (1)	Central Midwives' Board, England.
437	HEATH, Hilda Rowena Estelle	Norseman	13th Dec., 1911	255 (2)	In practice, June, 1909.
313	HEATH, Mary Ann	226 Hay Street, Kalgoorlie	29th Nov., 1911	255 (2)	In practice, June, 1909.
271	HELLWIG, Mary	Duke Street, East Northam	29th Nov., 1911	255 (2)	In practice, June, 1909.
294	HELSIN, Elizabeth Ann	Battle Street, Cottesloe Beach	29th Nov., 1911	255 (2)	In practice, June, 1909.
844	HEMBURY, Amelia	130 Parry Street, Perth	5th Sept., 1912	255 (2)	In practice, June, 1909.
282	HENDERSON, Ann	Tennyson Street, Leederville	29th Nov., 1911	255 (2)	In practice, June, 1909.
368	HERLIHY, Ellen	54 Moran Street, Boulder	8th Dec., 1911	255 (2)	In practice, June, 1909.

Registration No.	Name.	Address.	Date of Registration.	Section of Act under which Registration was effected.	Qualification.
891	HETTICH, Harriett Mary	Jarrahdale	20th Dec., 1912	255 (2)	In practice, June, 1909.
496	HEWLETT, Susan Ann	208 Piccadilly Street, Kalgoorlie	20th Dec., 1911	255 (2)	In practice, June, 1909.
836	HICKEY, Elizabeth	6 Montreal Street, East Fremantle	9th Aug., 1912	255 (2)	In practice, June, 1909.
447	HICKMMOTT, Fanny	Leonora	13th Dec., 1911	255 (2)	In practice, June, 1909.
661	HIGGINS, Rosalina	194 Stirling Street, Perth	5th Jan., 1912	255 (2)	In practice, June, 1909.
583	HIGGS, Esther Elizabeth	45 Evan Street, Boulder	29th Dec., 1911	255 (2)	In practice, June, 1909.
37	HILL, Gertrude Mary	Macdonald Street, Kalgoorlie	27th Sept., 1911	255 (2)	In practice, June, 1909.
340	HILL, Mary	Meelah Street, Sandstone	8th Dec., 1911	255 (2)	In practice, June, 1909.
490	HILLBRICH, Jessie	36 Hanover Street, North Perth	20th Dec., 1911	255 (2)	In practice, June, 1909.
154	HITCHCOCK, Martha Matilda	81 Jersey Street, Jolimont	8th Nov., 1911	255 (2)	In practice, June, 1909.
601	HOBBINS, Annie	Yarloop	29th Dec., 1911	255 (2)	In practice, June, 1909.
141	HOBLEY, Jane	2nd Avenue, North Perth	8th Nov., 1911	255 (2)	In practice, June, 1909.
577	HODGES, Frances	Merredin	29th Dec., 1911	255 (2)	In practice, June, 1909.
270	HOLCROFT, Ada Davey	50 Addis Street, Kalgoorlie	29th Nov., 1911	255 (2)	In practice, June, 1909.
759	HOLLAND, Emily Jane	Wedgegarrup, *via* Wagin	19th April, 1912	255 (2)	In practice, June, 1909.
740	HOLMES, Ann	"Helmewood," Williams	15th Mar., 1912	255 (2)	In practice, June, 1909.
554	HOLMES, Mary	"Marathon," Marmion Street, Cottesloe	29th Dec., 1911	255 (2)	In practice, June, 1909.
246	HOLST, Rose	Moora	22nd Nov., 1911	255 (2)	In practice, June, 1909.
4	HORNBY-BROWN, Jane	Mandurah Road, Fremantle	13th Sept., 1911	255 (1)	Central Midwives' Board, England.
149	HOSSACK, Margaret	Fingall Street, Day Dawn	20th Dec., 1911	255 (2)	In practice, June, 1909.
211	HOUGH, Emily	Princess Royal	22nd Nov., 1911	255 (2)	In practice, June, 1909.
878	HOULAHAN, Mary	Private Hospital, Powell Street, Boulder	22nd Nov., 1912	255 (2)	In practice, June, 1909.
757	HOUSE, Gertrude	Victoria Street, Bunbury	19th April, 1912	255 (2)	In practice, June, 1909.
450	HOWE, Elizabeth	Hubert Street, Guildford	20th Dec., 1911	255 (2)	In practice, June, 1909.
150	HOWELL, Mary	18 Wade Street, Perth	8th Nov., 1911	255 (2)	In practice, June, 1909.
311	HOWELL, Rebecca Jane	Egerton Street, Narrogin	29th Nov., 1911	255 (2)	In practice, June, 1909.
879	HUDSON, Louisa Matilda	"Birkdale," Hill Street, Fremantle	22nd Nov., 1912	261 (1)	Central Midwives' Board, England; **Birkenhead** Maternity Hospital.
384	HUNT, Elizabeth Jane	Eclipse Mine, Kallaroo, Kalgoorlie	8th Dec., 1911	255 (2)	In practice, June, 1909.
369	HUNT, Jane Elizabeth	York	8th Dec., 1911	255 (2)	In practice, June, 1909.
52	HUNTER, Harriet	Donnybrook	10th Oct., 1911	255 (2)	In practice, June, 1909.
858	HUNTER, Louisa	Holyoake	25th Oct., 1912	255 (2)	In practice, June, 1909.
227	HUSSEY, Emily	Hopkins Street, Boulder	22nd Nov., 1911	255 (2)	In practice, June, 1909.
634	HUTTON, Helena	194 Stirling Street, Perth	29th Dec., 1911	255 (2)	In practice, June, 1909.
365	HUXTABLE, Gertrude Isabel	Pinjarra	8th Dec., 1911	255 (2)	In practice, June, 1909.
623	INGLIS, Daisy	194 Stirling Street, Perth	29th Dec., 1911	255 (1)	Women's Hospital, Melbourne.
772	INGLIS, Sarah	Athelstan Street, Cottesloe	17th May, 1912	255 (2)	In practice, June, 1909.
729	IRVINE, Mary	Wharton Street, Cottesloe Beach	16th Feb., 1912	255 (2)	In practice, June, 1909.
196	ISAAC, Edith Lucy	Forrest Street, Beverley	22nd Nov., 1911	255 (1)	Central Midwives' Board, England.
134	JACKSON, Elizabeth Ann	Donnybrook	8th Nov., 1911	255 (2)	In practice, June, 1909.
880	JAMES, Alice Maud	Public Hospital, Perth	22nd Nov., 1912	261 (1)	Central Midwives' Board, England; **City of London** Lying-in Hospital.

448	JAMES, Eliza	Day Dawn	13th Dec., 1911	255	(2)	In practice, June, 1909.
395	JAMES, Jane	Morrison Road, Midland Junction	8th Dec., 1911	255	(2)	In practice, June, 1909.
131	JAMES, Theresa Adelaide	32 Windsor Street, Leederville	8th Nov., 1911	255	(2)	In practice, June, 1909.
426	JAMESON, Elizabeth Anne	Bunbury	13th Dec., 1911	255	(2)	In practice, June, 1909.
493	JEANES, Charlotte Christina	Lockyer Avenue, West Northam	20th Dec., 1911	255	(2)	In practice, June, 1909.
410	JECKS, Martha	Guildford	13th Dec., 1911	255	(2)	In practice, June, 1909.
198	JEFFREY, Janet	Silas Street, East Fremantle	22nd Nov., 1911	255	(1)	Fremantle Midwifery Training School.
546	JENKINS, Mary Eleanor	Government Hospital, Menzies	29th Dec., 1911	255	(1)	Rotunda Hospital, Dublin; Central Midwives' Board, England.
859	JENSEN, Laura	Newton House, Narrogin	25th Oct., 1912	255	(2)	In practice, June, 1909.
881	JOHNS, Ellen	7 Porter Street, Kalgoorlie	22nd Nov., 1912	255	(2)	In practice, June, 1909.
796	JOHNSON, Margaret Isabella	Sunnymead, Bunbury	7th June, 1912	255	(2)	In practice, June, 1909.
728	JOHNSON, Ellen Maria	South Bunbury	16th Feb., 1912	255	(2)	In practice, June, 1909.
715	JOHNSON, Jane Susan Sophia	93 Bourke Street, Leederville	16th Feb., 1912	255	(2)	In practice, June, 1909.
446	JOHNSON, Mary	Mason Street, North Fremantle	13th Dec., 1911	255	(2)	In practice, June, 1909.
169	JOHNSTON, Caroline	Jaloran Road, Wagin	15th Nov., 1911	255	(2)	In practice, June, 1909.
346	JONES, Elizabeth	James Street, Guildford	8th Dec., 1911	255	(2)	In practice, June, 1909.
385	JONES, Elizabeth	Rosebery Avenue, South Perth	8th Dec., 1911	255	(2)	In practice, June, 1909.
764	JONES, Elizabeth Ann	Brown Hill	19th April, 1912	255	(2)	In practice, June, 1909.
43	JONES, Ellen	Medice Street, Collie	10th Oct., 1911	255	(2)	In practice, June, 1909.
14	JONES, Emma Lydia	St. Peter's Hospital, Wagin	27th Sept., 1911	255	(1)	Central Midwives' Board, England.
11	JONES, Josephine Elizabeth	Napier Street, Cottesloe	13th Sept., 1911	255	(2)	In practice, June, 1909.
822	JONES, Olive	64 Millen Street, Boulder	9th Aug., 1912	255	(2)	In practice, June, 1909.
566	JORDAN, Henrietta Janet	86 Edward Street, Perth	29th Dec., 1911	255	(2)	In practice, June, 1909.
621	KALMUND, Hulda	30 North Terrace, Boulder	29th Dec., 1911	255	(2)	In practice, June, 1909.
770	KAZEA, Jane	19 South Terrace, Fremantle	19th April, 1912	255	(2)	In practice, June, 1909.
660	KEANE, Margaret Theresa	194 Stirling Street, Perth	5th Jan., 1912	255	(2)	In practice, June, 1909.
26	KEARNS, Emily	Kalgoorlie	27th Sept., 1911	255	(2)	In practice, June, 1909.
760	KELLIHER, Bessie Bertha	Narrogin	19th April, 1912	255	(2)	In practice, June, 1909.
5	KELLY, Georgina	22 Victoria Road, Fremantle	13th Sept., 1911	255	(2)	In practice, June, 1909.
685	KELLY, May	10 Carlton Street, Leederville	26th Jan., 1912	255	(2)	In practice, June, 1909.
808	KENNEDY, Martha	38 Coolgardie Street, Subiaco	5th July, 1912	255	(2)	In practice, June, 1909.
404	KENNEY, Rosina	Gwalia	13th Dec., 1911	255	(2)	In practice, June, 1909.
860	KENNY, Clare	330 Rokeby Road, Subiaco	25th Oct., 1912	255	(2)	In practice, June, 1909.
726	KIDD, Margaret Jane	Goodenough Farm, Nannup	16th Feb., 1912	255	(2)	In practice, June, 1909.
674	KIDSON, Polly	Kia Ora, Gill Street, Cottesloe Beach	12th Jan., 1912	255	(2)	In practice, June, 1909.
692	KILMURRAY, Bridget	Dongarra	26th Jan., 1912	255	(2)	In practice, June, 1909.
638	KILPIN, Louisa	Bunstey, Toodyay	5th Jan., 1912	255	(2)	In practice, June, 1909.
643	KINANE, Hanore	2881 Federal Road, Kalgoorlie	5th Jan., 1912	255	(2)	In practice, June, 1909.
892	KING, Florence	Rathay Street, Victoria Park	20th Dec., 1912	255	(2)	In practice, June, 1909.
574	KING, Harriett	Maninga Marley	29th Dec., 1911	255	(2)	In practice, June, 1909.
769	KING, Mary Jane	Post Office, Boulder	26th Jan., 1912	255	(2)	In practice, June. 1909.
333	KINSELLA, Susan Gabriel	Albany	8th Dec., 1911	255	(2)	In practice, June, 1909.
159	KIRWOOD, Annie May	194 South Terrace, Fremantle	15th Nov., 1911	255	(1)	Fremantle Midwifery Training School.
307	KITOVITZ, Rosa	335 Murray Street, Perth	29th Nov., 1911	255	(2)	In practice, June, 1909.
893	KNAPP, Elizabeth Margaret	Mundijong	20th Dec., 1912	255	(2)	In practice, June. 1909.
502	KNIGHT, Clara	329 Rokeby Road, Subiaco	20th Dec., 1911	255	(2)	In practice, June, 1909.
111	KNIGHT, Margaret Williamson	Women's Home, Fremantle	8th Nov., 1911	255	(1)	Fremantle Midwifery Training School.
100	KNIGHT, Rose Elizabeth	11 Lake Street, Perth	25th Oct., 1911	255	(2)	In practice, June, 1909.
589	KNIGHTS, Lydia	2 Marquis Street, Perth	29th Dec., 1911	255	(2)	In practice, June, 1909.

Registration No.	Name.	Address.	Date of Registration.	Section of Act under which Registration was effected.	Qualification.
695	KROENERT, Matilda Clara Alma	17 Hyde Street, Perth	26th Jan., 1912	255 (2)	In practice, June, 1909.
669	LANG, Georgianna	Lady Lawley Cottage by the Sea, Cottesloe	5th Jan., 1912	255 (2)	In practice, June, 1909.
327	LARKIN, Mary	283 Hay Street, Subiaco	8th Dec., 1911	255 (1)	Women's Hospital, Sydney.
372	LARSON, Christina May	Plummer Street, Williamstown, Kalgoorlie	8th Dec., 1911	255 (2)	In practice, June, 1909.
230	LAWSON, Jane	44 Thelbert Street, South Fremantle	22nd Nov., 1911	255 (2)	In practice, June, 1909.
610	LEE, Sadie	"Tredega," First Avenue, Mount Lawley, Perth	29th Dec., 1912	255 (2)	In practice, June, 1909.
850	LEE, Sophy	"Kilkerran," Shenton Road, Claremont	5th Sept., 1912	255 (2)	In practice, June, 1909.
269	LEIGHTON, Fanny Matilda	43 York Street, Subiaco	29th Nov., 1911	255 (2)	In practice, June, 1909.
413	LENNON, Margaret	Dart Street, Boulder	13th Dec., 1911	255 (2)	In practice, June, 1909.
188	LEONARD, Frances Mary	Wellington Street, Northam	15th Nov., 1911	255 (2)	In practice, June, 1909.
47	LESLIE, Elizabeth	252 Stirling Street, Perth	10th Oct., 1911	255 (2)	In practice, June, 1909.
173	LETHLEAN, Eliza Annie	43 Thomas Street, South Fremantle	15th Nov., 1911	255 (2)	In practice, June, 1909.
682	LEWIN, Amy Kathleen	Goomalling	26th Jan., 1912	255 (2)	In practice, June, 1909.
213	LEWIS, Annie	45 Tower Street, Leederville	22nd Nov., 1911	255 (2)	In practice, June, 1909.
644	LEWIS, Emily Elizabeth	Maylands	5th Jan., 1912	255 (2)	In practice, June, 1909.
217	LEWIS, Emma	Greenbushes	22nd Nov., 1911	255 (2)	In practice, June, 1909.
696	LILLIS, Alice Mary Maud	Meekatharra	26th Jan., 1912	255 (2)	In practice, June, 1909.
569	LINDLEY, Florence Lucy	Pickering Brook	29th Dec., 1911	255 (2)	In practice, June, 1909.
321	LINNDEBERG, Anne	192 Newcastle Street, Perth	8th Dec., 1911	255 (1)	Women's Hospital, Melbourne.
861	LISLE, May St. Clair	1018 Hay Street, West Perth	25th Oct., 1912	255 (2)	In practice, June, 1909.
258	LISTER, Emma	Battle Street, Cottesloe Beach	29th Nov., 1911	255 (1)	Clapham Maternity Hospital, London; Central Mid-wives' Board, England.
208	LLOYD, Minnie	23 Coolgardie Street, Subiaco	22nd Nov., 1911	255 (2)	In practice, June, 1909.
782	LONG, Emma	Palmerston Street, Cottesloe Beach	17th May, 1912	255 (2)	In practice, June, 1909.
800	LONGMORE, Isabel	Peak Hill	7th June, 1912	255 (2)	In practice, June, 1909.
371	LOVELAND, Elizabeth Ann	Cottesloe	8th Dec., 1911	255 (2)	In practice, June, 1909.
123	LUDGATE, Augusta Mary	19 Florence Street, Fremantle	8th Nov., 1911	255 (2)	In practice, June, 1909.
639	LUKEIS, Alice Louisa	Pingelly	5th Jan., 1912	255 (2)	In practice, June, 1909.
260	LUNNY, Bidget Agnes	70 Richmond Street, Leederville	29th Nov., 1911	255 (2)	In practice, June, 1909.
467	LUTH, Florence Vera	5 Bateman Street, Fremantle	20th Dec., 1911	255 (2)	In practice, June, 1909.
303	LYFORD, Charlotte Isabel	25 Olive Street, Subiaco	29th Nov., 1911	255 (2)	In practice, June, 1909.
798	LYNCH, Mary	194 Stirling Street, Perth	7th June, 1912	255 (2)	In practice, June, 1909.
305	MACAULAY, Susan Elizabeth	Collie	29th Nov., 1911	255 (2)	In practice, June, 1909.
689	MACKAY, Margaret	6 Cheriton Street, East Perth	26th Jan., 1912	255 (2)	In practice, June, 1909.
165	MACKIE, Ethel Jane	Clifford Street, York	15th Nov., 1911	255 (1)	Women's Hospital, Sydney.
466	MACLAGAN, Margaret Doris Beatrice	Chatsworth Terrace, Claremont	20th Dec., 1911	255 (2)	In practice, June, 1909.
407	MAIN, Margaret Annie	21 Outram Street, Perth	13th Dec., 1911	255 (2)	In practice, June, 1909.
25	MALE, Eleanor	Rockton Road, Claremont	27th Sept., 1911	255 (2)	In practice, June, 1909.
677	MALEY, Clara Mary	Government Road, Leederville	12th Jan., 1912	255 (2)	In practice, June, 1909.
619	MALONE, Maria	Rocky Bay, North Fremantle	29th Dec., 1911	255 (2)	In practice, June, 1909.
73	MALONEY, Annie	St. Cuthbert's Hospital, Northam	25th Oct., 1911	255 (1)	Royal Hospital for Women, Sydney.
231	MALTMAN, Sarah	110A Davis Street, Boulder	22nd Nov., 1911	255 (2)	In practice, June, 1909.

53	MANNING, Elvina	173 Carr Street, Perth	10th Oct., 1911	255 (2)	In practice, June, 1909.
835	MARKS, Mary Ann	7 Price Street, Fremantle	9th Aug., 1912	255 (2)	In practice, June, 1909.
226	MARSHALL, Ellen	Beach Road, South Bunbury	22nd Nov., 1911	255 (2)	In practice, June, 1909.
364	MARSHALL, Florence Maud	42 Vivian Street, Boulder	8th Dec., 1911	255 (2)	In practice, June, 1909.
254	MARSHALL, Jane Anne	Grosvenor Hospital, Fremantle	29th Nov., 1911	255 (1)	Fremantle Midwifery Training School.
124	MARSLAND, Charlotte Cameron	236 Rokeby Road, Subiaco	8th Nov., 1911	255 (2)	In practice, June, 1909.
863	MARTENS, Hannorah	Narrogin	25th Oct., 1912	255 (2)	In practice, June, 1909.
86	MARTIN, Annie	Elvira Street, Midland Junction	25th Oct., 1911	255 (2)	In practice, June, 1909.
463	MARTIN, Eliza Jane	Boulder	20th Dec., 1911	255 (2)	In practice, June, 1909.
474	MARTIN, Marion	Ravensthorpe	20th Dec., 1911	255 (2)	In practice, June, 1909.
138	MARTIN, Rose Alice	1038 Hay Street, Perth	8th Nov., 1911	255 (2)	In practice, June, 1909.
125	MASLIN, Elizabeth Janet	Bridgetown	8th Nov., 1911	255 (2)	In practice, June, 1909.
29	MASON, Elizabeth	Gresham Street, Victoria Park	27th Sept., 1911	255 (2)	In practice, June, 1909.
277	MAYS, Isabella	65 Johnston Street, Boulder	29th Nov., 1911	255 (2)	In practice, June, 1909.
58	McALINDEN, Alice Harriett	Hampton Street, Bridgetown	10th Oct., 1911	255 (2)	In practice, June, 1909.
259	McARTHUR, Marie	18 Clifton Street, Highgate Hill, Perth	29th Nov., 1911	255 (1)	Rotunda Hospital, Dublin.
828	McAULAY, Margaret	3 Marquis Street, Perth	9th Aug., 1912	255 (2)	In practice, June, 1909.
862	McCALLUM, Bessie	Hospital for the Insane, Claremont	25th Oct., 1912	255 (2)	In practice, June, 1909.
807	McCORMICK, Sophia Lillian Floyd	351 Lord Street, Perth	5th July, 1912	255 (2)	In practice, June, 1909.
367	McCROREY, Elizabeth Margaret	Nanga Brook	8th Dec., 1911	255 (2)	In practice, June, 1909.
626	McCUTCHEON, Grace	194 Stirling Street, Perth	29th Dec., 1911	255 (1)	Women's Hospital, Melbourne.
442	McDONALD, Elizabeth Marion	Forrest Street, Northam	13th Dec., 1911	255 (2)	In practice, June, 1909.
793	McDONALD, Flora	Frank Street, Boulder City	7th June, 1912	255 (2)	In practice, June, 1909.
139	McDONNELL, Maria	Beverley	8th Nov., 1911	255 (2)	In practice, June, 1909.
235	McDONOUGH, Catherine	237 Mueller Road, Subiaco	22nd Nov., 1911	255 (2)	In practice, June, 1909.
702	McGLADE, Elizabeth	Perth Road, Albany	26th Jan., 1912	255 (2)	In practice, June, 1909.
28	McGOWAN, Clara	316 Piccadilly Street, Kalgoorlie	27th Sept., 1911	255 (2)	In practice, June, 1909.
349	McGUCKIN, Helena	Bourke Street, Leederville	8th Dec., 1911	255 (2)	In practice, June, 1909.
528	McINNES, Amy	Bunbury	29th Dec., 1911	255 (1)	Fremantle Midwifery Training School.
598	McINTOSH, Minnie	Albany Road, Cannington	29th Dec., 1911	255 (2)	In practice, June, 1909.
200	McKAY, Amy Agnes	Northam	22nd Nov., 1911	255 (2)	In practice, June, 1909.
153	McKAY, Isabella	Cavendish Street, Perth	8th Nov., 1911	255 (2)	In practice, June, 1909.
755	McKENNAY, Helen	Brookside, Toodyay	19th April, 1912	255 (2)	In practice, June, 1909.
527	McKENZIE, Amelia Jane	21 Burt Street, Fremantle	29th Dec., 1911	255 (1)	Fremantle Midwifery Training School.
821	McKENZIE, Gwen	Lot 273, Hoover Street, Leonora	9th Aug., 1912	255 (2)	In practice, June, 1909.
237	McKINNEY, Elizabeth Ann	Parkerville	22nd Nov., 1911	255 (2)	In practice, June, 1909.
814	McLACHLAN, Annie Adelaide	Nanga Brook Mill, *via* Yarloop	9th Aug., 1912	255 (2)	In practice, June, 1909.
76	McLAREN, Emma	Cannington	25th Oct., 1911	255 (2)	In practice, June, 1909.
263	McLEAN, Eugene Eve	93 Railway Cottage, Broad Arrow	29th Nov., 1911	255 (2)	In practice, June, 1909.
894	McLEAN, Robina	1 Dart Street, Boulder	20th Dec., 1912	255 (2)	In practice, June, 1909.
826	McLERNON, Malvena Helena	Youanmi	9th Aug., 1912	255 (2)	In practice, June, 1909.
75	McMILLAN, Emma	33 Oxford Street, Leederville	25th Oct., 1911	255 (2)	In practice, June, 1909.
264	McMORRAN, Elizabeth	34 Charles Street, North Perth	29th Nov., 1911	255 (2)	In practice, June, 1909.
465	McMURRAY, Catherine	126 Grosvenor Road, North Perth	20th Dec., 1911	255 (2)	In practice, June, 1909.
337	McNABB, Julia	70 Davis Street, Boulder	8th Dec., 1911	255 (2)	In practice, June, 1909.
671	McNAMARA, Ellen May	Adelaide Terrace, Perth	12th Jan., 1912	255 (2)	In practice, June, 1909.
616	McNAMARA, Mary Ann	Moora	29th Dec., 1911	255 (2)	In practice, June, 1909.
319	McNERNEY, Margaret Hannah	22 King Street, Boulder	29th Nov., 1911	255 (2)	In practice, June, 1909.
424	McROHAN, Mary Ann	Duke Street, Subiaco	13th Dec., 1911	255 (2)	In practice, June, 1909.
730	McWHINNEY, May Alice	Gardener Street, Mount Lawley	16th Feb., 1912	255 (2)	In practice, June, 1909.
376	MEDLYN, Sarah	396 Beaufort Street, Perth	8th Dec., 1911	255 (2)	In practice, June, 1909.

Registration No.	Name.	Address.	Date of Registration.	Section of Act under which Registration was effected.	Qualification.
504	MENZIES, Grace	Yillimining, East Narrogin	20th Dec., 1911	255 (2)	In practice, June, 1909.
89	METTAM, Hannah	Kirkham Hill Terrace, Maylands	25th Oct., 1911	255 (2)	In practice, June, 1909.
212	MILES, Maggie Grace	173 Bourke Street, Kalgoorlie	22nd Nov., 1911	255 (2)	In practice, June, 1909.
363	MILES, Sarah Ann	517 Hannan Street, Kalgoorlie	8th Dec., 1911	255 (2)	In practice, June, 1909.
536	MILLEDGE, Mabel	194 Stirling Street, Perth	29th Dec., 1911	255 (1)	Women's Hospital, Melbourne.
526	MILLEN, Lydia	Kelmscott	29th Dec., 1911	255 (1)	Fremantle Midwifery Training School.
615	MILLER, Catherine Rachel	17 Stanmore Street, West Subiaco	29th Dec., 1911	255 (2)	In practice, June, 1909.
440	MILLS, Hannah	93 Bagot Road, Subiaco	13th Dec., 1911	255 (2)	In practice, June, 1909.
268	MILLWARD, Elizabeth	Brown Hill, Boulder	29th Nov., 1911	255 (2)	In practice, June, 1909.
777	MITCHELL, Alice	Hospital for the Insane, Claremont	17th May, 1912	255 (2)	In practice, June, 1909.
203	MITCHELL, Mary Catherine	Boulder	22nd Nov. 1911	255 (2)	In practice, June, 1909.
650	MOLAN, Emily	Nannine	5th Jan., 1912	255 (2)	In practice, June, 1909.
284	MOLISON-SMITH, Gertrude Ellen	Pennell Road, Claremont	29th Nov., 1911	255 (2)	In practice, June, 1909.
93	MOONEY, Bertha	7 Outridge Terrace, Kalgoorlie	25th Oct., 1911	255 (2)	In practice, June, 1909.
717	MOORE, Adeline	Grosvenor Hospital, Fremantle	16th Feb., 1912	261 (1)	Central Midwives' Board, England.
326	MOORE, Alice Forsyth	"Kareenya," St. George's Terrace, Perth	8th Dec., 1911	255 (1)	Women's Hospital, Melbourne.
718	MORESBY, Janet Caroline	Wongan	16th Feb., 1912	261 (1)	Central Midwives' Board England.
3	MORGAN, Charlotte	21 Jenkin Street, Fremantle	13th Sept., 1911	255 (1)	Fremantle Midwifery Training School.
170	MORGAN, Lucy Emma	William Street, North Perth	15th Nov., 1911	255 (2)	In practice, June, 1909.
241	MORLOCK, Alice Mary	Stirling Street, Perth	22nd Nov., 1911	255 (2)	In practice, June, 1909.
308	MORRIS, Gertrude Laura	11 Pirie Street, Boulder	29th Nov., 1911	255 (2)	In practice, June, 1909.
97	MORRIS, Sarah Ann	Crateris Street, Southern Cross	25th Oct., 1911	255 (2)	In practice, June, 1909.
403	MORRISON, Alice Catherine	"Royston," Elizabeth Terrace, Fremantle	13th Dec., 1911	255 (1)	Fremantle Midwifery Training School.
588	MORRISON, Jane Fothergill	Geraldton	29th Dec., 1911	255 (2)	In practice, June, 1909.
347	MOSLEY, Norah	Midland Junction	8th Dec., 1911	255 (2)	In practice, June, 1909.
285	MOTTERAM, Elizabeth	Dunbar Road, Claremont	29th Nov., 1911	255 (2)	In practice, June, 1909.
708	MUIR, Catherine	Menzies	26th Jan., 1912	255 (2)	In practice, June, 1909.
705	MUIR, Margaret	Southern Cross	26th Jan., 1912	255 (2)	In practice, June, 1909.
36	MULDER, Mary	191 Collins Street, Kalgoorlie	27th Sept., 1911	255 (2)	In practice, June, 1909.
359	MULLERY, Margaret	Newcastle Street, Perth	8th Dec., 1911	255 (2)	In practice, June, 1909.
784	MUNDAY, Miriam Grace	Marradong	17th May, 1912	255 (2)	In practice, June, 1909.
443	MURPHY, Elizabeth	Chidlow Street, Northam	13th Dec., 1911	255 (2)	In practice, June, 1909.
722	MURPHY, Sarah Jane	Doodennaning, *via* Green Hills	16th Feb., 1912	255 (2)	In practice, June, 1909.
816	MURRAY, Sarah Anne	32 Lacey Street, Perth	9th Aug., 1912	255 (2)	In practice, June, 1909.
611	NEEDLE, Mary Ann	Thompson Road, North Fremantle	29th Dec., 1911	255 (2)	In practice, June, 1909.
804	NELSON, Mary Jane	Vasse Road, South Bunbury	5th July, 1912	255 (2)	In practice, June, 1909.
117	NESS, Elizabeth Ann	Narrogin	8th Nov., 1911	255 (2)	In practice, June, 1909.
754	NEVE, Frances Swan	Niagara Road, Menzies	19th April, 1912	255 (2)	In practice, June, 1909.
461	NICHOLLS, Annie	67 King Street, Boulder	20th Dec., 1911	255 (2)	In practice, June, 1909.
309	NICHOLLS, Isabella	52 James Street, Fremantle	29th Nov., 1911	255 (2)	In practice, June, 1909.
179	NICKOLL, Elizabeth Harriet	Jarrahdale	15th Nov., 1911	255 (2)	In practice, June, 1909.
336	NILSSON, Eliza	Duke Street, Northam	8th Dec., 1911	255 (2)	In practice, June, 1909.
773	NORTHEY, Caroline	Boulder	17th May, 1912	255 (2)	In practice, June, 1909.
531	NYE, Eliza Constance	Cottesloe Beach	29th Dec., 1911	255 (1)	Fremantle Midwifery Training School.

794	OAKLANDS, Mary Anne	Norseman	7th June, 1912	255 (2)	In practice, June, 1909.
324	O'BRIEN, Mary Mildred	"Clareen," Coghlan Road, Subiaco	8th Dec., 1911	255 (1)	Rotunda Hospital, Dublin.
642	O'CALLAGHAN, Mary	Trained Nurses' Home, 194 Stirling Street, Perth	5th Jan., 1912	255 (2)	In practice, June, 1909.
356	O'CONNOR, Eliza	Dongarra	8th Dec., 1911	255 (2)	In practice, June, 1909.
699	O'CONNOR, Margaret	Hoffman Mill, Yarloop	26th Jan., 1912	255 (2)	In practice, June, 1909.
387	O'DEA, Margaret Ellen	Greenough Road, Geraldton	8th Dec., 1911	255 (2)	In practice, June, 1909.
15	O'FARRELL, Elizabeth	Private Hospital, Amherst Road, Midland Junction	27th Sept., 1911	255 (1)	Coombe Hospital, Dublin.
1	O'GRADY, Mary	Fremantle	13th Sept., 1911	255 (1)	Fremantle Midwifery Training School.
415	OLDHAM, Frances Maud	65 Hill Street, Perth	13th Dec., 1911	255 (2)	In practice, June, 1909.
106	OLDHAM, Mary Ellen	4 Canning Road, East Fremantle	8th Nov., 1911	255 (1)	Fremantle Midwifery Training School.
487	OLIVER, Elizabeth Lucy	Lukin Street, Beverley	20th Dec., 1911	255 (2)	In practice, June, 1909.
432	O'LOUGHLIN, Harriet Rachel	4 Davis Street, Boulder	13th Dec., 1911	255 (2)	In practice, June, 1909.
594	O'NEILL, Agnes Frances	1276 Hare Street, Kalgoorlie	29th Dec., 1911	255 (2)	In practice, June, 1909.
733	O'NEILL, Emily Gertrude	65 Hill Street, Perth	15th Mar., 1912	255 (2)	In practice, June, 1909.
780	O'NEILL, Mary Jane	Dardanup	17th May, 1912	255 (2)	In practice, June, 1909.
680	ORR, Maud Herrington	Greenbushes	12th Jan., 1912	255 (2)	In practice, June, 1909.
516	OSMOND, Marry Ellen	Mount Magnet	20th Dec., 1911	255 (2)	In practice, June, 1909.
675	OWENS, Ellen	116 Victoria Road, Fremantle	12th Jan., 1912	255 (2)	In practice, June, 1909.
215	PALMER, Elizabeth	208 Bagot Road, Subiaco	22nd Nov., 1911	255 (2)	In practice, June, 1909.
788	PARKER, Annie	Nita Vale, West Pingelly	17th May, 1912	255 (2)	In practice, June, 1909.
593	PARKER, Christina	Sandstone	29th Dec., 1911	255 (2)	In practice, June, 1909.
441	PARKER, Elizabeth	Caledonian Avenue, Maylands	13th Dec., 1911	255 (2)	In practice, June, 1909.
181	PARRY, Amelia Louisa	6 Moir Street, Perth	15th Nov. 1911	255 (2)	In practice, June, 1909.
701	PARSONS, Margaret Ann	115 Hubble Street, East Fremantle	26th Jan., 1912	255 (2)	In practice, June, 1909.
68	PATTERSON, Annie	Norseman	10th Oct., 1911	255 (2)	In practice, June, 1909.
693	PATTIESON, Henrietta C. F.	The Crescent, Midland Junction	26th Jan., 1912	255 (2)	In practice, June, 1909.
698	PAUL, Annetta	Eliot Street, Bunbury	26th Jan., 1912	255 (2)	In practice, June, 1909.
414	PAYNTER, Agnes Annie	Beverley	13th Dec., 1911	255 (2)	In practice, June, 1909.
189	PEACOCK, Susan	Cranbrook	15th Nov., 1911	255 (2)	In practice, June, 1909.
829	PEAKE, Jane	Northam (East)	9th Aug., 1912	255 (2)	In practice, June, 1909.
174	PEARSON, Annie	No. 6 Mill, Jarrahdale	15th Nov., 1911	255 (2)	In practice, June, 1909.
654	PEARSON, Barbara	Brown Hill	5th Jan., 1912	255 (2)	In practice, June, 1909.
618	PEAT, Jessie	192 Burt Street, Boulder	29th Dec., 1911	255 (2)	In practice, June, 1909.
563	PENDREIGH, Hannah	Laverton	29th Dec., 1911	255 (2)	In practice, June, 1909.
152	PENGLASE, Mary Ann	King Street, Coolgardie	8th Nov., 1911	255 (2)	In practice, June, 1909.
62	PENNY, Jenny	Pingelly	10th Oct., 1911	255 (2)	In practice, June, 1909.
233	PERKINS, Gertrude Maria	Leonora	22nd Nov., 1911	255 (2)	In practice, June, 1909.
587	PERRY, Catherine	Tammin	29th Dec., 1911	255 (2)	In practice, June, 1909.
544	PERRY, Isabella	Mt. Magnet	29th Dec., 1911	255 (1)	Women's Hospital, Melbourne.
300	PETERS, Ellen	Northam	29th Nov., 1911	255 (2)	In practice, June, 1909.
175	PETERSON, Emily	Horgan Street, Cottesloe Beach	15th Nov., 1911	255 (2)	In practice, June, 1909.
243	PETTERSON, Kate Louisa	Sandstone	22nd Nov., 1911	255 (2)	In practice, June, 1909.
507	PHILLIPS, Margaret	Sandstone	20th Dec., 1911	255 (2)	In practice, June, 1909.
602	PHILLIPS, Mary Louisa	Wilga	29th Dec., 1911	255 (2)	In practice, June, 1909.
747	PHILLIPS, Miriam	222 Egan Street, Kalgoorlie	15th Mar., 1912	255 (2)	In practice, June, 1909.
771	PHILLIPSON, Sarah Ann	25 Vincent Street, Leederville	19th April, 1912	255 (2)	In practice, June, 1909.
266	PHIN, William Jane	Montreal Road, Midland Junction	29th Nov., 1911	255 (2)	In practice, June, 1909.
721	PICKERING, Mary	Perth Street, Subiaco	16th Feb., 1912	255 (2)	In practice, June, 1909.
249	PLAYLE, Rose	Williams	22nd Nov., 1911	255 (2)	In practice, June, 1909.
559	PLEDGE, Elizabeth	"Brockhurst," Katanning	29th Dec., 1911	255 (2)	In practice, June, 1909.
70	PLUMMER, Lillian Susan	106 Charles Street, Perth	10th Oct., 1911	255 (2)	In practice, June, 1909.

Registration No.	Name.	Address.	Date of Registration.	Section of Act under which Registration was effected.	Qualification.
236	PODGER, Grace	Kelmscott	22nd Nov., 1911	255 (2)	In practice, June, 1909.
239	POLA, Mary	Day Dawn	22nd Nov., 1911	255 (2)	In practice, June, 1909.
423	POOLE, Jane	42A Moran Street, Boulder	13th Dec., 1911	255 (2)	In practice, June, 1909.
55	PORTER, Margaret	Amherst Street, Fremantle	10th Oct., 1911	255 (2)	In practice, June, 1909.
668	PORTER, May	1192 Charles Street, Kalgoorlie	5th Jan., 1912	255 (2)	In practice, June, 1909.
532	POTTER, Eleanor Annie	132 Lyall Street, Kalgoorlie	29th Dec., 1911	255 (1)	Women's Hospital, Melbourne.
801	POTTS, Emma	Grass Valley Farm, Pingelly	7th June, 1912	255 (2)	In practice, June, 1909.
85	POWELL, Ellen	Orchard Street, Albany	25th Oct., 1911	255 (2)	In practice, June, 1909.
267	PRESCOTT, Emily Jane	Henry Street, Cannington	29th Nov,. 1911	255 (2)	In practice, June, 1909.
30	QUARTERMAINE, Fanny Alice	Katanning	27th Sept., 1911	255 (2)	In practice, June, 1909.
229	QUIGLEY, Catherine	430 Newcastle Street, Perth	22nd Nov., 1911	255 (2)	In practice, June, 1909.
895	QUINN, Ada	Gwalia	20th Dec., 1912	255 (2)	In practice, June, 1909.
522	QUINN, Mary	May Avenue, Subiaco	20th Dec., 1911	255 (2)	In practice, June, 1909.
805	RAISON, Emily	129 Bulwer Street, Perth	5th July, 1912	255 (2)	In practice, June, 1909.
116	RANFORD, Sarah Agnes	Goomalling	8th Nov., 1911	255 (1)	City of London Lying-in Hospital; Central Midwives' Board, England.
33	RAUCH, Annie Marie	203 Barker Road Subiaco	27th Sept., 1911	255 (2)	In practice, June, 1909.
147	RAYMOND, Charlotte	47 Charles Street, Perth	8th Nov., 1911	255 (2)	In practice, June, 1909.
355	RAYNOR, Isabella	C/c Mrs. R. McRae, West Northam	8th Dec., 1911	255 (2)	In practice, June, 1909.
552	READ, Mary Ellen	54 Nicholson Road, Subiaco	29th Dec., 1911	255 (2)	In practice, June, 1909.
49	READER, Florence Emaline	22 Francis Street, Subiaco	10th Oct., 1911	255 (2)	In practice, June, 1909.
388	REED, Margaret Jane	Armadale	8th Dec., 1911	255 (2)	In practice, June, 1909.
707	REGAN, Hannah	Sandford Street, Geraldton	26th Jan., 1912	255 (2)	In practice, June, 1909.
882	RENNIE, Rachel	Watson Street, Mt. Magnet	22nd Nov., 1912	255 (2)	In practice, June, 1909.
469	REYNOLDS, Susanna	420 William Street, Perth	20th Dec., 1911	255 (2)	In practice, June, 1909.
354	RICHARDS, Edith Ellen	89 Chelmsford Road, North Perth	8th Dec., 1911	255 (2)	In practice, June, 1909.
706	RICHARDS, Elesa	Menzies	26th Jan., 1912	255 (2)	In practice, June, 1909.
679	RICHARDS, Eliza	Busselton	12th Jan., 1912	255 (2)	In practice, June, 1909.
219	RICHARDS, Martha	25 Dwyer Street, Boulder	22nd Nov., 1911	255 (2)	In practice, June, 1909.
647	RICHARDSON, Cicely Margaret	Lyall's Mills, Collie	5th Jan., 1912	255 (2)	In practice, June, 1909.
373	RICHARDSON, Jean Thomson	45 Outram Street, Perth	8th Dec., 1911	255 (2)	In practice, June, 1909.
191	RIDDELL, Alice Jane	Elewes Street, Geraldton	15th Nov., 1911	255 (2)	In practice, June, 1909.
416	RIX, Ethel Grace	66 Rupert Street, Subiaco	13th Dec., 1911	255 (2)	In practice, June, 1909.
61	ROATCH, Esther	Hill Street, Albany	10th Oct., 1911	255 (2)	In practice, June, 1909.
184	ROBERTS, Ann	Boulder	15th Nov., 1911	255 (2)	In practice, June, 1909.
540	ROBERTSON, Elizabeth Ann	Meekatharra	29th Dec., 1911	255 (1)	Women's Hospital, Melbourne.
547	ROBERTSON, Isabella	Comet Vale	29th Dec., 1911	255 (1)	Women's Hospital, Melbourne.
864	ROBOTTOM, Mary Annie	17 Hay Street, Subiaco	25th Oct., 1912	255 (2)	In practice, June, 1909.
278	RODDA, Catherine Morcom	119 Clancy Street, Boulder	29th Nov., 1911	255 (2)	In practice, June, 1909.
345	RODGERS, Elizabeth	Bunbury	8th Dec., 1911	255 (2)	In practice, June, 1909.
781	ROSS, Namoi Souter	C/o Nurse Loveland, Perth Street, Cottesloe	17th May, 1912	255 (2)	In practice, June, 1909.
209	ROSSER, Mary	Kalgoorlie	22nd Nov., 1911	255 (2)	In practice, June, 1909.
560	ROUTLEDGE, Flore[illegible]	C/o A. Francis, Kalgoorlie	29th Dec., 1911	255 (2)	In practice, June, 1909.

585	ROWE, Grace	James Street, Guildford	29th Dec., 1911	255 (2)	In practice, June, 1909.
571	RUDD. Alice	Duke Street, Northam	29th Dec., 1911	255 (2)	In practice, June, 1909.
578	RULE, Elizabeth	127 Fitzgerald Street, Perth	29th Dec., 1911	255 (2)	In practice, June, 1909.
275	RULE, Frances	62 Thomson Street, Boulder	29th Nov., 1911	255 (2)	In practice, June, 1909.
713	RUMBELLOW, Emily	Park Street, Subiaco	16th Feb., 1912	255 (2)	In practice, June, 1909.
712	RUSSELL, Emily Clara	144 Collins Street, Kalgoorlie	16th Feb., 1912	255 (2)	In practice, June, 1909.
280	RUST, Kate	123 Wellington Street, East Perth	29th Nov., 1911	255 (2)	In practice, June, 1909.
323	RYAN, Grace Josephine	Home of Peace, Subiaco	8th Dec., 1911	255 (1)	St. Margaret's Hospital, Sydney.
66	RYAN, Helena	9 Robinson Street, Subiaco	10th Oct., 1911	255 (2)	In practice, June, 1909.
455	RYAN, Josephine Mary	Public Hospital Malcolm	20th Dec., 1911	255 (1)	St. Margaret's Hospital, Sydney.
431	RYAN, Mary Jane	194 Vivian Street, Boulder	13th Dec., 1911	255 (2)	In practice, June, 1909.
452	RYDER, Louise	Pingelly	20th Dec., 1911	255 (1)	Central Midwives' Board, England.
635	RYRIE, Helen Blanche	Hillside, Benger, near Bunbury	30th Dec., 1911	255 (1)	Royal Hospital for Women, Sydney.
144	SALMON, Margaret Ann	Laverton	8th Nov., 1911	255 (2)	In practice, June, 1909.
193	SAMPSON, Anne Sarah Standfield	Kellerberrin	22nd Nov., 1911	255 (1)	London Obstetrical Society.
172	SANDS, Fanny Mercy	Surbiton Road, Victoria Park	15th Nov., 1911	255 (2)	In practice, June, 1909.
776	SAUNDERS, Phœbe Jean	South Bunbury	17th May, 1912	255 (2)	In practice, June, 1909.
637	SCALLY, Winifred	North Toodyay	5th Jan., 1912	255 (2)	In practice, June, 1909.
148	SCARFE, Clara Gertrude	88 John Street, Perth	8th Nov., 1911	255 (2)	In practice, June, 1909.
841	SCARFFE, Margaret Ann	"Birkdale," Hill Street, Fremantle	9th Aug., 1912	261 (1)	Central Midwives' Board, England.
716	SCOTT, Annie DeWitt	Northam	16th Feb., 1912	261 (1)	Alexandra Hospital, Hobart, Tasmania; **The Midwifery** Nurses' Act, 1901, Tasmania.
495	SCOTT, Elizabeth Harriet	Worsley	20th Dec., 1911	255 (2)	In practice, June, 1909.
472	SCOTT, Esther Jane	Boyanup	20th Dec., 1911	255 (2)	In practice, June, 1909.
57	SCOTT, Matilda	Otway Street, Claremont	10th Oct., 1911	255 (2)	In practice, June, 1909.
9	SCRIVENER, Eliza Ann	Gosnells	13th Sept., 1911	255 (2)	In practice, June, 1909.
444	SEABORN, Agnes	Trafalgar	13th Dec., 1911	255 (2)	In practice, June, 1909.
625	SEARL, Mary	Cargill Street, Victoria Park	29th Dec., 1911	255 (1)	Women's Hospital, Melbourne.
659	SEARLE, Annie	Garden Road, Geraldton	5th Jan., 1912	255 (2)	In practice, June, 1909.
257	SEARLES, Jean	"Anatoli," Brookman Street, Kalgoorlie	29th Nov., 1911	255 (1)	Royal Hospital for Women, Sydney.
105	SEFTON, Annie	246 Adelaide Terrace, Perth	8th Nov., 1911	255 (1)	Fremantle Midwifery Training School.
758	SELLIN, Ada	Rae Street, Leederville	19th April, 1912	255 (2)	In practice, June, 1909.
617	SHADDICK, Caroline	Mourambine	29th Dec., 1911	255 (2)	In practice, June, 1909.
832	SHARP, Jane Elizabeth	Wharf Street, Queen's Park	9th Aug., 1912	255 (2)	In practice, June, 1909.
792	SHARPE, Annie	McMillan Street, Victoria Park	7th June, 1912	255 (2)	In practice, June, 1909.
71	SHARPE, Frances Mary	281 Hamersley Road, Subiaco	10th Oct., 1911	255 (2)	In practice, June, 1909.
686	SHAW, Isabella	21 Derby Street, Leederville	26th Jan., 1912	255 (2)	In practice, June, 1909.
482	SHEEDY, Annie Jane	142 Alexander Road, South Fremantle	20th Dec., 1911	255 (2)	In practice, June, 1909.
484	SHELDON, Mary Ann	73 Dugan Street, Kalgoorlie	20th Dec., 1911	255 (2)	In practice, June, 1909.
406	SHIELDS, Florence Grace Goodall	Katanning	13th Dec., 1911	255 (1)	Women's Hospital, Melbourne.
405	SHIELDS, Margaret Evangeline	65 Hill Street, Perth	13th Dec., 1911	255 (1)	Women's Hospital, Melbourne.
790	SHORT, Susannah	24 Brookman Street, Perth	7th June, 1912	255 (2)	In practice, June, 1909.
103	SIEKMANN, Franziska Brinkworth	St. Cuthbert's Hospital, Northam	8th Nov., 1911	255 (1)	Queen's Home, Adelaide, South Australia.
434	SIEMONEIT, Anna	Edmund Street, Beaconsfield, Fremantle	13th Dec., 1911	255 (2)	In practice, June, 1909.
512	SIEVERS, Christina	Public Hospital, Nannine	20th Dec., 1911	255 (2)	In practice, June, 1909.
883	SIMCOCK, Isabel	Heidelberg, Darling Range	22nd Nov., 1912	255 (2)	In practice, June, 1909.
38	SIMMONS, Annie Palmer	Macdonald Street, Kalgoorlie	27th Sept., 1911	255 (2)	In practice, June, 1909.
541	SINCLAIR, Georgina	136 Chelmsford Road, North Perth	29th Dec., 1911	255 (1)	Central Midwives' Board, England.
562	SINCLAIR, Julia	Esperance	29th Dec., 1911	255 (2)	In practice, June, 1909.
658	SINCOCK, Isabella	Johnstone Street, Boulder	5th Jan., 1912	255 (2)	In practice, June, 1909.
195	SING, Louisa Emilie	"Ingleside," Walter Street, Claremont	22nd Nov., 1911	255 (1)	Central Midwives' Board, England.

Registration No.	Name.	Address.	Date of Registration.	Section of Act under which Registration was effected.	Qualification.
592	SIZER, Emma	Hainault Lease, Boulder	29th Dec., 1911	255 (2)	In practice, June, 1909.
317	SKENE, Mary	91 Jewell Street, Perth	29th Nov., 1911	255 (2)	In practice, June, 1909.
201	SKINNER, Elizabeth Maud	Federal Street, Narrogin	22nd Nov., 1911	255 (2)	In practice, June, 1909.
27	SKINNER, Jane Wilson	169 Charles Street, Perth	27th Sept., 1911	255 (2)	In practice, June, 1909.
194	SKINNER, Mary Louisa	Maternity Nursing Association, London, S.E.	22nd Nov., 1911	255 (1)	Central Midwives' Board, England.
114	SKOGLUND, Mary Amelie	50 Victoria Road, Fremantle	8th Nov., 1911	255 (1)	Queen's Home, Adelaide.
118	SLATER, Mary Eliza	37 Brewer Street, Perth	8th Nov., 1911	255 (2)	In practice, June, 1909.
186	SLATTERY, Teresa Anne	Holmesdale Road, West Midland	15th Nov., 1911	255 (2)	In practice, June, 1909.
823	SMALES, Sarah Frances	Pinjarra	9th Aug., 1912	255 (2)	In practice, June, 1909.
633	SMITH, Amelia Anne	John Street, North Fremantle	29th Dec., 1911	255 (2)	In practice, June, 1909.
896	SMITH, Amelia Victoria	Dangin	20th Dec., 1912	255 (2)	In practice, June, 1909.
498	SMITH, Annie Maria	Wellington Mills	20th Dec., 1911	255 (2)	In practice, June, 1909.
91	SMITH, Barbara	123 York Street, Subiaco	25th Oct., 1911	255 (2)	In practice, June, 1909.
851	SMITH, Bridget	17 Padbury Street, East Perth	5th Sept., 1912	255 (2)	In practice, June, 1909.
221	SMITH, Charlotte	York	22nd Nov., 1911	255 (2)	In practice, June, 1909.
665	SMITH, Eliza	Bridgetown	5th Jan., 1912	255 (2)	In practice, June, 1909.
604	SMITH, Elizabeth	Hayes Street, Kookynie	29th Dec., 1911	255 (2)	In practice, June, 1909.
843	SMITH, Elizabeth	23 Mile Camp, Dwellingup	5th Sept., 1912	255 (2)	In practice, June, 1909.
135	SMITH, Ellen	Yarloop	8th Nov. 1911	255 (2)	In practice, June, 1909.
98	SMITH, Emma	329 Hay Street, Kalgoorlie	25th Oct., 1911	255 (2)	In practice, June, 1909.
813	SMITH, Emma	Cue Hill, Cue	5th July, 1912	255 (2)	In practice, June, 1909.
119	SMITH, Emma Charity	First Avenue, Greylands, Claremont	8th Nov., 1911	255 (2)	In practice, June, 1909.
19	SMITH, Emma Elizabeth	564 Beaufort Street, Mount Lawley, Perth	27th Sept., 1911	255 (2)	In practice, June, 1909.
39	SMITH, Eveleen Maud Hayes	252 Barker Road, Subiaco	10th Oct., 1911	255 (1)	Central Midwives' Board, England.
817	SMITH, Margaret	Southern River, Gosnells	9th Aug., 1912	255 (2)	In practice, June, 1909.
265	SMITH, Maria	York	29th Nov., 1911	255 (2)	In practice, June, 1909.
655	SMITH, Maria	Morrell Street, West Northam	5th Jan., 1912	255 (2)	In practice, June, 1909.
736	SMITH, Marjory	Cue	15th Mar., 1912	255 (2)	In practice, June, 1909.
10	SMITH, Mary Ann	Francis Street, Geraldton	15th Sept., 1911	255 (2)	In practice, June, 1909.
180	SMITH, Myra King	Rozella Hospital, Geraldton	15th Nov., 1911	255 (2)	In practice, June, 1909.
109	SMITH, Marie Wilson	396 Beaufort Street, Perth	8th Nov., 1911	255 (1)	Fremantle Midwifery Training School.
501	SMITH, Rachel	Trafalgar Street, Trafalgar, Kalgoorlie	20th Dec., 1911	255 (2)	In practice, June, 1909.
137	SMITH, Susan	137 Lord Street, Perth	8th Nov., 1911	255 (2)	In practice, June, 1909.
865	SMOKER, Elizabeth Ann	Dangin	25th Oct., 1912	255 (2)	In practice, June, 1909.
737	SOMERS, Annie	26 Francis Street, Perth	15th Mar., 1912	255 (2)	In practice, June, 1909.
783	SPEEDY, Ellen Sarah	Narra Tarra, *via* Geraldton	17th May, 1912	255 (2)	In practice, June, 1909.
454	SPEERS, Eliza Emily	Old Men's Home, Claremont	20th Dec., 1911	255 (1)	Women's Hospital, Melbourne.
183	STAFFORD, Agnes	61 Wittenoom Street, Kalgoorlie	15th Nov., 1911	255 (2)	In practice, June, 1909.
795	STAFFORD, Margaret Maria	Wickepin	7th June, 1912	255 (2)	In practice, June, 1909.
738	STARICK, Henrietta	Gosnells	15th Mar., 1912	255 (2)	In practice, June, 1909.
678	STEVENS, Elizabeth	Armadale	12th Jan., 1912	255 (2)	In practice, June, 1909.
449	STEVENS, Sarah	Public Hospital, Laverton	20th Dec., 1911	255 (1)	London Obstetrical Society.
79	STEWART, Helen	Midland Junction	25th Oct., 1911	255 (2)	In practice, June, 1909.
609	STIRTON, Isabella	Holyoake	29th Dec., 1911	255 (2)	In practice, June, 1909.
653	STOBBS, Mabel	7 Price Street, Fremantle	5th Jan., 1912	255 (2)	In practice, June, 1909.

44	STOCKLEY, Alice Maud Mary	47 Newcastle Street, Perth	10th Oct., 1911	255 (2)	In practice, June, 1909.
402	STRANAGHAN, Jane	Waverley Private Hospital, Adelaide Terrace, Perth	13th Dec., 1911	255 (1)	Women's Hospital, Melbourne.
133	STREET, Elizabeth	Caledonian Avenue, Bayswater	8th Nov., 1911	255 (2)	In practice, June, 1909.
833	STUART, Catherine Mary	Guildford Post Office	9th Aug., 1912	255 (2)	In practice, June, 1909.
848	STURMAN, Agnes Mary	Marine Terrace, Geraldton	5th Sept., 1912	255 (2)	In practice, June, 1909.
129	STURT, Margaret	75 Brisbane Street, Perth	8th Nov., 1911	255 (2)	In practice, June, 1909.
370	SUMMERELL, Mary Elizabeth	117 Wellington Street, Perth	8th Dec., 1911	255 (2)	In practice, June, 1909.
88	SUMPTON, Mary Jane	Silas Street, East Fremantle	25th Oct., 1911	255 (2)	In practice, June, 1909.
897	SUTTON, Marian Elizabeth Margaret	Mandurah	20th Dec., 1912	261 (1)	Women's Hospital, Melbourne.
158	SWANNELL, Fanny Eliza	Lake Yealering, *via* Wickepin	15th Nov., 1911	255 (1)	Fremantle Midwifery Training School.
281	SWARBRICK, Elizabeth	Jolimont, Subiaco	29th Nov., 1911	255 (2)	In practice, June, 1909.
72	TAIT, Marky Minto	Harvest Terrace, Perth	25th Oct., 1911	255 (1)	Glasgow Maternity Hospital.
161	TALBOT, Ada Lucy	25 Quarry Street, Fremantle	15th Nov., 1911	255 (1)	Queen's Home, Adelaide.
160	TALBOT, Alice Mary Somerville	25 Quarry Street, Fremantle	15th Nov., 1911	255 (1)	Queen's Home, Adelaide.
168	TALBOT, Mabel Sophia	25 Quarry Street, Fremantle	15th Nov., 1911	255 (2)	In practice, June, 1909.
838	TATE, Irene	194 Stirling Street, Perth	9th Aug., 1912	261 (1)	Central Midwives' Board, England.
178	TAYLOR, Jessie	Gwalia	15th Nov., 1911	255 (2)	In practice, June, 1909.
238	TCHAN, Isabell	Midland Junction	22nd Nov., 1911	255 (2)	In practice, June, 1909.
651	TEASDALE, Mary Nicholson	Piesse Street, Boulder	5th Jan., 1912	255 (2)	In practice, June, 1909.
508	TETLOW, Elizabeth	Geraldton	20th Dec., 1911	255 (2)	In practice, June, 1909.
393	THIRLOWAY, Janet	Broad Arrow Road, Kalgoorlie	8th Dec., 1911	255 (2)	In practice, June, 1909.
898	THOMAS, Jane	Hepburn Street, Mt. Magnet	20th Dec., 1912	255 (2)	In practice, June, 1909.
797	THOMAS, Mary	Menzies	7th June, 1912	255 (2)	In practice, June, 1909.
120	THOMPSON, Laura	58 Ruth Street, Perth	8th Nov., 1911	255 (2)	In practice, June, 1909.
739	THOMPSON, Mary	48 Buller Street, Kalgoorlie	15th Mar., 1912	255 (2)	In practice, June, 1909.
664	THOMPSON, Mary Anne	29 Cheetham Street, Kalgoorlie	5th Jan., 1912	255 (2)	In practice, June, 1909.
216	THOMPSON, Mary Josephine	31 Davis Street, Boulder	22nd Nov., 1911	255 (2)	In practice, June, 1909.
763	TILLETT, Louisa	12 Forrest Street, Boulder City	19th April, 1912	255 (2)	In practice, June, 1909.
256	TINDALE, Eleanor Forrest	Public Hospital, Kookynie	29th Nov., 1911	255 (1)	Women's Hospital, Melbourne.
344	TRACEY, Eliza	64 Parry Street, Perth	8th Dec., 1911	255 (2)	In practice, June, 1909.
517	TRATHAM, Kathie	Tambellup	20th Dec., 1911	255 (2)	In practice, June, 1909.
101	TREBY, Sarah Avarilla	202 Bulwer Street, North Perth	25th Oct., 1911	255 (1)	The Lying-in Hospital, Melbourne.
411	TRIGWELL, Ellen	Donnybrook	13th Dec., 1911	255 (2)	In practice, June, 1909.
92	TRIGWELL, Lucy	Donnybrook	25th Oct., 1911	255 (2)	In practice, June, 1909.
596	TRUSCOTT, Annie	Elvira Street, Midland Junction	29th Dec., 1911	255 (2)	In practice, June, 1909.
622	TRUSLOVE, Sarah	Roebourne	29th Dec., 1911	255 (2)	In practice, June, 1909.
377	TURNER, Annie	Rason Parade, Bellevue	8th Dec., 1911	255 (2)	In practice, June, 1909.
90	TURNER, Elizabeth Anne	Balfour Street, Kalgoorlie	25th Oct., 1911	255 (2)	In practice, June, 1909.
13	TURNER, Susan	Broome Park Private Hospital, Tambellup	13th Sept., 1911	255 (2)	In practice, June, 1909.
132	TURTON, Mary Jane	80 Adelaide Street, Fremantle	8th Nov., 1911	255 (2)	In practice, June, 1909.
459	TWINE, Ethel Hannah	Toodyay	20th Dec., 1911	255 (2)	In practice, June, 1909.
401	TYERS, Lillian Rose	194 Stirling Street, Perth	13th Dec., 1911	255 (1)	Women's Hospital, Melbourne.
32	TYLOR, Annie Louisa	Piesse Street, Katanning	27th Sept., 1911	255 (2)	In practice, June, 1909.
422	UHE, Fanny Marie Helene	Colin Street, Perth	13th Dec., 1911	255 (2)	In practice, June, 1909.
545	UNDERHILL, Harriet	Waifs' Home, Parkerville	29th Dec., 1911	255 (2)	In practice, June, 1909.
503	UREN, Matilda Maud	130 Richardson Street, Boulder	20th Dec., 1911	255 (2)	In practice, June, 1909.
205	VAN HUERCK, Annie	79 Padbury Street, Perth	22nd Nov., 1911	255 (2)	In practice, June, 1909.
558	VIERK, Ernestine Sophia	45 Outram Street, Perth	29th Dec., 1911	255 (2)	In practice, June, 1909.
576	VINCENT, Mary Esther	Geraldton	29th Dec., 1911	255 (2)	In practice, June, 1909.

MIDWIVES' REGISTRATION BOARD—*continued.*

Registration No.	Name.	Address.	Date of Registration.	Section of Act under which Registration was effected.	Qualification.
409	WAITE, Sarah	242 Lake Street, Perth	13th Dec., 1911	255 (2)	In practice, June, 1909.
684	WAITE, Sarah Anne	Yeo Street, Woodlupine	26th Jan., 1912	255 (2)	In practice, June, 1909.
318	WAKEFORD, Ruth	Burracoppin	29th Nov., 1911	255 (2)	In practice, June, 1909.
299	WALKER, Ellen	10 Chatsworth Road, Perth	29th Nov., 1911	255 (2)	In practice, June, 1909.
899	WALKER, Margaret Ann	"Carlton," 17 Sanders Street, Leederville	20th Dec., 1912	261 (1)	Central Midwives' Board, England.
7	WALSH, Mary Ellen	Macdonald Street, Kalgoorlie	13th Sept., 1911	255 (2)	In practice, June, 1909.
762	WANSBROUGH, Mary	Beverley	19th April, 1912	255 (2)	In practice, June, 1909.
127	WANSBROUGH, Matilda	Forrest Street, Beverley	8th Nov., 1911	255 (2)	In practice, June, 1909.
297	WARD, Sarah Jane	19 Colin Crescent, West Perth	29th Nov., 1911	255 (2)	In practice, June, 1909.
473	WARMAN, Mary Jane	912 Wellington Street, West Perth	20th Dec., 1911	255 (2)	In practice, June, 1909.
65	WARNE, Wilhelmina	158 Mandurah Road, Fremantle	10th Oct., 1911	255 (2)	In practice, June, 1909.
666	WARNER, Bridget	Ludlow, near Busselton	5th Jan., 1912	255 (2)	In practice, June, 1909.
667	WARNER, Elizabeth	Busselton	5th Jan., 1912	255 (2)	In practice, June, 1909.
358	WASHER, Elizabeth	Walton Road, Victoria Park	8th Dec., 1911	255 (2)	In practice, June, 1909.
711	WATERS Mary	Toodyay	16th Feb., 1912	255 (2)	In practice, June, 1909.
34	WATKINS, Josephine Mary	Lancelot Street, North Fremantle	27th Sept., 1911	255 (2)	In practice, June, 1909.
334	WATSON, Henrietta	Grosvenor Hospital, Fremantle	8th Dec., 1911	255 (2)	In practice, June, 1909.
700	WATTS, Catherine	Johnston Street, Golden Gate, Boulde	26th Jan., 1912	255 (2)	In practice, June, 1909.
690	WATTS, Eliza Ann	C/o Mrs. Shackell, Nurses' Home, Stirling St., Perth	26th Jan., 1912	255 (2)	In practice, June, 1909.
511	WEAVER, Charlotte	108 Smith Street, Highgate Hill, Perth	20th Dec., 1911	255 (2)	In practice, June, 1909.
107	WEAVER, Hannah	Maylands	8th Nov., 1911	255 (1)	Fremantle Midwifery Training School.
775	WEBB, Harriett	48A Hopkins Street, Boulder	17th May, 1912	255 (2)	In practice, June, 1909.
745	WELLS, Amelia	525 Newcastle Street, Perth	15th Mar., 1912	255 (2)	In practice, June, 1909.
631	WELLS, Sarah	Fitzgerald Street, West Northam	29th Dec., 1912	255 (2)	In practice, June, 1909.
900	WEST, Charlotte	Beddingfield Road, Pinjarra	20th Dec., 1912	255 (2)	In practice, June, 1909.
279	WEST, Lavinia	Leonard Street, Victoria Park	29th Nov., 1911	255 (2)	In practice, June, 1909.
48	WESTBURY, Catherine Eliza	Bay Road, North Fremantle	10th Oct., 1911	255 (2)	In practice, June, 1909.
375	WHEELER, Madeline	Pennant Street, North Perth	8th Dec., 1911	255 (2)	In practice, June, 1909.
884	WHITE, Beatrice	Nurses' Home, 35 Hill Street, Perth	22nd Nov., 1912	261 (1)	Central Midwives' Board, England.
768	WHITE, Jane	1084 Hay Street, Perth	19th April, 1912	255 (2)	In practice, June, 1909.
339	WHITE, Margaret Ann	South Bunbury	8th Dec., 1911	255 (2)	In practice, June, 1909.
171	WHITE, Marie	Doodlakine	15th Nov., 1911	255 (2)	In practice, June, 1909.
16	WHITE, Priscilla Faith	Crawford Road, Maylands	27th Sept., 1911	255 (2)	In practice, June, 1909.
182	WHITTLESTON, Catherine	203 Royal Street, Perth	15th Nov., 1911	255 (2)	In practice, June, 1909.
525	WILDING, Mary	Railway Street, North Fremantle	29th Dec., 1911	255 (2)	In practice, June, 1909.
901	WILKINSON, Alice May	21 Hyde Street, North Perth	20th Dec., 1912	255 (2)	In practice, June, 1909.
902	WILKINSON, Mary Ann	226 Heytesbury Road, Subiaco	20th Dec., 1912	255 (2)	In practice, June, 1909.
167	WILLCOX-PLUMMER, Helena	33 Richardson Street, West Perth	15th Nov., 1911	255 (2)	In practice, June, 1909.
81	WILLIAMS, Dorothea Ann	Burbanks	25th Oct., 1911	255 (2)	In practice, June, 1909.
357	WILLIAMS, Emily	403 William Street, Perth	8th Dec., 1911	255 (2)	In practice, June, 1909.
811	WILLIAMS, Gertrude	194 Stirling Street, Perth	5th July, 1912	261 (1)	Central Midwives' Board, England.
744	WILLIAMS, Jane	Federal Road, Kalgoorlie	15th Mar., 1912	255 (2)	In practice, June, 1909.
714	WILLIAMS, Mary Elizabeth	86 Canning Road, East Fremantle	16th Feb., 1912	255 (2)	In practice, June, 1909.
293	WILLIAMSON, Mary	829 Wellington Street, West Perth	29th Nov., 1911	255 (2)	In practice, June, 1909.
557	WILLIS, Elizabeth	Cue	29th Dec., 1911	255 (2)	In practice, June, 1909.

435	WILLIS, Maud Alice	15 Moir Street, Perth	13th Dec., 1911	255	(2)	In practice, June, 1909.
104	WILLS, Emilie Charlotte	"Staplehurst," Hay Street, Perth	8th Nov., 1911	255	(1)	Queen Charlotte Lying-in Hospital, London.
670	WILLSON, Ruth	Claremont Avenue, Claremont	12th Jan., 1912	255	(2)	In practice, June, 1909.
64	WILSON, Annetta	74 Campbell Street, Kalgoorlie	10th Oct., 1911	255	(2)	In practice, June, 1909.
60	WILSON, Agnes	17 Charles Street, South Fremantle	10th Oct., 1911	255	(2)	In practice, June, 1909.
627	WILSON, Emily	108 Outram Street, Perth	29th Dec., 1911	255	(2)	In practice, June, 1909.
225	WILSON, Margaret	158 Oroya Street, Boulder	22nd Nov., 1911	255	(2)	In practice, June, 1909.
128	WILSON, Mary	Davis Street, South Fremantle	8th Nov., 1911	255	(2)	In practice, June, 1909.
176	WIGGETT, Annie	Keane Street, Cottesloe Beach	15th Nov., 1911	255	(2)	In practice, June, 1909.
471	WOOD, Mary Anne	Pinjarra	20th Dec., 1911	255	(2)	In practice, June, 1909.
310	WOODS, Julia Ann	Donnybrook	29th Nov., 1911	255	(2)	In practice, June, 1909.
94	WOODS, Sarah Elizabeth	Raymond Street, Collie	25th Oct., 1911	255	(2)	In practice, June, 1909.
418	WOODWORD, Ellen	109 Hope Street, Fremantle	13th Dec., 1911	255	(2)	In practice, June, 1909.
272	WOOLER, Annie	175 Vivian Street, Boulder	29th Nov., 1911	255	(2)	In practice, June, 1909.
151	WOOSNAM, Mary Ann	Day Dawn	8th Nov., 1911	255	(2)	In practice, June, 1909.
35	WRANKMORE, Sarah Alice	215 Brown Street, East Perth	27th Sept., 1911	255	(2)	In practice, June, 1909.
710	WRAY, Ernestine	Government Hospital, Collie	26th Jan., 1911	255	(2)	In practice, June, 1909.
866	WRIGHT, Adelaide	194 Stirling Street, Perth	25th Oct., 1912	261	(1)	St. Margaret's Maternity Hospital, Sydney.
735	WRIGHT, Margaret	Sandstone	15th Mar., 1912	255	(2)	In practice, June, 1909.
457	WRIGHT, Martha Annie	Miller Street, Boulder	20th Dec., 1911	255	(1)	Central Midwives' Board, England.
244	WYATT, Sarah	Kulyaling	22nd Nov., 1911	255	(2)	In Practice, June, 1909.
389	WYLDE, Sara	Bayswater	8th Dec., 1911	255	(2)	In practice, June, 1909.
190	YEOMAN, Florence	St. Leonard's Avenue, Leederville	15th Nov., 1911	255	(2)	In practice, June, 1909.
8	YURACKA, Ctherine	119 Wellington Street, Perth	13th Sept., 1911	255	(2)	In practice, June, 1909.

APPENDIX III

A.T.N.A. RULES AND REGULATIONS & SCHEDULE OF STUDY

Objects.

The Association was founded in the year 1899, and its objects were briefly set forth as follows :—

1. To promote the interests of Trained Nurses—male and female—in all matters affecting their work as a class.

2. To establish a system of registration for Trained Nurses.

3. To afford opportunities for discussing subjects bearing on the work of Nursing.

4. To initiate and control schemes that will afford to Nurses a means of providing an allowance during incapacity for work caused by sickness, accident, age, or other necessitous circumstances.

Rules.

Constitution and Management.

(i.) The governing body of the Association shall be a Council, which shall consist of the President, the Vice-President, Hon. Treasurer, two Hon. Secretaries, and twenty Members (of whom five shall be duly qualified Medical Practitioners, five Matrons and Superintendents of Nurses, five Sisters and Nurses, three Representatives of the Midwifery Branch, and two may be Honorary Members), who shall be elected as hereinafter directed, and of whom five shall form a quorum.

(ii) The management of the Association shall be entrusted to the governing body, who will have power to appoint such Committees as may from time to time be deemed necessary in order to carry out the objects of the Association.

Election of Officers

(iii.) The election of a President, Vice-President, Hon. Treasurer, and Hon. Secretaries and Members of Council shall be vested in the general body of Members of the Association, and, except as hereinafter mentioned, shall be made in the Annual Meeting or at a Special Meeting of the Members then present.

(iv.) Until the first Annual Meeting shall be held, the following shall form a Council :—Dr. Manning, President ; Dr. Goode, Vice-President ; Mr. J. Oswald Fairfax, Honorary Treasurer ; Dr. Mills, Miss McGahey, Honorary Secretaries ; Dr. Clubbe. Dr. Fiaschi, Dr. Thring, Dr. James Graham ; Miss Spencer, Miss Creal, Miss McMaster, Miss Venables, Miss Gould, Mrs. Joseph Graham, Matrons ; Miss Ryrie, Private Hospital ; Miss Sanders, Miss Johnston, Sisters ; Miss Davies, Miss Wilson, Miss Godson, Nurses' Homes ; Mrs. J. T. Wilson, Honorary Member.

(v.) The Council shall have power to temporarily fill any vacancy if they think it indispensable to do so.

QUALIFICATIONS AND PRIVILEGES OF MEMBERS.

(xiii.) The Association shall consist of Members and Honorary Members.

(xiv.) Members shall be—

(*a*) Nurses on the Register or Roll of the Association ; or

(*b*) Duly qualified Medical Practitioners elected by the Council,

who in each case have paid for the current year the annual subscription fixed by the Council.

(xv.) Honorary Members shall be elected from those who have identified themselves with the work of public Hospitals and kindred institutions.

(xvi.) Honorary Members shall have no voice in the management of the Association, except when elected as Members of the Council under the provisions of Rule i.

(xvii.) Every Member shall pay to the Association an annual subscription of such amount as shall be from time to time determined by the Council.

(xviii.) Candidates for registration must produce proof that they have been trained by a Matron or Nurse who holds a certificate from a Training School for Nurses recognised by the Council of this Association, and who, if the Hospital be situate in States in which the training of Nurses is controlled by the Association, is a Member of the Australasian Trained Nurses' Association ; and

(*a*) That they have been engaged for three years in a general Hospital recognised by the Council, and having an average of not less than 40 beds occupied daily ; or

(*b*) That they have been engaged for four years in a

country, district, or suburban Hospital recognised by the Council, and having an average of not less than 20 beds occupied daily ; or

(*c*) That they have been engaged for five years in a private, country, district, or suburban Hospital recognised by the Council, and having an average of not less than 10 beds occupied daily.

(*d*) That they have obtained their certificate as Mental Nurses and have been registered as such by this Association under rule 1 (*a*) (2) and have subsequently been engaged for two years in a General Hospital recognised by the Council having an average of not less than 40 beds daily occupied, or for a proportional period in a four or a five years' training school.

Furthermore, all candidates must give references as to their moral character, produce certificates of competency from the Hospitals in which they have been engaged, and account for any interval of time in their nursing career when not engaged in Hospitals or Nursing Associations.

In the case of all Nurses completing their training after June 30th, 1906, it will be necessary to pass the examination for membership of the Association, except in the case of candidates presenting certificates from those other States or countries with which the Australasian Trained Nurses' Association has a reciprocal agreement.

(xix.) Any Nurse who has been trained for a period of two years at a Training School for Nurses deemed worthy of recognition by the Council, and has obtained her certificate as a Nurse from that Training School prior to March 31st, 1900, shall be eligible for registration.

(xx.) (OBSOLETE) Any Nurse who has been trained in a private Hospital, containing not less than 10 beds, for a period of five years, and who has been trained at that Hospital under a Matron who holds a certificate from a Training School for Nurses, and who can produce certificates of competency from two reputable Medical Practitioners, shall be eligible for registration up to 31st March, 1900, subject to the approval of the Council of the Association.

(xxi.) (OBSOLETE) Any Nurse who can show to the satisfaction of the Council that she has been engaged for not less than three years in the *bona fide* work of medical and surgical nursing, either in Hospitals or in private nursing, and can produce certificates of competency and good conduct satisfactory to the Council from at least three reputable Medical Practitioners as to her attainments and repute, shall be eligible for registration up to March 31st, 1900, subject to the approval of the Council. Provided always that the Council shall have power in any case to direct that any candidate under this Rule may be examined in practical nursing by three examiners appointed by the Council, and, provided further, that in the case of Nurses registered under this Rule the qualification in the Register shall stand as "Admitted by the Council under the provisions of Rule xxi."

(xxiA.) In the case of any Nurse who, prior to March 31st, 1900, has been engaged for a period of three years in nursing in a Hospital or Hospitals recognised by, or deemed worthy of recognition by the Council of the Australasian Trained Nurses' Association, and who can produce satisfactory evidence to that effect, together with certificates of competency from three reputable Medical Practitioners, the Council shall have power to consider the claims of such Nurse to membership, and may if they consider them adequate, admit her as a Member, either after examination or not, as they see fit. Such decision must be ratified at the next succeeding Council Meeting, and Members so admitted are to be entered in the Register as admitted under Rule xxiA.

[All cases of Nurses under concessional clauses applying to qualify for Matronships must be individually considered by the Central Council, and they should have received a training in a Hospital deemed worthy of recognition by the Council, and present certificates of Invalid Cookery.]

(xxii.) The Council shall cause to be kept a Register in which shall be entered the names, addresses, qualifications, training, &c., of all Nurses who have been approved of by the Council, and who have paid the prescribed fee.

(xxiii.) The Council shall have power to remove from the Register the name of any Nurse who, after full inquiry, may prove herself hereafter to be unworthy of trust. Provided always that before any name be so removed due notice of the Council's intention shall be given to the Nurse, who shall have the opportunity of making any personal explanation that she may deem desirable.

(xxiiiA.) No General Nurse, unless trained in Midwifery, shall undertake the care of obstetric cases. A Nurse who has been proved to the satisfaction of the Council to have violated this rule shall be liable to have her name removed from the Register.

(The Council may exercise its discretionary power to relax this rule in the case of General Nurses in country districts where no Midwifery Nurse is at the time available.)

(xxiv.) The Council shall also have the right to restore any name removed from the Register on satisfactory proof being given that the causes which led to the removal no longer exist.

Schedule of Study to be Accepted as Minimum Course for Registration by the A.T.N.A.

PRACTICAL INSTRUCTION TO BE GIVEN BY MATRON.

LECTURES BY RESIDENT AND HONORARY STAFF.

SUGGESTED ATTENDANCE.

First Year:

12 Anatomy and Physiology. 12 General Nursing.

Second Year:

12 Medical Nursing. 12 Surgical Nursing.

Third Year:

6 Invalid Cookery, practical. Urine Testing Housekeeping.

This is to be accepted as a Minimum Course, but all teachers to be urged to make such Course as complete as possible.

ANATOMY AND PHYSIOLOGY—12 LECTURES TO BE GIVEN.

The structural composition of the human body—bone, ligament, muscles, arteries, veins, nerves, glands, lymphatics, organs of assimilation, of secretion and excretion.

The skeleton, names and functions of various bones—joints, nature of, chief varieties, functions, ball and socket, hinge, &c.

Muscles, anatomical description of, action of, names of most important, physiology of muscle.

Arteries and veins—structure and functions, names of, position of chief arteries and veins.

Nervous system – brief sketch of: – Brain—structure and functions; spinal cord structure and functions; motor nerves, structure and functions.

The heart, structure and functions, its position.

The circulation.

The blood, its constitution and use.

The lungs, structure, position, functions. Respiration.

The larnyx—speech.

Animal heat.

Digestion and absorption.

Mastication the teeth.

Saliva, and salivary glands.

The stomach, its position, structure and functions.

The small intestine, position, structure and functions.

The colon, structure and functions, position.

Defœcation.

The liver, position, structure and functions.

The pancreas, position, structure and functions.

The kidneys, position, structure and functions.

Secretion of urine. The ureters.

The bladder, its position and functions. Excretion.

The urine, its composition and quantity.

The spleen, its position and functions.

The thyroid, supra-renals.

The skin, its structure and functions. The sweat.

The organs of special sense. The eye, nose, ear, taste.

GENERAL NURSING—12 LECTURES.

Qualifications of a Nurse.

Distinction between the Doctor's work and that of the Nurse. Hospital etiquette.

The Nurse's general work—

(*a*) Bedmaking, management of helpless patients.

(*b*) Hygiene of the sick room. Ventilation, lighting, temperature, &c.

(*c*) Baths (different kinds), sponging.

(*d*) Cleansing and padding splints.

(*e*) Prevention of infection.

Use of clinical thermometer.

The pulse, its variations and method of record.

Respiration, its method of record.

External applications—Preparation of fomentations and poultices, local application of heat and cold, cold and hot packs, hot-air bath, counter-irritation, leeches, blisters.

Various methods of administering drugs, enemata, subcutaneous injections (hypodermic), saline, &c.

Lotions in common use, preparation of in varying strengths.

Hypnotics, doses and actions of more commonly used, and methods of administration.

Poison, dosage and effects. Symptoms of poisoning by morphia, strychnine, arsenic, belladonna, alcohol, chloroform, mercury, iodoform, carbolic acid, &c.

What to use in case of poisoning.

Drug rashes.

Methods of observing symptoms, and manner of reporting same to doctor.

Dressings and their preparation.

Operation case—Preparation of patient and room.

Instruments—Their care and use.

Disinfectants and antiseptics.

Administration of food.

MEDICAL NURSING—12 LECTURES.

General symptoms in disease—Value of close observation.

Temperature, rigors, pain, dyspnœa, expectoration.

Hæmoptysis, state of pulse, collapse, cyanosis, sweating, vomiting.

Hæmatemesis, diarrhœa, malæna, abdominal distention.

Delirium, œdema, tenderness.

Specific fevers, characteristics—Incubation, infection, contagion, disinfection.

Emergencies—Poisoning. Drowning. Fainting. Fits—epileptic, apoplectic, hysterical. Coma. Paralytic cases—special care of. Prevention of bedsores.

Urine testing.

Nursing of special cases—Bright's Disease—Urine, pyuria, hæmaturia. Cardiac, pulmonary—Pneumonia, phthisis, bronchitis, &c. Nervous cases—Cerebral hæmorrhage, neuritis, epilepsy, mania, sciatica, meningitis, &c. Rheumatic fever. Chorea. Alcoholism. Dropsy. Gastric ulcer. Skin disease. Nursing and feeding of sick children, &c.

SURGICAL NURSING—12 LECTURES, WITH DEMONSTRATIONS.

Inflammation, suppuration, ulceration, gangrene, and septicæmia.

Healing and dressing of wounds, burns, and scalds.

Hæmorrhage and its arrest.

Bedsores—prevention and treatment.

Fractures and splints.

Bandaging.

Operation cases—Preparation of patient in general and for special operations.

Disinfection and antiseptics.

Nursing of special cases—Tracheotomy. Jaw operations. Amputations, resections. Empyæma. Tapping abdomen or chest. Operations on nose, head, tongue, throat, neck, eye, pelvic organs. Hare lip. Cleft palate. Caries of spine. Tubercular joints, &c. Management of abdominal operations. Catheterisation. Preparation of salines.

INVALID COOKERY—6 PRACTICAL LESSONS.

Instruction should be given in the preparation of invalid drinks, the cooking of beef tea, broths, poultry, fish, meats, eggs, light puddings, jellies, vegetables, and fruits.

Invalid drinks—Barley water, toast water, lemonade, apple water, gruel, white wine, whey, &c.

Beef juice.

Beef tea—Various methods.

Broths—Chicken, mutton, &c.

Fish—Filleting. Various methods of cooking.

Poultry—Method of baking and boiling.

Chops and steak—Various methods of cooking.

Brains and sweetbreads—Various methods of cooking.

Custards and light puddings—Baked and boiled custard, baked rice, rice custard, tapioca pudding, &c.

Eggs—Various methods of cooking.

Jellies—Wine and lemon.

---

‡ FORM OF CERTIFICATE.

This is to Certify *that* *has regularly attended the prescribed course of Lectures at this Hospital, and completed her years of training. She has passed her examinations and her practical work has been*

Signed

Medical Supt. or Hon. Sec.

Signed

Signed

Examiners.

Matron.

Signature of Nurse.

Text Books Suggested.

Foster and Shore's Physiology for Beginners.

General Nursing—Lücke's General Nursing; Lewis' Nursing, its Theory and Practice; Stewart and Cuffs' Practical Nursing.

Medical Nursing—Cuffs' Lectures on Medicine to Nurses.

Gynæcological Nursing Fullerton's Nursing in Abdominal Surgery.

APPENDIX IV

WAGE SCALES FROM W.A.N.A. FIRST AWARD COURT OF ARBITRATION 1935

Metropolitan Area.

(Note:- The years mentioned hereunder shall be construed to mean years of experience.)

	Basis from which calculations made Per Annum.	Cash			Board and Lodging			Total per Week			Margin		
	£	£	s.	d.	£	s.	d.	£	s.	d.	£	s.	d.
NURSES													
1st. Year	95	1	16	5	1	0	0	2	16	5		18	1
2nd. Year	105	2	0	3	1	0	0	3	0	3	1	1	11
3rd. Year	115	2	4	1	1	0	0	3	4	1	1	5	9
SISTERS													
1st. Year	130	2	9	10	1	0	0	3	9	10	1	11	6
2nd. Year	140	2	13	8	1	0	0	3	13	8	1	15	4
3rd. Year	150	2	17	6	1	0	0	3	17	6	1	19	2
MATRONS Where daily average of occupied beds is :-													
Less than 1 :-													
1st. Year	130	2	9	10	1	0	0	3	9	10	1	11	6
2nd. Year	140	2	13	8	1	0	0	3	13	8	1	15	4
3rd. Year	150	2	17	6	1	0	0	3	17	6	1	19	2
1 & less than 3:-													
1st. Year	140	2	13	8	1	0	0	3	13	8	1	15	4
2nd. Year	150	2	17	6	1	0	0	3	17	6	1	19	2
3rd. Year	160	3	1	4	1	0	0	4	1	4	2	3	0
3 & less than 5:-													
1st. Year	160	3	1	4	1	0	0	4	1	4	2	3	0
2nd. Year	170	3	5	2	1	0	0	4	5	2	2	6	10
3rd. Year	180	3	9	0	1	0	0	4	9	0	2	10	8
5& less than 10:-													
1st. Year	170	3	5	2	1	2	6	4	7	8	2	9	4
2nd Year	180	3	9	0	1	2	6	4	11	6	2	13	2
3rd. Year	190	3	12	11	1	2	6	4	15	5	2	17	1
10&less than15:-													
1st. Year	180	3	9	0	1	2	6	4	11	6	2	13	2
2nd. Year	190	3	12	11	1	2	6	4	15	5	2	17	1
3rd. Year	200	3	16	9	1	2	6	4	19	3	3	0	11

	Basis from which calculations made Per Annum.	Cash			Board and Lodging			Total per Week			Margin		
	£	£	s.	d.	£	s.	d.	£	s.	d.	£	s.	d.
15&less than20:-													
1st. Year	190	3	12	11	1	5	0	4	17	11	2	19	7
2nd. Year	200	3	16	9	1	5	0	5	1	9	3	3	5
3rd. Year	210	4	0	7	1	5	0	5	5	7	3	7	3
20&less than40:-													
1st. Year	220	4	4	5	1	7	6	5	11	11	3	13	7
2nd. Year	230	4	8	3	1	7	6	5	15	9	3	17	5
3rd. Year	235	4	10	2	1	7	6	5	17	8	3	19	4
40 & less than 100:-													
1st. Year	230	4	8	3	1	7	6	5	15	9	3	17	5
2nd. ,,	240	4	12	1	1	7	6	5	19	7	4	1	3
3rd. ,,	250	4	15	11	1	7	6	6	3	5	4	5	1
100 & less than 200:-													
1st. Year	250	4	15	11	1	10	0	6	5	11	4	7	7
2nd. ,,	265	5	1	8	1	10	0	6	11	8	4	13	4
3rd, ,,	280	5	7	5	1	10	0	6	17	5	4	19	1
200 & upwards:-													
1st. Year	350	6	14	3	1	15	0	8	9	3	6	10	11
2nd. ,,	375	7	3	10	1	15	0	8	18	10	7	0	6
3rd. ,,	400	7	13	5	1	15	0	9	8	5	7	10	1
As/st Matrons Perth Hospital and Infectious Diseases branch Subiaco :-													
1st. Year	190	3	12	11	1	5	0	4	17	11	2	19	7
2nd. ,,	200	3	16	9	1	5	0	5	1	9	3	3	5
3rd. ,,	210	4	0	7	1	5	0	5	5	7	3	7	3
Other Assistant Matrons :-													
1st. Year	160	3	1	4	1	0	0	4	1	4	2	3	0
2nd. ,,	170	3	5	2	1	0	0	4	5	2	2	6	10
3rd. ,,	180	3	9	0	1	0	0	4	9	0	2	10	8
Women's Home Fremantle :- If and when position of Matron is held by a Nurse, the salary shall be as under:													
1st. Year	220	4	4	5	1	7	6	5	11	11	3	13	7
2nd. ,,	230	4	8	3	1	7	6	5	15	9	3	17	5
3rd. ,,	240	4	12	1	1	7	6	5	19	7	4	1	3
4th. ,,	250	4	15	11	1	7	6	6	3	5	4	5	1

NOTES

ABBREVIATIONS

A.N.F.	Australian Nurses Federation
A.T.N.A.	Australasian Trained Nurses Association
B.L.	Battye Library
C.S.O.	Colonial Secretary's Office Records
C.S.R.	Colonial Secretary's Office, Inward Correspondence
Gov. Gaz.	*Government Gazette*
J.W.A.N.	*Journal of the Western Australian Nurses* 1935-45; *Journal of the West Australian Nurses* 1945-71
R.W.A.H.S.	Royal Western Australian Historical Society
V. & P.	Western Australia, *Minutes, Votes and Proceedings of the Parliament*
W.A.N.A.	*Western Australian Nurses' Association*

1. NINETEENTH CENTURY NURSING

1. Colonial secretary to Dr Creighton, colonial surgeon, 15 November 1840, reproduced in the Royal Perth Hospital Milligan Society *News Bulletin* 1, 2 (September 1970).
2. A. S. Ellis, 'Montgomery of Claremont—first fifteen years', *Early Days, Journal and Proceedings of the Royal Western Australian Historical Society* VII, 7 (1975).
3. C. T. Stannage (ed.), *Local History in Western Australia* (Nedlands, 1974); J. T. Reilly, *Reminiscences of Fifty Years in Western Australia* (Perth, 1903).
4. J. H. Stubbe, *Medical Background, being a history of Fremantle hospitals and doctors* (Nedlands, 1969).
5. Interview with Mrs E. de Moulin, who was one of the first five probationers, April 1971.
6. C.S.R. 377/55.
7. Blue Book 1853, p. 94.
8. 'An afternoon at the Colonial Hospital', *Herald* 8.3.1884; 'As it is', 'As it should be', *Inquirer* 15.12.1886.
9. *The Sisters of the People: their mission and work in Western Australia* (Perth, 1897); records held by Sunset Hospital, Dalkeith.
10. Mrs Edward Millett, *An Australian Parsonage* (London, 1872); 'West Australian Hospital System' (Public Health & Medical Department, 1960).
11. C.S.R. 3578/86.
12. *V. & P.* 1886-87, 31.12.1886.
13. Margaret Walpole diary, original held by relatives, microfilm copy B.L. 585A.
14. *Blue Book* 1891.
15. 'Nursing Past and Present', *The Magazine* (1930), p. 13. This journal was put out by the nursing staff of the Children's Hospital.
16. *Blue Books* 1890-1896.

17. C.S.O. 1290/91 (2), 1824/91 (2).
18. Interview in the *West Australian* 4.8.1937; sketch of Florence Nightingale, *J. W.A.N.* 2, 9 (15.6.1937), p. 14.
19. Home of Peace records, held by the Home of Peace; *Blue Book* 1896, part XIII.
20. Mary Pittman Monk, report of the voyage of *Echuca*, in matrons' diaries and reports, AN3 Arc. Acc. 504, B.L.
    Elizabeth Agnes Sadleir, née Seymour, 'Reminiscences', August 1947, RWAHS; copy held by author; part published in *J. W.A.N.* 19 (1953), p. 14.
21. Jessie Hurnall, Notes, 1893-1904, typescript held by author.
22. Australasian Trained Nurses Association *Register of Members* 1910 (Sydney). Two registers of members for Western Australia have been consulted: one is the official A.T.N.A. *Register of Members*, which first included a section on Western Australia in 1908, and was published annually till 1924; the other is an unpublished Western Australian Register of Members, held by the author, comprising cuttings from the official A.T.N.A. *Register*, as well as handwritten material.
23. Correspondence with the British Ministry of Defence, London, 1978.
24. Sadleir Reminiscences.
25. Ibid.
26. Taped interview with Mrs Penglase's daughter, Mrs Hughes; Arthur Reid, *Those Were the Days* (Perth, 1933).
27. The South Australian Trained Nurses' Centenary Committee, *Nursing in South Australia: The First Hundred Years 1837-1937* (Adelaide, 1938); correspondence from relatives and interviews; Pioneer Nurses file, held by the author.
28. Sadleir Reminiscences.
29. Reid, *Those Were the Days.*
30. Ibid.; Sadleir Reminiscences.
31. Sadleir Reminiscences.
32. Letters of James Francis Marks, 2424A/30 B.L.
33. Reid, *Those Were the Days.*
34. *The Wesley Story: Centenary of the Wesley Church, Perth, 1870-1970* (Perth, n.d.); *Sisters of the People*; Sadleir Reminiscences; Correspondence and interviews with relatives; Pioneer Nurses file.
35. *Centenary of the Foundation of the Sisters of St John of God 1871-1971* (Perth, n.d.); records of St John of God Hospital, Subiaco; 'A century of helping the sick', *West Australian* 8.10.1971; 'Broome not like the old days', *Sunday Times* 30.8.70; interview with Sisters Ignatius and Magdalen of St John of God order, 1970.
36. *Gov. Gaz.* 1895.
37. Reid, *Those Were the Days.*
38. Dr Roberta Jull, *The Story of the Alexandra Home for Women* (Perth, n.d.); records at Ngal-A.
39. Hurnall, Notes; *Blue Books* from 1896.
40. *Blue Book* 1896; *Nursing in South Australia.*
41. *Blue Book* 1895; de Moulin interview.
42. *Blue Book* 1897; Royal Victorian Trained Nurses Association, *Register of Members.*
43. Mrs A. H. Garnsey, *Scarlet Pillows* (Melbourne, n.d.); Reid, *Those Were the Days.*
44. Reid, *Those Were the Days; Nursing in South Australia.*

45. Notes from Margaret Edis, held by the author; *Blue Book* 1898.
46. *Blue Books* from 1900 onward.
47. Papers, letters, certificates from Steers relatives; Pioneer Nurses file.
48. The use of the term 'nurse' by Mrs Bedford Fenwick is quoted in Gerald Bowman, *The Lamp and the Book* (London, 1967), p. 4.

2. THE BEGINNING OF THE TWENTIETH CENTURY

1. *Albany Advertiser* 24.3.1900; Dr Ignatius J. Flynn to Annie May-Steers, letter held by author; J. Burridge, *Western Australian Contingents to the South African War* (Perth, 1972).
2. Interview with Miss Masters and Mrs Stannage re Sister Elizabeth Bole (aunt), 1977, and documents and certificates of her nursing service.
3. A.T.N.A. *Register of Members* 1900-1905 (Sydney, n.d.).
4. Daisy Caroline Bridges, *A History of the International Council of Nurses 1899-1964: The first sixty-five years* (London, 1967).
5. An illustration of the badge is reproduced on the cover of the *Journal of the Western Australian Nurses* (1936).
6. *Register of Members* 1900-1905.
7. De Moulin interview; taped interviews with Miss Helena Hutton, 1973-79.
8. *Report of the Select Committee of the Legislative Assembly appointed to inquire into the conditions of Perth Public Hospital*, A22 (Perth, 1900).
9. Interview with Ruth Bottle, 1975. Tapes are held by the author and B.L.
10. Letters and interviews with the relatives of pioneer nurses; birth entries and certificates.
11. *Register of Members* 1900-1905.
12. *Register of Members* 1908; Minutes of the inaugural meeting of the W.A. branch of A.T.N.A., Minutes Book 1, 1907, pp. 1-2.
13. *Register of Members* 1900-1905.
14. A.T.N.A. Minutes Book 1, pp. 1-3.
15. *Registers of Members* from 1908 onwards; letters from relatives and interviews with colleagues; subsequent A.T.N.A. minutes.
16. Taped interviews with elderly nurses and their relatives; also author's correspondence re pioneer nurses.
17. Minutes Book 1, pp. 8-11, 12-15.
18. Ibid. pp. 37-42.
19. *Statistical Registers of Western Australia*; see also Appendix 1.
20. Minutes Book 1, 1.5.1908, pp. 12-25.
21. Ibid. p. 26; *West Australian* 25.7.1908.
22. Minutes Book 1, pp. 37-47.
23. Ibid.
24. Ibid. 4.9.1908, pp. 33-6.
25. Ibid. pp. 37-47.
26. Ibid. 7.8.1908, pp. 27-32.
27. Ibid.
28. Ibid. 23.7.1909, pp. 91-4.
29. Ibid. 21.5.1909, pp. 76-84.
30. Annual Report of the P.M.O. Dr Hope, 1909.
31. Minutes Book 1, 18.6.1909, pp. 55-9; *Report of the Children's Hospital, Perth* (Perth, 1909).
32. Minutes Book 1, 23.7.1909, pp. 91-4.
33. *West Australian* 6.7.1909.
34. Minutes Book 1, 7.8.1909, pp. 95-6.

35. Ibid. 7.9.1909, pp. 101-5.
36. Ibid. 19.8.1910, pp. 135-6.
37. *V. & P.* 1910-11.
38. Interviews with old North Fremantle residents living in the vicinity.
39. Certificates of O'Grady and Appleton, B.L.; Appleton, textbook and examination papers; information from Miss O'Grady, Miss Appleton and Mrs Simm; early Registers of Midwives, in *Gov. Gaz.* 1912-1918.
40. Taped interviews with Elizabeth Grover and Clara Padbury Rutherford, 1971.
41. *Report of the Children's Hospital*; Minutes Book 1, 18.6.1909, pp. 85-90.
42. Minutes Book 1, 18.11.1909, pp. 109-10.
43. Ibid. 17.12.1909, pp. 111-17.
44. Ibid. 13.1.1911, pp. 147-9.
45. Ibid.
46. Ibid. 7.2.1911, pp. 152-5.
47. Ibid. 24.3.1911, pp. 156-8.
48. Minutes Book of the Midwives Registration Board, 1.7.1911, Nurses' Board, Perth.
49. Ibid.
50. Ibid.
51. *Register of Members* 1910.
52. E. L. Grant Watson, *Journey under the Southern Stars* (London, 1968).
53. Minutes Book 2, 19.4.1912, pp. 3-5.
54. Ibid. 19.7.1912, pp. 12-13.
55. Ibid. p. 9: Special meeting.
56. *West Australian* 7.12.1912.
57. *Gov. Gaz.* 6.12.1912, p. 6848.
58. Minutes Book 2, 17.5.1912, pp. 6-8.
59. Ibid. 19.8.1913, pp. 41-2, 46-8.
60. Ibid. 20.12.1912, pp. 20-1.
61. Ibid. 13.10.1914, pp. 84-6.
62. 'A mole-hill and a mountain', *Medical Journal of Australia* 10.10.1914; 'Children's Hospital, Perth, Western Australia', in ibid. 12.9.1914; 'Hospital Management', in ibid. 28.11.1914.
63. 'Official History of the Royal Australian Army Nursing Corps', copy held by author; Grace M. Wilson, *The Story of the Royal Australian Army Nursing Service* (Melbourne, 1949); May (Mary?) Ashton, 'Early Reminiscences', *R.P.H. Journal* (1956); Elizabeth Bole, Certificate of Efficiency; Christian Shackell, Certificate of Appointment, 1911, held by her daughter, Mrs Moira Ward.
64. Letter from the High Commissioner, Minutes Book 2, 1915, p. 104.
65. Minutes Book 2, 10.8.1915, pp. 116-19.

3. FIRST WORLD WAR AND AFTERMATH

1. Minutes Book 2, 14.12.1915, pp. 128-9.
2. Ibid. 19.1.1915, pp. 95-6.
3. Ibid. 9.2.1915, pp. 98-102.
4. Bertram Clarence Cohen and R. L. Hutchinson, *History of the King Edward Memorial Hospital for Women: First Fifty Years 1916-1966* (Subiaco, 1966).

5. Minutes Book 2, 7.11.1916, pp. 162-5.
6. Interview with Ruth Bottle; interview with Margaret Edis, 1975, tape held by author.
7. Interview with Lizzie Faram, 1970, tape held by author.
8. Minutes Book 2, 10.8.1915, pp. 116-19.
9. Minutes of the special meeting, in ibid., 18.8.1916, p. 153.
10. Minutes Book 2, 12.6.1917, pp. 189-92.
11. Dr Gertrude Mead, Report, in ibid. 10.9.1918, pp. 233-5.
12. Woodman Point records; W.A. Branch of the Commonwealth Archives; Stella Willis, née Morris, Reminiscences, held by the author; press cuttings of articles by 'R.E.L.', source unknown, held by the author; Pioneer Nurses file.
13. Interview with Clarice Wintle, tape held by the author.
14. Minutes of the special meeting, Book 2, 30.6.1920, pp. 306-8; 14.7.1920, pp. 309-10.
15. Ibid. 20.8.1920, pp. 321-4.
16. Ibid. pp. 314-16.
17. Ibid. 27.4.1920, pp. 295-7.
18. Grover interview.
19. Bottle interview.
20. Minutes Book 2, 20.4.1920, pp. 291-4.
21. *Gov. Gaz.* 20.7.1922. In the *Gazette* the appointment of the board is dated 19.7.1922.
22. Ibid. 3.11.1922, p. 2046.
23. *Register of Members* 1908.
24. See Appendix III.
25. *Rules and Regulations of the Australasian Trained Nurses Association* (Sydney, 1920); *Gov. Gaz.* 3.11.1922.
26. *Gov. Gaz.* 1.2.1924, p. 156.
27. *Rules of the Trained Nurses' Guild* (Melbourne, n.d.), Sect. 25, the first Committee of Management and members (the original meeting was 27.1.1921); Minutes Book 3, 13.12.1921, pp. 39-42; ibid. 17.11.1925, pp. 175-8; 'The Evolution of the A.U.N.A.,*J. W.A.N.* 17, 7 (July 1951).
28. Minutes Book 3, 10.6.1921, pp. 11-14; ibid. 9.8.1921 and 13.9.1921.
29. Ibid. 24.1.1922, pp. 43-4.
30. Ibid. 9.10.1923, pp. 116-18; Correspondence and reports, A.T.N.A.-A.N.F., 30.5.1924 (typescript, R.A.N.F.); *Australian Nursing Federation Constitution and By Laws, 1.7.1924* (Sydney, 1926).
31. Dr R. H. Crisp, 'The Early History of Infant Health Services and Training in W.A.' (typescript of lecture given to W.A. Infant Health Refresher Course, 1964), copy held by author.
32. Ruth Allen, *Life in her Hands: the Matron Walsh Story* (Melbourne, 1955); Cohen and Hutchinson, *History of K.E.M.H.*; interviews with Bottle and Edis.
33. Interview with Eileen Ivy Curwood, 1971, tape held by author.
34. Minutes Book 3, 13.5.1924, pp. 131-2.
35. Minutes Book 4, 12.6.1928, pp. 22-4.
36. Minutes Book 3, 24.1.1922, pp. 43-4; *Register of Members* 1923.
37. Ibid. 27.1.1925, pp. 148-9.
38. Ibid. 10.8.1926, p. 201; Book 4, 9.1.1929, pp. 54-7; 10.2.1931, pp. 119-31.
39. Minutes Book 3, 13.12.1927, pp. 253-6.
40. Ibid. 9.8.1927, pp. 232-4.
41. Cohen and Hutchinson, *History of K.E.M.H.*

4. THE THIRTIES

1. M. Balding, matron Fremantle Hospital, to A.T.N.A. (W.A.), Minutes Book 4, 10.12.1929, pp. 79-82.
2. Ibid. 16.7.1929, pp. 64-6.
3. Ibid. 10.7.1931, pp. 133-5.
4. Evans to secretary A.T.N.A. (W.A.), correspondence and reports file R.A.N.F.; Minutes Book 4, 9.6.1931, pp. 131-2.
5. Minutes Book 4, 9.2.1932, pp. 157-60.
6. Ibid. 9.8.1932, pp. 172-4.
7. Ibid. 10.10.1933, pp. 205-6.
8. Ibid. 13.6.1933, pp. 191-3; 12.9.1933, pp. 203-4.
9. Ibid. 12.3.1935, pp. 255-7; 8.5.1934, pp. 218-20.
10. Ibid. 12.6.1934, pp. 221-3.
11. Ibid. 14.6.1934, p. 224.
12. Ibid. 25.6.1934, p. 227.
13. Ibid. 9.7.1934, p. 228.
14. Inaugural meeting, W.A.N.A. Minutes Book 1 (held by R.A.N.F.); Certificate of Registration and Incorporation, 19.9.1934.
15. A.T.N.A. Minutes Book 4, 6.7.1934, p. 226.
16. Press cuttings, A.T.N.A. Scrapbook, held by author.
17. *J. W.A.N.* 1, 1 (15.10.1935).
18. Ibid.
19. Report of the special meeting, Minutes Book 4, 11.2.1936, p. 291; also in the *J. W.A.N.* (25.2.1936).
20. Minutes Book 4, 11.2.1936, p. 290.
21. 'Opening of the Florence Nightingale Club', *J. W.A.N.* 1, 8 (19.5.1936), p. 14.
22. *J. W.A.N.* from Vol. 1, No. 8 onwards.
23. 'Official opening of new rooms', ibid. 4, 1 (October 1938).
24. *The Florence Nightingale International Foundation* (London, 1937).
25. Minute Book 4, 12.2.1935, pp. 250-4.
26. Ibid.
27. Ibid. 14.5.1935, pp. 260-1; Editorial, *J. W.A.N.* 1, 7 (21.4.1936), p. 1.
28. 'Florence Nightingale Sunday', ibid. 1, 8 (19.5.1936), p. 10.
29. 'Florence Nightingale International Foundation. "White Angel" Ball', ibid. 2, 1 (20.10.1936), p. 14.
30. 'Farewell to Miss Campbell', ibid. 4, 10 (18.7.1939), p. 9.
31. See Appendix IV.
32. Hutton interviews.
33. *The Optimist*, magazine of the nursing staff of the Children's Hospital (1931), p. 23.
34. *J. W.A.N.* 1, 12 (15.9.1936), p. 4.
35. Ibid. p. 8.
36. Ibid. 2, 7 (20.4.1937), p. 13.
37. Evidence given in the Arbitration Court by Dr K. Aberdeen, *Daily News* 18.7.1935; Minutes Book 4, 13.8.1934, pp. 236-7; 7.8.1934, pp. 234-5; 11.12.1934, p. 238.
38. 'Training School for Nurses', *West Australian* June 1935.
39. Mary Brady gave information about the school and identified the people in photographs.
40. Minutes Book 4, 10.12.1935, pp. 285-6.

41. Ibid. 10.8.1937, pp. 349-51.
42. Ibid. 7.7.1937, pp. 344-5; 'Thirteenth Annual Report', *J. W.A.N.* 2, 10 (20.7.1937); 'Australian Nursing Federation', *Australasian Nurses' Journal* (15.7.1937), p. 151.
43. Nurses' Registration Act, No. 14 of 1937; *Gov. Gaz.* 2.8.1940.
44. Twenty pages of cuttings from the *West Australian* and the *Daily News*, some undated, A.T.N.A. Scrapbook, 1935.
45. Verbal accounts of nurses there at the time, including Dora Isaacs, née Culmsee.
46. A.T.N.A. Scrapbook, May 1935.
47. A.T.N.A. University Correspondence file; Minutes Book 5, 8.3.1938, pp. 5-7.
48. Minutes Book, 5, 9.8.1938, pp. 26-31.
49. Ibid. 14.6.1938, pp. 15-19.
50. Ibid. 14.2.1939, pp. 48-53.
51. 'Off Duty', *J. W.A.N.* 5, 1 (17.10.1939).

5. THE WAR YEARS

1. Army Central Records Office, Melbourne.
2. Ibid.
3. Annette Wellesley-Smith and E. L. Shaw, *Lest We Forget: 'Centaur' Memorial Scholarships, Australian Army Nursing Service* (Melbourne, 1944); Jessie Elizabeth Simons, *While History Passed* (Adelaide, 1954); Betty Jeffrey, *White Coolies* (Sydney, 1954).
4. Information from Audrey Ingram, formerly Bennett.
5. The following paragraphs are based on the minutes of the A.T.N.A. and the W.A.N.A. during the wartime years, 1939-45; and *J. W.A.N.* Volumes 5 to 10.
6. *J. W.A.N.* 7, 4 (Jan. 1942); 7, 6 (March 1942); 8, 6 (March 1943): and the Jubilee issue (July 1951).
7. Documents, Minutes, Constitution, etc. held by the War Nurses Memorial Association.
8. Documents, Minutes, Constitution, etc. held by the honorary secretary of the Society for the Care of Aged and Incapacitated Nurses; *J. W.A.N.* 8, 12 (Sept. 1943).
9. Bottle interview.
10. Hutton interviews.
11. Minutes Book 5, 8.11.1938, pp. 41-5.
12. A.T.N.A. correspondence.
13. Thirty-seventh Annual Report, A.T.N.A. Minutes Book 6, 5.7.1944, pp. 74-5.
14. Minutes Book 6, 8.8.1944, pp. 80-2; 10.8.1944, pp. 83-7; numerous press cuttings, many undated, A.T.N.A. Scrapbook, 1944.
15. Nurses' Registration Act 1921-1924, No. 14 of 1944, No. 14 of 1946; *Gov. Gaz.* 10.2.1947.
16. *J. W.A.N.* 10, 5 (20.2.1945); Minutes W.A.N.A., November 1944; A.T.N.A. Minutes Book 6, 14.11.1944, pp. 97-8.
17. Minutes Book 6, 31.1.1945, pp. 103-6.
18. Report of meetings (typescript); Conference of the A.T.N.A., A.N.F. and T.N.G., Melbourne 1947, R.A.N.F. file.

19. Numerous press cuttings from the *Mirror, Daily News, West Australian* and others, A.T.N.A. Scrapbook.
20. Reports of visits to many country hospitals by the secretary of the W.A.N.A., typescript attached to the W.A.N.A. Minutes, 6.12.1951, p. 218.
21. 'Male Nurses' Association' 1946-52, in the A.T.N.A. correspondence file; *J. W.A.N.* 12, 7 (July 1947), and 16, 12 (July 1950).
22. 'Green Diamond News', Army Educational Service, 71 Camp Hospital, Northam (typescript, 1946); experience of the author in the A.A.N.S.
23. Correspondence file of the Tuberculosis Association Inc. and the Anti-Tuberculosis Association, 1947-48, R.A.N.F.
24. Bridges, *History of the International Council of Nurses.*
25. For the scholarship holders see the Minutes of the Florence Nightingale Committee (W.A.), held by the R.A.N.F.
26. Minutes Book, 7, 8.11.1949, pp. 89-93.
27. Ibid. 12.4.1949, pp. 46-50.
28. Minutes Book 6, 10.12.1948, p. 331.
29. *Radio Salutes the Nurses* (Melbourne, 1948), copy held by author.
30. *Conference: Journal of the First Australian Nursing Conference* (Melbourne, 1950).
31. 'Education Officer to the Nurses' Registration Board', *J. W.A.N.* July 1960; 'A Recipe for Retirement', *West Australian* 30.10.1975.
32. These and the following paragraphs are based on the Reports of the Commissioner of Public Health, 1947 to 1951, in the *Votes and Proceedings*; discussions with Helen Bailey and other personnel connected with the school; 'Short History of Government School of Nursing' (typescript), held by the author; press cuttings in the A.T.N.A. Scrapbook.
33. *Gov. Gaz.* No. 8, 1947.
34. Minutes Book 6, 10.2.1948, pp. 325-31.
35. Nurses' Registration Act No. 7 of 1922, and amendments to 1952: Nos 32 of 1939, 14 of 1946, 38 of 1948, 30 of 1951, and 41 of 1952.

6. THE FIFTIES

1. Minutes Book 7, 12.1.1954, pp. 265-6; 'Professional and Industrial Units Become One', *J. W.A.N.* 20, 2 (Feb. 1954).
2. Annual Report 1955-56, *J. W.A.N.* 22, 8 (Aug. 1956).
3. 'Possibility of providing a Centre', *J. W.A.N.* 24, 12 (Dec. 1958).
4. 'Nurses' Memorial Centre—Proposed Aim and Function', *J. W.A.N.* 5, 5 (Nov. 1959).
5. 'College of Nursing, Australia', *J. W.A.N.* Jubilee issue, 17, 7 (July 1951).
6. Minutes of the Sister Tutor Section of A.N.F., 1954-1957, R.A.N.F. archives.
7. 'New Government School of Nursing', *J. W.A.N.* 22, 4 (April 1956); and an unpublished 'Short History' by the author.
8. Nurses' Registration Act 1921-1952; *Gov. Gaz.* 4.7.1952, p. 1673.
9. 'First Colombo Plan Nurses Graduate', *J. W.A.N.* 23, 3 (March 1957).
10. Registered as a Training School in September 1958, Records of the Nurses' Registration Board.
11. *J. W.A.N.* 24, 6 (June 1958).
12. Nurses' Registration Act 1921-1959 Amendment No. 61 of 1953.
13. Nurses' Registration Act Amendment No. 41 of 1952.
14. *J. W.A.N.* 25, 5 (May 1959).

7. THE SIXTIES

1. The Male Nurses' Association of W.A. was founded 5 July 1946, and had its office in Cecil Buildings, Sherwood Court.
   'Welcome to Male Nurses: Membership of Federation', *J. W.A.N.* 24, 6 (June 1958), p. 14.
2. *Gov. Gaz.* No. 97, 25.10.1960.
3. Nurses' Registration Act 1921-1952; Health Act 1911-1956 Amendment 1957; *Gov. Gaz.* No. 2, 7.1.1958.
4. 'Education Officer to the Nurses' Registration Board', *J. W.A.N.* 26, 7 (July 1960), p. 13.
5. *J. W.A.N.* 26, 12 (Dec. 1960); also the issues of January to March, and May, 1961.
6. Ibid. 27, 11 (Nov. 1961).
7. Robin Miller, 'Conquest of Loneliness', *J. W.A.N.* 27, 12 (Dec. 1961); and Robin Miller, *Flying Nurse* (Adelaide, 1971).
8. 'Sir Charles Gairdner Hospital', *J. W.A.N.* 19, 6 (June 1963), p. 19.
9. Information in these paragraphs is from the minutes and reports of the College of Nursing, held by the R.A.N.F.
10. *J. W.A.N.* 30, 1 (Jan. 1964).
11. Nurses' Registration Act 1921-1959; Regulations, *Gov. Gaz.* No. 56, 10.6.1965.
12. Cohen and Hutchinson, *History of K.E.M.H.*
13. Vicki Hobbs, 'Short History of the Nurses' Memorial Centre' (M.S.), abridged version pending publication in a brochure.
14. *J. W.A.N.* 32, 7 (July 1966).
15. Ibid. 29, 12 (Dec. 1963).
16. Ibid. 32, 2 (Feb. 1966); 32, 4 (April 1966); 32, 5 (May 1966).
17. Ibid. 32, 10 (Oct. 1966).
18. 'Pioneer Women's Memorial Fountain', ibid. p. 14; Report of the Subcommittee, August 1967, held by the author.

8. THE SEVENTIES

1. '100 patients evacuated in R.P.H. blaze', *West Australian* 15.10.1970.
2. 'Bachelor of Applied Science (Nursing) W.A.I.T.', *Australian Nurses Journal,* March 1979.
3. Catherine Martin, 'If the cap fits, the nurse should wear it', *West Australian* 25.11.1977.
4. *Australian Nurses Journal* Feb. 1979.
5. Nurses Board of Western Australia, 'Jubilee Celebrations 1922-1972', commemorative brochure (typescript), copy held by author.
6. 'Change of Name—A.N.F.E.S. to A.N.F.', *J. W.A.N.* 37, 4 (April 1971).
7. 'Farewell . . . To the Journal of the West Australian Nurses', ibid. 37, 6 (June 1971).
8. The typescript index is in the R.A.N.F. archives. The indexers were Jess Terry, Hilda Jury, Foreste Williams and Vicki Hobbs.
9. *Australian Nurses Journal* July 1979.
10. Ibid. June 1977, p. 5; Catherine Martin, interview with the president, in ibid. July 1977.
11. Shirley Donaghue, 'Goals in Nursing Practice', review in the *Australian Nurses Journals* Dec./Jan. and Feb. 1978.

BIBLIOGRAPHY

GOVERNMENT SOURCES

Blue Books of Western Australia 1834-69 (MSS.); *Blue Books of Western Australia* 1872- .

Government Gazettes.

Public Service List.

Statistical Registers of Western Australia.

Western Australia. *Minutes, Votes and Proceedings of the Parliament.*

OFFICIAL DOCUMENTS

Minutes

Minutes of the Australasian Trained Nurses Association: (i) Western Australia, as branch of A.T.N.A. New South Wales, October 1907 to 1924; and (ii) as branch (W.A.) of the Australian Nursing Federation, 1924 to 1954, both held by the R.A.N.F.

Minutes of the Florence Nightingale Committee (W.A. Branch).

Minutes of the Midwives Registration Board. 1912- .

Minutes of the Nurses' Memorial Centre Committee (W.A.).

Minutes of the Nurses' Registration Board, 1922-1968; and of the Nurses Board, 1968- .

Minutes of the Society for the Care of the Aged or Incapacitated Nurses. Held by R.A.N.F. (W.A.).

Minutes of the State Committee (W.A.) of the College of Nursing, Australia.

Minutes of the Western Australian Nurses' Association, 1935-1954. Held by R.A.N.F. (W.A.).

Reports

Annual Reports of the Australian Nursing Federation W.A. Branch Industrial Union of Workers, 1954-1979, in the Minutes of the Western Australian Nurses' Association.

Annual Reports of the Australasian Trained Nurses Association, W.A., as branch of the A.T.N.A. (N.S.W.), 1907-1924, in A.T.N.A. Minutes for the period; and as branch of the Australian Nursing Federation, 1924-1954, typescript copies held by the author.

Annual Reports of the College of Nursing, Australia. Melbourne, 1953-1979.

Annual Reports and Statements of Receipts and Payments of Fremantle Hospital.

Annual Reports of the Nurses Board of Western Australia.

Annual Reports of Royal Perth Hospital.

Annual Reports of the Sisters of the People, 1895-1897. Perth Central Mission.

Correspondence and Reports of the Tuberculosis Association, the Male Nurses' Association, and the Trained Nurses' Guild, all held by the author.

'History of the Home of Peace', *Annual Report of the Home of Peace 1955*. Perth.

Report of Select Committee Inquiring into Conditions of Perth Public Hospital. Perth, 1900.

Rules and Constitutions

Australasian Trained Nurses Association Rules and Constitution, 1900, 1904, 1913, 1920. Sydney.
Australian Nursing Federation Constitution and By-Laws 1924. Sydney, 1926.
Australian Nursing Federation Constitution 1937. Sydney, 1938.
The Florence Nightingale International Foundation. London, 1937.
The Florence Nightingale International Foundation By-Laws. London, n.d.
Rules of the Western Australian Nurses' Association Industrial Union of Workers. Perth [1934].
Rules, Trained Nurses' Guild. Melbourne [1921].
Rules, Royal Australian Nursing Federation Industrial Union of Workers. Perth [1954].
Constitution of the Society for the Care of Aged or Incapacitated Nurses. Perth, n.d.

Rolls and Registers

Australasian Trained Nurses Association Registers of Members, 1904, 1907, 1909, 1913, 1923. Sydney.
A.T.N.A. Register of W.A. Branch, 1910-1916 (incomplete). Held by R.A.N.F.
A.T.N.A. Life Membership Roll (incomplete), closed 1932. Typescript, held by R.A.N.F.
Nurses Board, Registers and Records of all categories of trained nurses.
(First) Register of General Nurses. *Government Gazette* 1.2.1924. Registers of nurses were published annually in the *Government Gazettes* from 1923 to the late 1960s.
(First) Register of Midwives. Supplement to the *Government Gazette* 7.2.1913. Registers of midwives were published annually in the *Government Gazettes.*

BOOKS

Allen, Ruth. *Life in her Hands: The Matron Walsh Story.* Melbourne, 1955.
Ashdown, Millicent A. *A Complete System of Nursing.* London, 1917.
Bowman, Gerald. *The Lamp and the Book: The Story of the R.C.N. 1916-1966.* London, 1967.
Bridges, Daisy Caroline. *A History of the International Council of Nurses 1899-1964: The First Sixty-Five Years.* London, 1967.
Cohen, B. C. *A History of Medicine in Western Australia: Biographical and Historical Account to 1900.* Perth, 1965.
Cohen, B. C. and R. L. Hutchinson, *History of the King Edward Memorial Hospital for Women: First Fifty Years 1916-1966.* Subiaco, 1966.
Cygnet. *Swan River Booklets,* 1-12. Perth, 1935.
Garnsey, Mrs Arthur H. *Scarlet Pillows: An Australian Nurse's Tales of Long Ago.* Melbourne, n.d.
Hammond, Jesse E. Western Pioneers: The Battle Well Fought. Perth, n.d. [1936].

Hawtrey, C. L. M. *The Availing Struggle: Record of the Planning and Development of the Church of England in Western Australia,* n.d.

Hector, Winifred. *The Work of Mrs Bedford Fenwick and the Rise of Professional Nursing.* London, 1973.

Jeffrey, Betty. *White Coolies.* London, 1954.

Luckes, Eva C. *General Nusring.* 5th ed., London, 1905.

Miller, Robin. *Flying Nurse.* Adelaide, 1971.

Millett, Mrs E. *An Australian Parsonage, or, The Settlers and the Savage in Western Australia.* London, 1872.

Reid, Arthur. *Those Were the Days.* Perth, 1933.

Reilly, J. T. *Reminiscences of Fifty Years in Western Australia.* Perth, 1903.

Rischbieth, Bessie M. *March of Australian Women.* Perth, 1964.

Simons, Jessie Elizabeth. *While History Passed: the story of the Australian nurses who were prisoners of the Japanese for three and a half years.* London, 1954.

Skinner, M. L. *The Fifth Sparrow: An Autobiography.* Sydney, 1972.

South Australian Trained Nurses Centenary Committee. *Nursing in South Australia: The First Hundred Years 1837-1937.* Adelaide, 1938.

Stannage, C. T. (ed.). *Local History in Western Australia: A Guide to Research.* Perth, n.d.

Stewart, Noel. *Little But Great: Saga of the Silver Chain (1905-1965).* Perth, 1968.

Stubbe, J. H. *Medical Background: being a History of Fremantle Hospitals and Doctors.* Nedlands, 1969.

Watson, E. L. Grant. *Journey Under the Southern Stars.* London, 1968.

Watson, J. K. *A Handbook for Nurses.* 4th ed., London, 1908.

Wesley Story: Centenary of the Wesley Church, Perth 1870-1970. Perth, n.d.

West, D. P. *The First Hundred Years: Albany, Western Australia.* Albany, 1932.

Wrench, G. T. *Rotunda, Midwifery for Nurses.* London, 1908.

PAMPHLETS

Centenary of the Foundation of the Sisters of St John of God 1871-1971. Perth, n.d.

D., L. N. & M. M. K. *The Lamp Radiant: The Story of an Association of Nurses from Many Lands.* Switzerland, 1955.

Jull, Roberta. *The Story of the Alexandra Home for Women.* Perth, n.d.

Radio Salutes the Nurses. Souvenir Programme of the Nurses War Memorial Appeal. Melbourne, 1948.

Souvenir Programme of the Nurses' Memorial Centre Appeal. Perth, 1960. Contains a short history of the teaching hospitals.

Subcommittee of R.A.N.F. Nursing Education Section. *An assessment of the nurse teacher as an educationalist.* Perth, 1968.

Wellesley-Smith, Annette E. & E. L. Shaw. *Lest We Forget. 'Centaur' Memorial Scholarship, A.A.N.S.* Melbourne, 1944.

Wilson, Grace. *The Royal Australian Army Nursing Service.* Melbourne, 1949.

NEWSPAPERS

Daily News.

Inquirer.

Kalgoorlie Miner.
Mirror.
Sunday Times.
West Australian.
Western Argus.
Western Mail.

JOURNALS

Australasian Nurses Journal, 1935-1945.
Australian Nurses Journal, 1971-1979.
Civil Service Journal, July 1929.
Conference: Journal of the First Australian Nursing Conference, Melbourne, 1950.
Early Days, Journal and Proceedings of the Royal Western Australian Historical Society.
Journal of the Western Australian Nurses, 1935-1945; *Journal of the West Australian Nurses*, 1945-1971.
The Magazine, 1930; *The Optimist*, 1931 (nursing staff of the Children's Hospital, Perth).
Medical Journal of Australia, 1914.
Perth Hospital Review, August 1924 to 1925.
Perth Hospital Journal, 1938-1946; *Royal Perth Hospital Journal*, 1946-1975.

DIARIES, LETTERS AND TAPES

Diary of Miss Mary Pittman Monk, the matron in charge of immigrant girls on the *Echuca*, 1892, B.L. AN3 Acc. 504.
Diary of Mrs Margaret Walpole, Albany, B.L. 585A.
Letters from relatives and colleagues of pioneer nurses sent to the A.N.F. in connection with the Women's Memorial in Kings Park, 1966, held by the author.
Pioneer Nurses' File, including personal correspondence sent to the author re pioneer nurses, held by the author.
Reminiscences of Elizabeth Agnes Sadleir, née Seymour (Sister Agnes), August 1947 (typescript), R.W.A.H.S.; part published in *J. W.A.N.* 19 (1953).
Tapes of interviews with many older members of the nursing profession: 1970: Miss Lizzie Faram; 1971: Misses Ruth Bottle, Ivy Curwood, M. D. Edis, Elizabeth Grover, Milne Robinson, Taylor, Wiley; Mesdames de Moulin, Freman, Hughes (née Penglase), E. King (née Daniels), Pat Morris, C. P. Rutherford, Smith (née King); 1975: Miss Helena Hutton.

MANUSCRIPTS AND LECTURE NOTES

Beard, M. E. Origin and development of all nurse training schools in Western Australia. Lecture notes, n.d., held by author.
Cox, John R. The History of the Royal Perth Hospital 1829-1895. Archives, R.P.H.
Crisp, R. N. The early history of infant health services and training in W.A. Child Health, 1964.
Lee, P. F. The development of the nursing service under the control of the Medical Department of Western Australia. Public Health Library.

Public Health and Medical Department. The Western Australian Hospital System. 1960.
Woolcott, J. F. Progress in Public Health since 1900. Public Health Library.

MISCELLANEOUS

Assortment of early examination question papers, held by the author.
Nurses' Certificates, Hospital and Registration Board.
Ward reports and patients' records, House of Mercy, Alexandra Home, Ngal-A, held by Ngal-A.
Wellcome's Professional Nurses' Diary, 1905-1906, 1911-1912.

INDEX

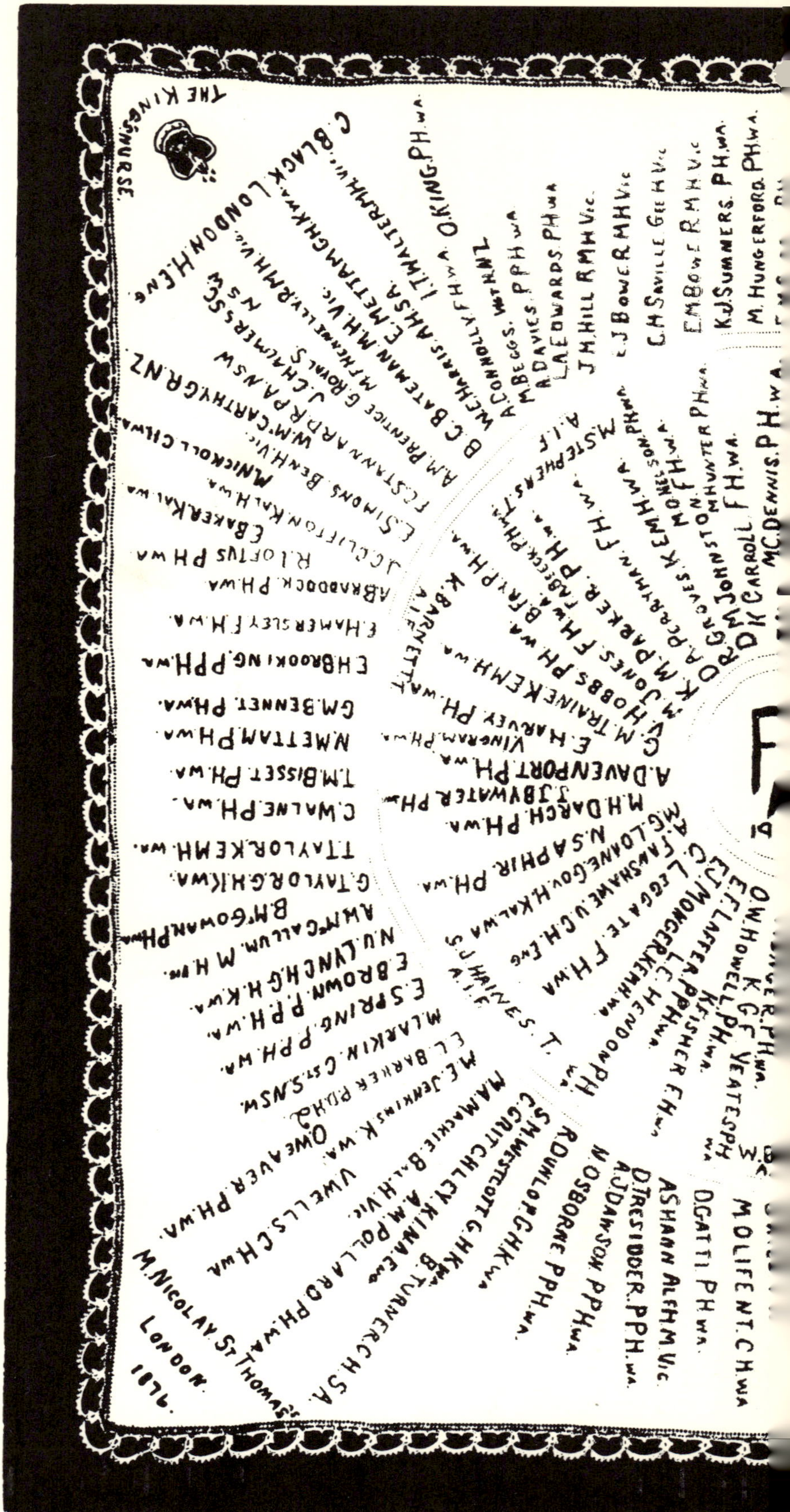
THE KING'S NURSE
C. BLACK LONDON H. Eng
O. KING P.H. WA
M. BEGGS
A. DAVIES P.P.H. WA
L.A. EDWARDS P.H. WA
J.M. HILL R.M.H. Vic
E.J. BOWE R.M.H. Vic
C.H. SAVILLE
E.M. BOWE R.M.H. Vic
K.J. SUMMERS P.H. WA
M. HUNGERFORD P.H. WA
B.C. BATEMAN M.H. Vic
M.M'CARTHY G.R.N.Z.
M. NICKOLL
E. BAKER
R. LOFTUS P.H. WA
A. BRADDOCK P.H. WA
E. HAMERSLEY F.H. WA
E.H. BROOKING P.P.H. WA
G.M. BENNET P.H. WA
N. METTAM P.H. WA
T.M. BISSETT P.H. WA
C. WALNE P.H. WA
T. TAYLOR K.E.M.H. WA
G. TAYLOR G.H.K. WA
B.M'GOWAN P.H. WA
E. BROWN P.P.H. WA
E. SPRING P.P.H. WA
M. LARKIN P.P.H. WA
O. WEAVER P.H. WA
V. WELLS C.H. WA
A.M. POLLARD P.H. WA
B. TURNER C.H. S.A.
M. NICOLAY St THOMAS'S LONDON 1917
M. OSBORNE P.P.H. WA
A.J. DAWSON P.P.H. WA
D. TRESIDDER P.P.H. WA
D. GATTI P.H. WA
M. OLIFENT C.H. WA
A. DAVENPORT P.H.
J. BYWATER P.H.
M.H. DARCH P.H. WA
N. SAPHIR P.H. WA
E. HARVEY P.H. WA
G.M. TRAINE K.E.M.H.
M. STEPHENS T. A.I.F.
K. BARNETT T. A.I.F.
D.K. CARROLL F.H. WA
M.C. DENNIS P.H. WA